# Student Solutions Manual

AF816873

# Mathematics:
## with Allied Health Applications

**Richard N. Aufmann**
Palomar College

**Joanne S. Lockwood**
Nashua Community College

with additional contributions by

**Catherine W. Johnson**
Alamance Community College

Prepared by

**Pat Foard**
South Plains College

BROOKS/COLE
CENGAGE Learning

Australia • Brazil • Japan • Korea • Mexico • Singapore • Spain • United Kingdom • United States

BROOKS/COLE
CENGAGE Learning

© 2013 Brooks/Cole, Cengage Learning

ALL RIGHTS RESERVED. No part of this work covered by the copyright herein may be reproduced, transmitted, stored, or used in any form or by any means graphic, electronic, or mechanical, including but not limited to photocopying, recording, scanning, digitizing, taping, Web distribution, information networks, or information storage and retrieval systems, except as permitted under Section 107 or 108 of the 1976 United States Copyright Act, without the prior written permission of the publisher.

For product information and technology assistance, contact us at **Cengage Learning Customer & Sales Support, 1-800-354-9706**

For permission to use material from this text or product, submit all requests online at **www.cengage.com/permissions**
Further permissions questions can be emailed to **permissionrequest@cengage.com**

ISBN-13: 978-1-133-11230-3
ISBN-10: 1-133-11230-7

**Brooks/Cole**
20 Davis Drive
Belmont, CA 94002-3098
USA

Cengage Learning is a leading provider of customized learning solutions with office locations around the globe, including Singapore, the United Kingdom, Australia, Mexico, Brazil, and Japan. Locate your local office at: **www.cengage.com/global**

Cengage Learning products are represented in Canada by Nelson Education, Ltd.

To learn more about Brooks/Cole, visit **www.cengage.com/brookscole**

Purchase any of our products at your local college store or at our preferred online store **www.cengagebrain.com**

Printed in the United States of America
1 2 3 4 5 6 7 15 14 13 12 11

# Contents





© 2013 Cengage Learning. All Rights Reserved. May not be scanned, copied or duplicated, or posted to a publicly accessible website, in whole or in part.

# Chapter 1: Whole Numbers

## Prep Test

**1.** 8

**2.** 1 2 3 4 5 6 7 8 9 10

**3.** a and D; b and E; c and A; d and B; e and F; f and C

## Section 1.1

### Objective A Exercises

**1.** 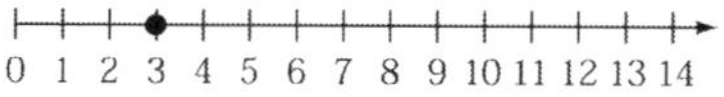


**3.** 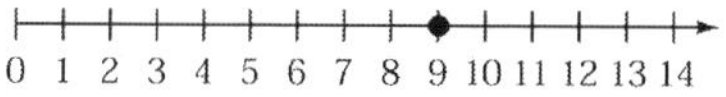


**5.** 37 < 49

**7.** 101 > 87

**9.** 2701 > 2071

**11.** 107 > 0

**13.** Yes

### Objective B Exercises

**15.** Millions

**17.** Hundred-thousands

**19.** Three thousand seven hundred ninety

**21.** Fifty-eight thousand four hundred seventy-three

**23.** Four hundred ninety-eight thousand five hundred twelve

**25.** Six million eight hundred forty-two thousand seven hundred fifteen

**27.** 357

**29.** 63,780

**31.** 7,024,709

### Objective C Exercises

**33.** 5000 + 200 + 80 + 7

**35.** 50,000 + 8000 + 900 + 40 + 3

**37.** 200,000 + 500 + 80 + 3

**39.** 400,000 + 3000 + 700 + 5

**41.** No

### Objective D Exercises

**43.** 850

**45.** 4000

**47.** 53,000

**49.** 630,000

**51.** 250,000

**53.** 72,000,000

### Applying the Concepts

**55.** The results are different. 3846 rounded to the nearest ten is 3850, and 3850 rounded to the nearest hundred is 3900. But 3846 rounded to the nearest hundred is 3800, which is the correct method.

## Section 1.2

### Objective A Exercises

**1.** 28

**3.** 125

**5.** 102

**7.** 154

**9.** 1489

**11.** 828

© 2013 Cengage Learning. All Rights Reserved. May not be scanned, copied or duplicated, or posted to a publicly accessible website, in whole or in part.

**13.**
$$\begin{array}{r} {\scriptstyle 1\phantom{00}} \\ 859 \\ +\ 725 \\ \hline 1584 \end{array}$$

**15.**
$$\begin{array}{r} {\scriptstyle 1\phantom{00}} \\ 470 \\ +\ 749 \\ \hline 1219 \end{array}$$

**17.**
$$\begin{array}{r} {\scriptstyle 1\,1\,1\phantom{00}} \\ 36,925 \\ +\ 65,392 \\ \hline 102,317 \end{array}$$

**19.**
$$\begin{array}{r} {\scriptstyle 1\,\,1\phantom{000}} \\ 50,873 \\ +\ 28,453 \\ \hline 79,326 \end{array}$$

**21.**
$$\begin{array}{r} {\scriptstyle 2\,2\phantom{0}} \\ 878 \\ 737 \\ +\ 189 \\ \hline 1804 \end{array}$$

**23.**
$$\begin{array}{r} {\scriptstyle 1\phantom{00}} \\ 319 \\ 348 \\ +\ 912 \\ \hline 1579 \end{array}$$

**25.**
$$\begin{array}{r} {\scriptstyle 1\,2\phantom{0}} \\ 9409 \\ 3253 \\ +\ 7078 \\ \hline 19,740 \end{array}$$

**27.**
$$\begin{array}{r} {\scriptstyle 1\,2\phantom{0}} \\ 2038 \\ 2243 \\ +\ 3139 \\ \hline 7420 \end{array}$$

**29.**
$$\begin{array}{r} {\scriptstyle 1\,1\,\,1\,1\phantom{0}} \\ 67,428 \\ 32,171 \\ +\ 20,971 \\ \hline 120,570 \end{array}$$

**31.**
$$\begin{array}{r} {\scriptstyle 1\,1\,\,1\phantom{00}} \\ 76,290 \\ 43,761 \\ +\ 87,402 \\ \hline 207,453 \end{array}$$

**33.**
$$\begin{array}{r} {\scriptstyle 1\,1\,1\phantom{0}} \\ 20,958 \\ 3,218 \\ +\ 42 \\ \hline 24,218 \end{array}$$

**35.**
$$\begin{array}{r} {\scriptstyle 1\,\,1\,1\phantom{0}} \\ 392 \\ 37 \\ 10,924 \\ +\ 621 \\ \hline 11,974 \end{array}$$

**37.**
$$\begin{array}{r} {\scriptstyle 1\,2\,2\phantom{0}} \\ 294 \\ 1029 \\ 7935 \\ +\ 65 \\ \hline 9323 \end{array}$$

**39.**
$$\begin{array}{r} {\scriptstyle 1\,1\,\,2\,1\phantom{0}} \\ 97 \\ 7,234 \\ 69,532 \\ +\ 276 \\ \hline 77,139 \end{array}$$

**41.**
$$\begin{array}{r} {\scriptstyle 1\,\,\,1\phantom{0}} \\ 9874 \\ +\ 4509 \\ \hline 14,383 \end{array}$$

**43.**
$$\begin{array}{r} {\scriptstyle 1\,1\,1\phantom{0}} \\ 3487 \\ +5986 \\ \hline 9473 \end{array}$$

**45.**
$$\begin{array}{r} {\scriptstyle 1\,\,\,1\,1\,1\phantom{0}} \\ 9678 \\ +23,569 \\ \hline 33,247 \end{array}$$

**47.**
$$\begin{array}{r} {\scriptstyle 1\,1\,1\phantom{0}} \\ 4579 \\ +479 \\ \hline 5058 \end{array}$$

© 2013 Cengage Learning. All Rights Reserved. May not be scanned, copied or duplicated, or posted to a publicly accessible website, in whole or in part.

**49.**
$$\begin{array}{r} \scriptstyle{1\,2} \\ 659 \\ 55 \\ +1278 \\ \hline 1992 \end{array}$$

**51.**
$$\begin{array}{r} \scriptstyle{1\,1\,2} \\ 34 \\ 329 \\ 8 \\ +67,892 \\ \hline 68,263 \end{array}$$

**53.**
$$\begin{array}{rcr} 1234 & \approx & 1200 \\ 9780 & \approx & 9800 \\ +\ 6740 & \approx & +\ 6700 \\ \text{Cal.: } 17,754 & & \text{Est.: } 17,700 \end{array}$$

**55.**
$$\begin{array}{rcr} 241 & \approx & 200 \\ 569 & \approx & 600 \\ 390 & \approx & 400 \\ +\ 1672 & \approx & +\ 1700 \\ \text{Cal.: } 2872 & & \text{Est.: } 2900 \end{array}$$

**57.**
$$\begin{array}{rcr} 32,461 & \approx & 32,000 \\ 9,844 & \approx & 10,000 \\ +\ 59,407 & \approx & +\ 59,000 \\ \text{Cal.: } 101,712 & & \text{Est.: } 101,000 \end{array}$$

**59.**
$$\begin{array}{rcr} 25,432 & \approx & 25,000 \\ 62,941 & \approx & 63,000 \\ +\ 70,390 & \approx & +\ 70,000 \\ \text{Cal.: } 158,763 & & \text{Est.: } 158,000 \end{array}$$

**61.**
$$\begin{array}{rcr} 67,421 & \approx & 70,000 \\ 82,984 & \approx & 80,000 \\ 66,361 & \approx & 70,000 \\ 10,792 & \approx & 10,000 \\ +\ 34,037 & \approx & +\ 30,000 \\ \text{Cal.: } 261,595 & & \text{Est.: } 260,000 \end{array}$$

**63.**
$$\begin{array}{rcr} 281,421 & \approx & 280,000 \\ 9,874 & \approx & 10,000 \\ 34,394 & \approx & 30,000 \\ 526,398 & \approx & 530,000 \\ +\ 94,631 & \approx & +\ 90,000 \\ \textit{Cal.: } 946,718 & & \textit{Est.: } 940,000 \end{array}$$

**65.** Commutative Property of Addition

## Objective B Exercises

**67.** **Strategy** To find the total number of multiple births, add the four amounts (110,670, 6919, 627, and 79).

**Solution**
$$\begin{array}{r} 110,670 \\ 6,919 \\ 627 \\ +\quad 79 \\ \hline 118,295 \end{array}$$

There were 118,295 multiple births during the year.

**69.** **Strategy** To estimate the total income from *Patch Adams* and *The Awakening*, add the income from each movie (135,026,902 and 8,415,112).

**Solution**
$$\begin{array}{r} \scriptstyle{1\quad\ 1\,1\quad} \\ 135,026,902 \\ +\ 8,415,112 \\ \hline 143,442,014 \end{array}$$

The total income from *Patch Adams* and *The Awakening* was \$143,442,014.

**71.** **Strategy** To find the total income from the two movies with the lowest box-office incomes, add the incomes from *The Awakening* (\$8,415,112) and *The Doctor* (\$38,120,905).

**Solution**
$$\begin{array}{r} \scriptstyle{1\quad\ 1\quad} \\ 8,415,112 \\ +\ 38,120,905 \\ \hline 46,536,017 \end{array}$$

The income from the two movies with the lowest box-office returns is \$46,536,017.

© 2013 Cengage Learning. All Rights Reserved. May not be scanned, copied or duplicated, or posted to a publicly accessible website, in whole or in part.

**73a.** **Strategy** To find the total number of miles walked during the three days, add the three amounts (3, 4, and 4 miles).

**Solution**

$$\begin{array}{r} 3 \\ 4 \\ +\ 4 \\ \hline 11 \end{array}$$

The orderly walked 11 in mi from Monday to Wednesday.

**75.** **Strategy** To find the total miles, add the number of miles of each leg of the trip (75, 178, and 146).

**Solution**

$$\begin{array}{r} {}^{1\,1} \\ 75 \\ 178 \\ +146 \\ \hline 399 \end{array}$$

The total length of the trip was 399 miles.

## Applying the Concepts

**77.** There are 6 possible outcomes for each die (1, 2, 3, 4, 5, and 6).

The smallest sum on two dice is 1 + 1 = 2. The largest sum on two dice is 6 + 6 = 12. There are 11 different sums from 2 to 12 (2, 3, 4, 5, 6, 7, 8, 9, 10, 11, and 12).

**79.** No; 0 + 0 = 0

**81.** Ten numbers that are less than 100 end in a 7. They are 7, 17, 27, 37, 47, 57, 67, 77, 87, and 97.

# Section 1.3

## Objective A Exercises

**1.** 4

**3.** 4

**5.** 10

**7.** 4

**9.** 9

**11.** 22

**13.** 60

**15.** 66

**17.** 31

**19.** 901

**21.** 791

**23.** 1125

**25.** 3131

**27.** 47

**29.** 925

**31.** 4561

**33.** 3205

**35.** 1222

## Objective B Exercises

**37.**

$$\begin{array}{r} {}^{6\ 11} \\ \not{7}\not{1} \\ -\ 18 \\ \hline 53 \end{array}$$

**39.**

$$\begin{array}{r} {}^{3\ 17} \\ \not{4}\not{7} \\ -\ 18 \\ \hline 29 \end{array}$$

**41.**

$$\begin{array}{r} {}^{2\ 17} \\ \not{3}\not{7} \\ -\ 29 \\ \hline 8 \end{array}$$

**43.**

$$\begin{array}{r} {}^{6\ 10} \\ \not{7}\not{0} \\ -\ 33 \\ \hline 37 \end{array}$$

© 2013 Cengage Learning. All Rights Reserved. May not be scanned, copied or duplicated, or posted to a publicly accessible website, in whole or in part.

**45.**
$$\begin{array}{r} \scriptstyle 14 \\ \scriptstyle 1\ 4\ 10 \\ 250 \\ -\ 192 \\ \hline 58 \end{array}$$

**47.**
$$\begin{array}{r} \scriptstyle 6\ 16 \\ 768 \\ -\ 194 \\ \hline 574 \end{array}$$

**49.**
$$\begin{array}{r} \scriptstyle 6\ 14 \\ 674 \\ -\ 337 \\ \hline 337 \end{array}$$

**51.**
$$\begin{array}{r} \scriptstyle 10 \\ \scriptstyle 6\ 0\ 12 \\ 1712 \\ -\ \ 289 \\ \hline 1423 \end{array}$$

**53.**
$$\begin{array}{r} \scriptstyle 16\ 9 \\ \scriptstyle 0\ 6\ 1012 \\ 1702 \\ -\ 948 \\ \hline 754 \end{array}$$

**55.**
$$\begin{array}{r} \scriptstyle 12 \\ \scriptstyle 8\ 2\ 13 \\ 5933 \\ -\ 3754 \\ \hline 2179 \end{array}$$

**57.**
$$\begin{array}{r} \scriptstyle 13\ 9 \\ \scriptstyle 8\ 3\ 10\ 17 \\ 9407 \\ -\ 2918 \\ \hline 6489 \end{array}$$

**59.**
$$\begin{array}{r} \scriptstyle 15\ 9 \\ \scriptstyle 7\ 5\ 1015 \\ 8605 \\ -7716 \\ \hline 889 \end{array}$$

**61.**
$$\begin{array}{r} \scriptstyle 9 \\ \scriptstyle 7\ 10\ 2\ 1015 \\ 80{,}305 \\ -\ 9{,}176 \\ \hline 71{,}129 \end{array}$$

**63.**
$$\begin{array}{r} \scriptstyle 9\ 9\ 9 \\ \scriptstyle 0\ 10\ 10\ 10\ 14 \\ 10{,}004 \\ -\ 9{,}306 \\ \hline 698 \end{array}$$

**65.**
$$\begin{array}{r} \scriptstyle 6\ 10 \\ 70{,}618 \\ -41{,}213 \\ \hline 29{,}405 \end{array}$$

**67.**
$$\begin{array}{r} \scriptstyle 9 \\ \scriptstyle 6\ 10\ 6\ 1010 \\ 70{,}700 \\ -21{,}076 \\ \hline 49{,}627 \end{array}$$

**69.**
$$\begin{array}{r} \scriptstyle 15\ 9 \\ \scriptstyle 1\ 5\ 10\ 10 \\ 2600 \\ -1972 \\ \hline 628 \end{array}$$

**71.**
$$\begin{array}{r} \scriptstyle 9 \\ \scriptstyle 8\ 1010 \\ 9003 \\ -2471 \\ \hline 6532 \end{array}$$

**73.**
$$\begin{array}{r} \scriptstyle 11\ 9 \\ \scriptstyle 7\ 1\ 10\ 12 \\ 8202 \\ -3916 \\ \hline 4286 \end{array}$$

**75.**
$$\begin{array}{r} \scriptstyle 9 \\ \scriptstyle 6\ 1011 \\ 7015 \\ -2973 \\ \hline 4042 \end{array}$$

**77.**
$$\begin{array}{r} \scriptstyle 9\ 9 \\ \scriptstyle 6\ 10\ 10\ 15 \\ 7005 \\ -1796 \\ \hline 5209 \end{array}$$

**79.**
$$\begin{array}{r} \scriptstyle 9\ 9\ 9 \\ \scriptstyle 1\ 10\ 10\ 1015 \\ 20{,}005 \\ -\ 9{,}627 \\ \hline 10{,}378 \end{array}$$

**81.** (ii) and (iii)

**83.**
$$\begin{array}{r} \scriptstyle 6\ \ 91211 \\ 17{,}031 \\ -5{,}792 \\ \hline 11{,}239 \end{array}$$

**85.**
$$\begin{array}{r} \scriptstyle 7\ 17 \\ 29{,}874 \\ -21{,}392 \\ \hline 8{,}482 \end{array}$$

© 2013 Cengage Learning. All Rights Reserved. May not be scanned, copied or duplicated, or posted to a publicly accessible website, in whole or in part.

**87.**
$$\begin{array}{r} {}^{6\ 9\ \ 9\ 9\ 14} \\ \not{7}\not{0},\not{0}\not{0}\not{4} \\ -69,379 \\ \hline 625 \end{array}$$

**89.**
$$\begin{array}{r} {}^{7\ 15\ \ 16\ 9\ 11} \\ \not{8}\not{6},\not{7}\not{0}\not{1} \\ -9,976 \\ \hline 76,725 \end{array}$$

**91. Strategy** To find the amount that completes the statement, subtract the addend (67) from the sum (90).

**Solution**
$$\begin{array}{r} 90 \\ -67 \\ \hline 23 \end{array}$$

Therefore 23 completes the statement, 67 + 23 = 90.

**93. Strategy** To find the amount that completes the statement, subtract the addend (253) from the sum (4901).

**Solution**
$$\begin{array}{r} 4901 \\ -\ 253 \\ \hline 4648 \end{array}$$

Therefore 4648 completes the statement, 253 + 4648 = 4901.

**95.**
$$\begin{array}{rcr} 90,765 & \approx & 90,000 \\ -60,928 & \approx & -60,000 \\ \hline \text{Cal.}: 29,837 & & \text{Est.}: 30,000 \end{array}$$

**97.**
$$\begin{array}{rcr} 96,430 & \approx & 100,000 \\ -59,762 & \approx & -60,000 \\ \hline \text{Cal.}: 36,668 & & \text{Est.}: 40,000 \end{array}$$

**99.**
$$\begin{array}{rcr} 300,712 & \approx & 300,000 \\ -198,714 & \approx & -200,000 \\ \hline \text{Cal.}: 101,998 & & \text{Est.}: 100,000 \end{array}$$

## Objective C Exercises

**101a. Strategy** To find the number of units sold in New York, California, and Quebec, add the number sold in each area (289, 391, and 234).

**Solution**
$$\begin{array}{r} 289 \\ 391 \\ +234 \\ \hline 914 \end{array}$$

The total sold in New York, California, and Quebec is 914 units.

**b. Strategy** To find difference in the amounts sold in the United States and Canada

- Add to find the total units sold in the United States (289, 53, 167, 175, and 391).
- Subtract the number of units sold in Quebec from the total number of units sold in the United States.

**Solution**
$$\begin{array}{r} 289 \\ 53 \\ 167 \\ 175 \\ +391 \\ \hline 1075 \end{array} \qquad \begin{array}{r} 1075 \\ -234 \\ \hline 841 \end{array}$$

There were 841 more units sold in the United States than in Quebec.

**c. Strategy** To find how many more units were sold in California than in Florida, subtract the number of units sold in Florida (167) from the number of units sold in New York (391).

**Solution**
$$\begin{array}{r} 391 \\ -167 \\ \hline 224 \end{array}$$

224 more units were sold in New York than in Florida.

**d. Strategy** To find the total number of units sold, add the units for each area (289, 53, 167, 175, 391, and 234).

© 2013 Cengage Learning. All Rights Reserved. May not be scanned, copied or duplicated, or posted to a publicly accessible website, in whole or in part.

**Solution**

$$\begin{array}{r} 289 \\ 53 \\ 167 \\ 175 \\ 391 \\ +234 \\ \hline 1309 \end{array}$$

A total of 1309 units were sold.

**103. Strategy** To find the amount you still owe:

• Add (125, 457, and 87) to find the total of your purchases.

• Add the total amount of your purchases to the balance before the purchase ($398).

• Subtract your payment ($650) from the new balance.

**Solution** Purchases :

$$\begin{array}{r} 125 \\ 457 \\ +87 \\ \hline 669 \end{array}$$

$$\begin{array}{r} 398 \\ +669 \\ \hline 1067 \end{array} \qquad \begin{array}{r} 1067 \\ -650 \\ \hline 417 \end{array}$$

The new balance is $417.

**105. Strategy** To find how many more women than men earned a bachelor's degree, subtract number of men (573,079) who earned a degree from the number of women (775,424) who earned a degree.

**Solution**

$$\begin{array}{r} 775{,}424 \\ -573{,}079 \\ \hline 202{,}345 \end{array}$$

202,345 more women than men earned a bachelor's degree.

**107a. Strategy** To find which 2-year period has the smallest expected increase, find the difference for each of the 2-year periods and determine which is the smallest difference.

**Solution** For 2010 – 2012:

$$\begin{array}{r} 146{,}000 \\ -129{,}000 \\ \hline 17{,}000 \end{array}$$

For 2012 – 2014:

$$\begin{array}{r} 166{,}000 \\ -146{,}000 \\ \hline 20{,}000 \end{array}$$

For 2014 – 2016:

$$\begin{array}{r} 187{,}000 \\ -166{,}000 \\ \hline 21{,}000 \end{array}$$

For 2016 – 2018:

$$\begin{array}{r} 208{,}000 \\ -187{,}000 \\ \hline 21{,}000 \end{array}$$

For 2018 – 2020:

$$\begin{array}{r} 235{,}000 \\ -208{,}000 \\ \hline 27{,}000 \end{array}$$

The smallest expected 2-year increase is 17,000 for 2010–2012.

**b. Strategy** To find which 2-year period has the greatest increase, find the difference for each of the 2-year periods and determine which is the greatest difference.

**Solution** Using the calculations from 116a, the greatest expected 2-year increase is 27,000 for 2018–2020.

**109. Strategy** To find number of calories remaining:

• Add (375, 450 and 630) to find the total of calories consumed.

• Subtract the calories consumed from 1500.

• See from the list what snack

© 2013 Cengage Learning. All Rights Reserved. May not be scanned, copied or duplicated, or posted to a publicly accessible website, in whole or in part.

you can have.

**Solution**

$$\begin{array}{r} 375 \\ 450 \\ +630 \\ \hline 1455 \end{array} \qquad \begin{array}{r} 1500 \\ -1455 \\ \hline 45 \end{array}$$

You can have one cup of air-popped popcorn.

## Applying the Concepts

**111.** Answers will vary. For example:

Pat has earned 15 college credits, and Leslie has earned 8 college credits. How many more college credits has Pat earned? 7 college credits.

# Section 1.4

## Objective A Exercises

**1.** $6 \times 2$ or $6 \cdot 2$

**3.** $4 \times 7$ or $4 \cdot 7$

**5.** 12

**7.** 35

**9.** 25

**11.** 0

**13.** 72

**15.** $$\begin{array}{r} {}^{1}\phantom{6} \\ 66 \\ \times 3 \\ \hline 198 \end{array}$$

**17.** $$\begin{array}{r} {}^{3}\phantom{7} \\ 67 \\ \times\ 5 \\ \hline 335 \end{array}$$

**19.** $$\begin{array}{r} {}^{1}\phantom{23} \\ 623 \\ \times\ \ 4 \\ \hline 2492 \end{array}$$

**21.** $$\begin{array}{r} {}^{6}\phantom{07} \\ 607 \\ \times\ \ 9 \\ \hline 5463 \end{array}$$

**23.** $$\begin{array}{r} 600 \\ \times\ \ 7 \\ \hline 4200 \end{array}$$

**25.** $$\begin{array}{r} {}^{2}\phantom{3} \\ 703 \\ \times\ \ 9 \\ \hline 6327 \end{array}$$

**27.** $$\begin{array}{r} 632 \\ \times\ \ 3 \\ \hline 1896 \end{array}$$

**29.** $$\begin{array}{r} {}^{2\,1}\phantom{2} \\ 632 \\ \times\ \ 8 \\ \hline 5056 \end{array}$$

**31.** $$\begin{array}{r} {}^{1\,3}\phantom{7} \\ 337 \\ \times\ \ 5 \\ \hline 1685 \end{array}$$

**33.** $$\begin{array}{r} {}^{4\ \ 6}\phantom{9} \\ 6709 \\ \times\ \ \ 7 \\ \hline 46,963 \end{array}$$

**35.** $$\begin{array}{r} {}^{3\,4\,5}\phantom{8} \\ 8568 \\ \times\ \ \ 7 \\ \hline 59,976 \end{array}$$

**37.** $$\begin{array}{r} {}^{3\,3}\phantom{80} \\ 4780 \\ \times\ \ \ 4 \\ \hline 19,120 \end{array}$$

**39.** $$\begin{array}{r} {}^{1\,1\,1}\phantom{5} \\ 9895 \\ \times\ \ \ 2 \\ \hline 19,790 \end{array}$$

**41.** $5 \times 7 \times 4 = 140$

**43.** $$\begin{array}{r} 3208 \\ \times\ \ \ 7 \\ \hline 22,456 \end{array}$$

**45.** $$\begin{array}{r} 3105 \\ \times\ \ \ 6 \\ \hline 18,630 \end{array}$$

© 2013 Cengage Learning. All Rights Reserved. May not be scanned, copied or duplicated, or posted to a publicly accessible website, in whole or in part.

## Objective B Exercises

**47.** $$\begin{array}{r} 16 \\ \times\ 21 \\ \hline 16 \\ 32\phantom{0} \\ \hline 336 \end{array}$$

**49.** $$\begin{array}{r} 35 \\ \times\ 26 \\ \hline 210 \\ 70\phantom{0} \\ \hline 910 \end{array}$$

**51.** $$\begin{array}{r} 693 \\ \times\ 91 \\ \hline 693 \\ 6237\phantom{0} \\ \hline 63{,}063 \end{array}$$

**53.** $$\begin{array}{r} 419 \\ \times\ \ 80 \\ \hline 33{,}520 \end{array}$$

**55.** $$\begin{array}{r} 8279 \\ \times\ \ 46 \\ \hline 49674 \\ 33116\phantom{0} \\ \hline 380{,}834 \end{array}$$

**57.** $$\begin{array}{r} 6938 \\ \times\ \ 78 \\ \hline 55504 \\ 48566\phantom{0} \\ \hline 541{,}164 \end{array}$$

**59.** $$\begin{array}{r} 7035 \\ \times\ \ 57 \\ \hline 49245 \\ 35175\phantom{0} \\ \hline 400{,}995 \end{array}$$

**61.** $$\begin{array}{r} 3009 \\ \times\ \ 35 \\ \hline 15045 \\ 9027\phantom{0} \\ \hline 105{,}315 \end{array}$$

**63.** $$\begin{array}{r} 809 \\ \times\ \ 530 \\ \hline 24270 \\ 4045\phantom{00} \\ \hline 428{,}770 \end{array}$$

**65.** $$\begin{array}{r} 800 \\ \times\ \ 325 \\ \hline 4000 \\ 1600\phantom{0} \\ 2400\phantom{00} \\ \hline 260{,}000 \end{array}$$

**67.** $$\begin{array}{r} 987 \\ \times\ 349 \\ \hline 8883 \\ 3948\phantom{0} \\ 2961\phantom{00} \\ \hline 344{,}463 \end{array}$$

**69.** $$\begin{array}{r} 312 \\ \times\ 134 \\ \hline 1248 \\ 936\phantom{0} \\ 312\phantom{00} \\ \hline 41{,}808 \end{array}$$

**71.** $$\begin{array}{r} 379 \\ \times\ \ 500 \\ \hline 189{,}500 \end{array}$$

**73.** $$\begin{array}{r} 985 \\ \times\ \ 408 \\ \hline 7880 \\ 39400\phantom{0} \\ \hline 401{,}880 \end{array}$$

**75.** $$\begin{array}{r} 3407 \\ \times\ \ 309 \\ \hline 30663 \\ 102210\phantom{0} \\ \hline 1{,}052{,}763 \end{array}$$

**77.** $$\begin{array}{r} 4258 \\ \times\ 986 \\ \hline 25548 \\ 34064\phantom{0} \\ 38322\phantom{00} \\ \hline 4{,}198{,}388 \end{array}$$

© 2013 Cengage Learning. All Rights Reserved. May not be scanned, copied or duplicated, or posted to a publicly accessible website, in whole or in part.

**79.** Answers will vary. For example, 5 and 20

$$\begin{array}{r} 20 \\ \times 5 \\ \hline 100 \end{array}$$

**81.**

$$\begin{array}{r} 7349 \\ \times \quad 27 \\ \hline 51443 \\ 14698\phantom{0} \\ \hline 198{,}423 \end{array}$$

**83.** $6 \times 73 = 438$

$$\begin{array}{r} 438 \\ \times \quad 43 \\ \hline 1314 \\ 1752\phantom{0} \\ \hline 18{,}834 \end{array}$$

**85.**

$$\begin{array}{r} 842 \\ \times \quad 309 \\ \hline 7578 \\ 2526\phantom{00} \\ \hline 260{,}178 \end{array}$$

**87.**

$$\begin{array}{rcr} 4732 & \approx & 5000 \\ \times \quad 93 & \approx & \times \quad 90 \\ \hline \text{Cal.: } 440{,}076 & & \text{Est.: } 450{,}000 \end{array}$$

**89.**

$$\begin{array}{rcr} 8941 & \approx & 9000 \\ \times \quad 726 & \approx & \times \quad 700 \\ \hline \text{Cal.: } 6{,}491{,}166 & & \text{Est.: } 6{,}300{,}000 \end{array}$$

**91.**

$$\begin{array}{rcr} 6379 & \approx & 6000 \\ \times \quad 2936 & \approx & \times \quad 3000 \\ \hline \text{Cal.: } 18{,}728{,}744 & & \text{Est.: } 18{,}000{,}000 \end{array}$$

**93.**

$$\begin{array}{rcr} 62{,}504 & \approx & 60{,}000 \\ \times \quad 923 & \approx & \times \quad 900 \\ \hline \text{Cal.: } 57{,}691{,}192 & & \text{Est.: } 54{,}000{,}000 \end{array}$$

## Objective C Exercises

**95. Strategy** To find the number of milligrams in a day, multiply the number of milligrams per dose (25) times the number of doses per day (4).

**Solution**

$$\begin{array}{r} 25 \\ \times 4 \\ \hline 100 \end{array}$$

The total daily dose is 100 milligrams.

**97. Strategy** To find miles driven, multiply the number of gallons (20) by the number of miles per gallon (28).

**Solution**

$$\begin{array}{r} 28 \\ \times 20 \\ \hline 560 \end{array}$$

You drove 560 miles.

**99. Strategy** To cost, multiply the number of cases (12) by the cost per case (25).

**Solution**

$$\begin{array}{r} 25 \\ \times 12 \\ \hline 50 \\ 25\phantom{0} \\ \hline 300 \end{array}$$

The cost for 12 cases is $300.

**101. Strategy** To find cost:

- Multiply the number of cases of gloves (2) by the cost per case (57).
- Multiply the number of boxes of tongue depressors (10) by the cost per box (7).
- Multiply the number of cases of prep pads (1) by the cost per case (35).
- Add the costs together.

**Solution** Gloves: $\begin{array}{r} 57 \\ \times 2 \\ \hline 114 \end{array}$ Depressors: $\begin{array}{r} 10 \\ \times 7 \\ \hline 70 \end{array}$

Prep pads: 35 x 1 = 35

$$\begin{array}{r} 114 \\ 70 \\ +35 \\ \hline 219 \end{array}$$

© 2013 Cengage Learning. All Rights Reserved. May not be scanned, copied or duplicated, or posted to a publicly accessible website, in whole or in part.

The total bill is \$219.

**103. Strategy** To find the number of rolls in one case, multiply the number of rolls per box (12) by the number of boxes per case (24).

**Solution**

$$\begin{array}{r} 24 \\ \underline{\times 12} \\ 48 \\ \underline{24\phantom{0}} \\ 288 \end{array}$$

There are 288 rolls in one case.

**Strategy** To find the cost of one case, multiply the number of rolls per case (24) by the cost per roll (18).

**Solution**

$$\begin{array}{r} 24 \\ \underline{\times 18} \\ 192 \\ \underline{24\phantom{0}} \\ 432 \end{array}$$

The cost of a case is \$432.

## Applying the Concepts

**105.** There is one accidental death every 5 minutes.

There are 60 minutes in an hour.

$5 \times 12 = 60$

There are 12 accidental deaths in an hour.

There are 24 hours per day.

$12 \times 24 = 288$

There are 288 accidental deaths in a day.

There are 365 days in a year.

$288 \times 365 = 105,120$

There are 105,120 accidental deaths in a year.

# Section 1.5

## Objective A Exercises

**1.** 2

**3.** 6

**5.** 7

**7.**

$$\begin{array}{r} 16 \\ 6\overline{)96} \\ \underline{-6}\phantom{0} \\ 36 \\ \underline{-36} \\ 0 \end{array}$$

**9.**

$$\begin{array}{r} 210 \\ 4\overline{)840} \\ \underline{-8}\phantom{00} \\ 04\phantom{0} \\ \underline{-4}\phantom{0} \\ 00 \\ \underline{-0} \\ 0 \end{array}$$

**11.**

$$\begin{array}{r} 44 \\ 7\overline{)308} \\ \underline{-28}\phantom{0} \\ 28 \\ \underline{-28} \\ 0 \end{array}$$

**13.**

$$\begin{array}{r} 703 \\ 9\overline{)6327} \\ \underline{-63}\phantom{00} \\ 02\phantom{0} \\ \underline{-0}\phantom{0} \\ 27 \\ \underline{-27} \\ 0 \end{array}$$

**15.**

$$\begin{array}{r} 910 \\ 8\overline{)7280} \\ \underline{-72}\phantom{00} \\ 08\phantom{0} \\ \underline{-8}\phantom{0} \\ 00 \\ \underline{-0} \\ 0 \end{array}$$

© 2013 Cengage Learning. All Rights Reserved. May not be scanned, copied or duplicated, or posted to a publicly accessible website, in whole or in part.

**17.**
$$\begin{array}{r} 21{,}560 \\ 3\overline{)64{,}680} \\ -6\phantom{4{,}680} \\ \hline 04\phantom{{,}680} \\ -3\phantom{{,}680} \\ \hline 16\phantom{80} \\ -15\phantom{80} \\ \hline 18\phantom{0} \\ -18\phantom{0} \\ \hline 00 \\ -0 \\ \hline 0 \end{array}$$

**19.**
$$\begin{array}{r} 3{,}580 \\ 6\overline{)21{,}480} \\ -18\phantom{{,}480} \\ \hline 34\phantom{80} \\ -30\phantom{80} \\ \hline 48\phantom{0} \\ -48\phantom{0} \\ \hline 00 \\ -0 \\ \hline 0 \end{array}$$

**21.**
$$\begin{array}{r} 1075 \\ 7\overline{)7525} \\ -7\phantom{525} \\ \hline 05\phantom{25} \\ -0\phantom{25} \\ \hline 52\phantom{5} \\ -49\phantom{5} \\ \hline 35 \\ -35 \\ \hline 0 \end{array}$$

**23.** 1

**25.**
$$\begin{array}{r} 47 \\ 8\overline{)376} \\ -32\phantom{6} \\ \hline 56 \\ -56 \\ \hline 0 \end{array}$$

**27.**
$$\begin{array}{r} 23 \\ 4\overline{)92} \\ -8\phantom{2} \\ \hline 12 \\ -12 \\ \hline 0 \end{array}$$

## Objective B Exercises

**29.**
$$\begin{array}{r} 3 \text{ r1} \\ 2\overline{)7} \\ -6 \\ \hline 1 \end{array}$$

**31.**
$$\begin{array}{r} 9 \text{ r7} \\ 9\overline{)88} \\ -81 \\ \hline 7 \end{array}$$

**33.**
$$\begin{array}{r} 16 \text{ r1} \\ 6\overline{)97} \\ -6\phantom{7} \\ \hline 37 \\ -36 \\ \hline 1 \end{array}$$

**35.**
$$\begin{array}{r} 10 \text{ r4} \\ 5\overline{)54} \\ -5\phantom{4} \\ \hline 04 \\ -0 \\ \hline 4 \end{array}$$

**37.**
$$\begin{array}{r} 90 \text{ r3} \\ 4\overline{)363} \\ -36\phantom{3} \\ \hline 03 \\ -0 \\ \hline 3 \end{array}$$

**39.**
$$\begin{array}{r} 120 \text{ r5} \\ 7\overline{)845} \\ -7\phantom{45} \\ \hline 14\phantom{5} \\ -14\phantom{5} \\ \hline 05 \\ -0 \\ \hline 5 \end{array}$$

**41.**
$$\begin{array}{r} 309 \text{ r3} \\ 5\overline{)1548} \\ -15\phantom{48} \\ \hline 04\phantom{8} \\ -0\phantom{8} \\ \hline 48 \\ -45 \\ \hline 3 \end{array}$$

© 2013 Cengage Learning. All Rights Reserved. May not be scanned, copied or duplicated, or posted to a publicly accessible website, in whole or in part.

**43.** 1160 r4
$7\overline{)8124}$
−7
11
−7
42
−42
04
− 0
4

**45.** 708 r2
$5\overline{)3542}$
−35
04
− 0
42
−40
2

**47.** 3,825 r1
$4\overline{)15,301}$
−12
33
−32
10
− 8
21
−20
1

**49.** 9,044 r2
$8\overline{)72,354}$
−72
03
−0
35
−32
34
−32
2

**51.** 11,434 r2
$4\overline{)45,738}$
−4
05
−4
17
−16
13
−12
18
−16
2

Round to 11,430.

**53.** 510 r2
$7\overline{)3572}$
−35
07
−7
02
−0
2

Round to 510.

**55.** False

## Objective C Exercises

**57.** 1 r38
$44\overline{)82}$
−44
38

**59.** 1 r26
$67\overline{)93}$
−67
26

**61.** 21 r21
$32\overline{)693}$
−64
53
−32
21

**63.** 30 r22
$25\overline{)772}$
− 75
22
− 0
22

**65.** 5 r40
$92\overline{)500}$
− 460
40

**67.** 9 r17
$50\overline{)467}$
−450
17

© 2013 Cengage Learning. All Rights Reserved. May not be scanned, copied or duplicated, or posted to a publicly accessible website, in whole or in part.

**69.**
$$\begin{array}{r} 200 \text{ r21} \\ 44\overline{)8821} \\ -88 \\ \hline 02 \\ -0 \\ \hline 21 \\ -0 \\ \hline 21 \end{array}$$

**71.**
$$\begin{array}{r} 303 \text{ r1} \\ 32\overline{)9697} \\ -96 \\ \hline 09 \\ -0 \\ \hline 97 \\ -96 \\ \hline 1 \end{array}$$

**73.**
$$\begin{array}{r} 67 \text{ r13} \\ 92\overline{)6177} \\ -552 \\ \hline 657 \\ -644 \\ \hline 13 \end{array}$$

**75.**
$$\begin{array}{r} 176 \text{ r13} \\ 27\overline{)4765} \\ -27 \\ \hline 206 \\ -189 \\ \hline 175 \\ -162 \\ \hline 13 \end{array}$$

**77.**
$$\begin{array}{r} 1{,}086 \text{ r7} \\ 77\overline{)83{,}639} \\ -77 \\ \hline 66 \\ -0 \\ \hline 662 \\ -616 \\ \hline 469 \\ -462 \\ \hline 7 \end{array}$$

**79.**
$$\begin{array}{r} 403 \\ 78\overline{)31{,}434} \\ -312 \\ \hline 23 \\ -0 \\ \hline 234 \\ -234 \\ \hline 0 \end{array}$$

**81.**
$$\begin{array}{r} 12 \text{ r456} \\ 504\overline{)6504} \\ -504 \\ \hline 1464 \\ -1008 \\ \hline 456 \end{array}$$

**83.**
$$\begin{array}{r} 4 \text{ r160} \\ 546\overline{)2344} \\ -2184 \\ \hline 160 \end{array}$$

**85.**
$$\begin{array}{r} 160 \text{ r27} \\ 53\overline{)8507} \\ -53 \\ \hline 320 \\ -318 \\ \hline 27 \end{array}$$

**87.**
$$\begin{array}{r} 1{,}669 \text{ r14} \\ 46\overline{)76{,}788} \\ -46 \\ \hline 307 \\ -276 \\ \hline 318 \\ -276 \\ \hline 428 \\ -414 \\ \hline 14 \end{array}$$

**89.**
$$\begin{array}{r} 7{,}948 \text{ r17} \\ 43\overline{)341{,}781} \\ -301 \\ \hline 407 \\ -387 \\ \hline 208 \\ -172 \\ \hline 361 \\ -344 \\ \hline 17 \end{array}$$

Round to 7950.

**91.** Cal.: $76\overline{)389{,}804}$ = 5,129 Est.: $80\overline{)400{,}000}$ = 5,000

**93.** Cal.: $29\overline{)637{,}072}$ = 21,968 Est.: $30\overline{)600{,}000}$ = 20,000

**95.** Cal.: $38\overline{)934{,}684}$ = 24,596 Est.: $40\overline{)900{,}000}$ = 22,500

© 2013 Cengage Learning. All Rights Reserved. May not be scanned, copied or duplicated, or posted to a publicly accessible website, in whole or in part.

**97.** Cal.: $309\overline{)876,324}$ = 2,836  Est.: $300\overline{)900,000}$ = 3,000

**99.** Cal.: $209\overline{)632,016}$ = 3,024  Est.: $200\overline{)600,000}$ = 3,000

**101.** Cal.: $179\overline{)5,734,444}$ = 32,036  Est.: $200\overline{)6,000,000}$ = 30,000

## Objective D Exercises

**103. Strategy** To find the average claim for hip replacement surgery, divide the yearly cost (879,000) by the number of months in a year (12).

**Solution**

$$\begin{array}{r} 73,250 \\ 12\overline{)879,000} \\ -84\phantom{0,000} \\ \hline 39\phantom{,000} \\ -36\phantom{,000} \\ \hline 30\phantom{00} \\ -24\phantom{00} \\ \hline 60\phantom{0} \\ -60\phantom{0} \\ \hline 00 \end{array}$$

The average monthly claim for hip replacement is $73,250.

**105. Strategy** To find the average claim for fracture repair, divide the yearly cost (684,000) by the number of months in a year (12).

**Solution**

$$\begin{array}{r} 57,000 \\ 12\overline{)684,000} \\ -60\phantom{0,000} \\ \hline 84\phantom{,000} \\ -84\phantom{,000} \\ \hline 0\phantom{,000} \end{array}$$

The average monthly claim for fracture repair is $57,000.

**107. Strategy** To find the approximate number of permits per person, divide the number of pennies in circulation (114,000,000,000) by the number of people (300,000,00).

**Solution** $114,000,000,000 \div 300,000,000 = 380$

380 pennies are in circulation for each person.

**109. Strategy** To find the average number of bills, divide the total number of bills (11,520) by the number of months in a year (12).

**Solution**

$$\begin{array}{r} 960 \\ 12\overline{)11,520} \\ -108\phantom{0} \\ \hline 72\phantom{0} \\ -72\phantom{0} \\ \hline 0\phantom{0} \end{array}$$

There were an average of 960 bills per month.

**111.** (i) and (ii)

## Applying the Concepts

**113. Strategy** To find the total of the three deductions, add the three deductions.

**Solution**

| | |
|---|---|
| $225 | Savings |
| 98 | Taxes |
| 27 | Insurance |
| $350 | |

The total of the three deductions is $350.

**115. Strategy** To find the cost per year for one, multiply the monthly cost for one (432) time the number of months in a year (12).

**117. Strategy** To find the total amount spent annually, add all the expenses.

© 2013 Cengage Learning. All Rights Reserved. May not be scanned, copied or duplicated, or posted to a publicly accessible website, in whole or in part.

**Solution**

$$\begin{array}{r} \$11{,}713 \\ 5366 \\ 1746 \\ 1903 \\ 3381 \\ 4810 \\ +\,6616 \\ \hline \$35{,}535 \end{array}$$

The total amount spent annually is $35,535.

**119. Strategy** To find a dental hygienists monthly pay, divide the annual pay by the number of months in a year (12).

**Solution**

$$\begin{array}{r} 5{,}571 \\ 12\overline{)66{,}852} \\ \underline{-60}\phantom{{,}852} \\ 68\phantom{52} \\ \underline{-60}\phantom{52} \\ 85\phantom{2} \\ \underline{-84}\phantom{2} \\ 12 \\ \underline{-12} \\ 0 \end{array}$$

The monthly pay for a dental hygienist is $5571.

**121. Strategy** To find the total amount paid for the car:

• Multiply $195 by 48 to find the amount paid in monthly payments.

• Add the total for the monthly payments to the down payment ($2500).

**Solution**

$$\begin{array}{r} 195 \\ \times\ 48 \\ \hline 1560 \\ 780\phantom{0} \\ \hline 9360 \end{array} \qquad \begin{array}{r} 2500 \\ +9360 \\ \hline 11{,}860 \end{array}$$

The total amount paid for the car was $11,860.

## Section 1.6

### Objective A Exercises

**1.** $2^3$

**3.** $6^3 \cdot 7^4$

**5.** $2^3 \cdot 3^3$

**7.** $5 \cdot 7^5$

**9.** $3^3 \cdot 6^4$

**11.** $3^3 \cdot 5 \cdot 9^3$

**13.** $2 \cdot 2 \cdot 2 = 8$

**15.** $2 \cdot 2 \cdot 2 \cdot 2 \cdot 5 \cdot 5 = 16 \cdot 25 = 400$

**17.** $3 \cdot 3 \cdot 10 \cdot 10 = 9 \cdot 100 = 900$

**19.** $6 \cdot 6 \cdot 3 \cdot 3 \cdot 3 = 36 \cdot 27 = 972$

**21.** $5 \cdot 2 \cdot 2 \cdot 2 \cdot 3 = 5 \cdot 8 \cdot 3 = 120$

**23.** $2 \cdot 2 \cdot 3 \cdot 3 \cdot 10 = 4 \cdot 9 \cdot 10 = 360$

**25.** $0 \cdot 0 \cdot 4 \cdot 4 \cdot 4 = 0 \cdot 64 = 0$

**27.** $3 \cdot 3 \cdot 10 \cdot 10 \cdot 10 \cdot 10 = 9 \cdot 10{,}000 = 90{,}000$

**29.** $2 \cdot 2 \cdot 3 \cdot 3 \cdot 3 \cdot 5 = 4 \cdot 27 \cdot 5 = 540$

**31.** $2 \cdot 3 \cdot 3 \cdot 3 \cdot 3 \cdot 5 \cdot 5 = 2 \cdot 81 \cdot 25 = 4050$

**33.** $5 \cdot 5 \cdot 3 \cdot 3 \cdot 7 \cdot 7 = 25 \cdot 9 \cdot 49 = 11{,}025$

**35.** $3 \cdot 3 \cdot 3 \cdot 3 \cdot 2 \cdot 2 \cdot 2 \cdot 2 \cdot 2 \cdot 2 \cdot 5$
$= 81 \cdot 64 \cdot 5$
$= 25{,}920$

**37.** $4 \cdot 4 \cdot 3 \cdot 3 \cdot 3 \cdot 10 \cdot 10 \cdot 10 \cdot 10$
$= 16 \cdot 27 \cdot 10{,}000$
$= 4{,}320{,}000$

### Objective B Exercises

**39.** $4 - 2 + 3 = 2 + 3 = 5$

**41.** $6 \div 3 + 2 = 2 + 2 = 4$

**43.** $6 \cdot 3 + 5 = 18 + 5 = 23$

© 2013 Cengage Learning. All Rights Reserved. May not be scanned, copied or duplicated, or posted to a publicly accessible website, in whole or in part.

**45.** $3^2 - 4 = 9 - 4 = 5$

**47.** $4 \cdot (5 - 3) + 2 = 4 \cdot 2 + 2 = 8 + 2 = 10$

**49.** $5 + (8 + 4) \div 6 = 5 + 12 \div 6$
$= 5 + 2 = 7$

**51.** $16 \cdot (3 + 2) \div 10 = 16 \cdot 5 \div 10$
$= 80 \div 10 = 8$

**53.** $10 - 2^3 + 4 = 10 - 8 + 4$
$= 2 + 4 = 6$

**55.** $16 + 4 \cdot 3^2 = 16 + 4 \cdot 9$
$= 16 + 36 = 52$

**57.** $16 + (8 - 3) \cdot 2 = 16 + 5 \cdot 2$
$= 16 + 10 = 26$

**59.** $2^2 + 3 \cdot (6 - 2)^2 = 2^2 + 3 \cdot 4^2$
$= 4 + 3 \cdot 16$
$= 4 + 48 = 52$

**61.** $2^2 \cdot 3^2 + 2 \cdot 3 = 4 \cdot 9 + 2 \cdot 3$
$= 36 + 2 \cdot 3$
$= 36 + 6 = 42$

**63.** $16 - 2 \cdot 4 = 16 - 8 = 8$

**65.** $3 \cdot (6 - 2) + 4 = 3 \cdot 4 + 4 = 12 + 4 = 16$

**67.** $8 - (8 - 2) \div 3 = 8 - 6 \div 3 = 8 - 2 = 6$

**69.** $8 + 2 - 3 \cdot 2 \div 3 = 8 + 2 - 6 \div 3$
$= 8 + 2 - 2$
$= 10 - 2 = 8$

**71.** $3 \cdot (4 + 2) \div 6 = 3 \cdot 6 \div 6 = 18 \div 6 = 3$

**73.** $20 - 4 \div 2 \cdot (3 - 1)^3 = 20 - 4 \div 2 \cdot 2^3$
$= 20 - 4 \div 2 \cdot 8$
$= 20 - 2 \cdot 8$
$= 20 - 16 = 4$

**75.** $(4 - 2) \cdot 6 \div 3 + (5 - 2)^2 = 2 \cdot 6 \div 3 + 3^2$
$= 2 \cdot 6 \div 3 + 9$
$= 12 \div 3 + 9$
$= 4 + 9 = 13$

**77.** $100 \div (2 + 3)^2 - 8 \div 2 = 100 \div 5^2 - 8 \div 2$
$= 100 \div 25 - 8 \div 2$
$= 4 - 8 \div 2$
$= 4 - 4 = 0$

**79.** $8 - 2 \cdot (3 + 1) = 0$

## Applying the Concepts

**81.** In part a, the expression $(14 - 2)$ is first divided by 2 and then multiplied by 3. In part b, the same expression is divided by the product of 2 and 3.

$(14 - 2) \div 2 \cdot 3 = 12 \div 2 \cdot 3 = 6 \cdot 3 = 18$

$(14 - 2) \div (2 \cdot 3) = 12 \div 6 = 2$

The difference between the two answers is $18 - 2 = 16$.

# Section 1.7

## Objective A Exercises

**1.** $4 \div 1 = 4$
$4 \div 2 = 2$
Factors are 1, 2, and 4.

**3.** $10 \div 1 = 10$
$10 \div 2 = 5$
$10 \div 5 = 2$
Factors are 1, 2, 5, and 10.

**5.** $7 \div 1 = 7$
$7 \div 7 = 1$
Factors are 1 and 7.

**7.** $9 \div 1 = 9$
$9 \div 3 = 3$
Factors are 1, 3, and 9.

**9.** $13 \div 1 = 13$
$13 \div 13 = 1$
Factors are 1 and 13.

© 2013 Cengage Learning. All Rights Reserved. May not be scanned, copied or duplicated, or posted to a publicly accessible website, in whole or in part.

**11.** $18 \div 1 = 18$
$18 \div 2 = 9$
$18 \div 3 = 6$
$18 \div 6 = 3$
Factors are 1, 2, 3, 6, 9, and 18.

**13.** $56 \div 1 = 56$
$56 \div 2 = 28$
$56 \div 4 = 14$
$56 \div 7 = 8$
$56 \div 8 = 7$
Factors are 1, 2, 4, 7, 8, 14, 28, and 56.

**15.** $45 \div 1 = 45$
$45 \div 3 = 15$
$45 \div 5 = 9$
Factors are 1, 3, 5, 9, 15, and 45.

**17.** $29 \div 1 = 29$
$29 \div 29 = 1$
Factors are 1 and 29.

**19.** $22 \div 1 = 22$
$22 \div 2 = 11$
$22 \div 11 = 2$
Factors are 1, 2, 11, and 22.

**21.** $52 \div 1 = 52$
$52 \div 2 = 26$
$52 \div 4 = 13$
$52 \div 13 = 4$
Factors are 1, 2, 4, 13, 26, and 52.

**23.** $82 \div 1 = 82$
$82 \div 2 = 41$
$82 \div 41 = 2$
Factors are 1, 2, 41, and 82.

**25.** $57 \div 1 = 57$
$57 \div 3 = 19$
$57 \div 19 = 3$
Factors are 1, 3, 19, and 57.

**27.** $48 \div 1 = 48$
$48 \div 2 = 24$
$48 \div 3 = 16$
$48 \div 4 = 12$
$48 \div 6 = 8$
$48 \div 8 = 6$
Factors are 1, 2, 3, 4, 6, 8, 12, 16, 24, and 48.

**29.** $95 \div 1 = 95$
$95 \div 5 = 19$
$95 \div 19 = 5$
Factors are 1, 5, 19, and 95.

**31.** $54 \div 1 = 54$
$54 \div 2 = 27$
$54 \div 3 = 18$
$54 \div 6 = 9$
$54 \div 9 = 6$
Factors are 1, 2, 3, 6, 9, 18, 27, and 54.

**33.** $66 \div 1 = 66$
$66 \div 2 = 33$
$66 \div 3 = 22$
$66 \div 6 = 11$
$66 \div 11 = 6$
Factors are 1, 2, 3, 6, 11, 22, 33, and 66.

**35.** $80 \div 1 = 80$
$80 \div 2 = 40$
$80 \div 4 = 20$
$80 \div 5 = 16$
$80 \div 8 = 10$
$80 \div 10 = 8$
Factors are 1, 2, 4, 5, 8, 10, 16, 20, 40, and 80.

**37.**

$96 \div 1 = 96$
$96 \div 2 = 48$
$96 \div 3 = 32$
$96 \div 4 = 24$
$96 \div 6 = 16$
$96 \div 8 = 12$
$96 \div 12 = 8$
Factors are 1, 2, 3, 4, 6, 8, 12, 16, 24, 32, 48, and 96.

© 2013 Cengage Learning. All Rights Reserved. May not be scanned, copied or duplicated, or posted to a publicly accessible website, in whole or in part.

**39.**

$90 \div 1 = 90$
$90 \div 2 = 45$
$90 \div 3 = 30$
$90 \div 5 = 18$
$90 \div 6 = 15$
$90 \div 9 = 10$
$90 \div 10 = 9$
Factors are 1, 2, 3, 4, 6, 8, 12, 16, 24, 32, 48, and 96.

**41.** True

## Objective B Exercises

**43.**

| 6 | |
|---|---|
| 2 | 3 |
| 3 | 1 |

$6 = 2 \cdot 3$

**45.** 17 is prime.

**47.**

| 24 | |
|---|---|
| 2 | 12 |
| 2 | 6 |
| 2 | 3 |
| 3 | 1 |

$24 = 2 \cdot 2 \cdot 2 \cdot 3$

**49.**

| 27 | |
|---|---|
| 3 | 9 |
| 3 | 3 |
| 3 | 1 |

$27 = 3 \cdot 3 \cdot 3$

**51.**

| 36 | |
|---|---|
| 2 | 18 |
| 2 | 9 |
| 3 | 3 |
| 3 | 1 |

$36 = 2 \cdot 2 \cdot 3 \cdot 3$

**53.** 19 is prime.

**55.**

| 90 | |
|---|---|
| 2 | 45 |
| 3 | 15 |
| 3 | 5 |
| 5 | 1 |

$90 = 2 \cdot 3 \cdot 3 \cdot 5$

**57.**

| 115 | |
|---|---|
| 5 | 23 |
| 23 | 1 |

$115 = 5 \cdot 23$

**59.**

| 18 | |
|---|---|
| 2 | 9 |
| 3 | 3 |
| 3 | 1 |

$18 = 2 \cdot 3 \cdot 3$

**61.**

| 28 | |
|---|---|
| 2 | 14 |
| 2 | 7 |
| 7 | 1 |

$28 = 2 \cdot 2 \cdot 7$

**63.** 31 is prime.

**65.**

| 62 | |
|---|---|
| 2 | 31 |
| 31 | 1 |

$62 = 2 \cdot 31$

**67.**

| 22 | |
|---|---|
| 2 | 11 |
| 11 | 1 |

$22 = 2 \cdot 11$

**69.** 101 is prime.

**71.**

| 66 | |
|---|---|
| 2 | 33 |
| 3 | 11 |
| 11 | 1 |

$66 = 2 \cdot 3 \cdot 11$

**73.**

| 74 | |
|---|---|
| 2 | 37 |
| 37 | 1 |

$74 = 2 \cdot 37$

**75.** 67 is prime.

**77.**

| 55 | |
|---|---|
| 5 | 11 |
| 11 | 1 |

$55 = 5 \cdot 11$

© 2013 Cengage Learning. All Rights Reserved. May not be scanned, copied or duplicated, or posted to a publicly accessible website, in whole or in part.

**79.**
$$\begin{array}{r|r} & 120 \\ \hline 2 & 60 \\ 2 & 30 \\ 2 & 15 \\ 3 & 5 \\ 5 & 1 \end{array}$$
$120 = 2 \cdot 2 \cdot 2 \cdot 3 \cdot 5$

**81.**
$$\begin{array}{r|r} & 160 \\ \hline 2 & 80 \\ 2 & 40 \\ 2 & 20 \\ 2 & 10 \\ 2 & 5 \\ 5 & 1 \end{array}$$
$160 = 2 \cdot 2 \cdot 2 \cdot 2 \cdot 2 \cdot 5$

**83.**
$$\begin{array}{r|r} & 216 \\ \hline 2 & 108 \\ 2 & 54 \\ 2 & 27 \\ 3 & 9 \\ 3 & 3 \\ 3 & 1 \end{array}$$
$216 = 2 \cdot 2 \cdot 2 \cdot 3 \cdot 3 \cdot 3$

**85.**
$$\begin{array}{r|r} & 625 \\ \hline 5 & 125 \\ 5 & 25 \\ 5 & 5 \\ 5 & 1 \end{array}$$
$625 = 5 \cdot 5 \cdot 5 \cdot 5$

**87.** False; the prime factorization of 102 is $2 \cdot 3 \cdot 17$.

## Applying the Concepts

**89.** 2 is the *only* even prime number because all other even numbers have 2 as a factor and thus cannot be prime.

# Chapter 1 Concept Review

**1.** The symbol < means "is less than." A number that appears to the left of a given number on the number line is less than (<) the given number. For example, 4 < 9. The symbol > means "is greater than." A number that appears to the right of a given number on the number line is greater than (>) the given number. For example, 5 > 2.

**2.** To round a four-digit number to the nearest hundred, look at the digit in the tens place. If the digit in the tens place is less than 5, that digit and the digit in the ones place are replaced by zeros. If the digit in the tens place is greater than or equal to 5, increase the digit in the hundreds place by 1 and replace the digit in the tens place and the ones place by zeros.

**3.** The Commutative Property of Addition states that two numbers can be added in either order; the sum is the same. For example, 3 + 5 = 5 + 3. The Associative Property of Addition states that changing the grouping of three or more addends does not change their sum. For example, 3 + (4 + 5) = (3 + 4) + 5. Note that in the Commutative Property of Addition, the order in which the numbers appear changes, while in the Associative Property of Addition, the order in which the numbers appear does not change.

**4.** To estimate the sum of two numbers, round each number to the same place value. Then add the

© 2013 Cengage Learning. All Rights Reserved. May not be scanned, copied or duplicated, or posted to a publicly accessible website, in whole or in part.

numbers. For example, to estimate the sum of 562,397 and 41,086, round the numbers to 560,000 and 40,000. Then add 560,000 + 40,000 = 600,000.

**5.** It is necessary to borrow when performing subtraction if, in any place value, the lower digit is larger than the upper digit.

**6.** The Multiplication Property of Zero states that the product of a number and zero is zero. For example, $8\times0=0$. The Multiplication Property of One states that the product of a number and one is the number. For example, $8\times1=8$.

**7.** To multiply a whole number by 100, write two zeros to the right of the number. For example, $64\times100=6400$.

**8.** To estimate the product of two numbers, round each number so that it contains only one nonzero digit. Then multiply. For example, to estimate the product of 87 and 43, round the two numbers to 90 and 40; then multiply $90\times40=3600$.

**9.** $0\div9=0$. Zero divided by any whole number except zero is zero. $9\div0$ is undefined. Division by zero is not allowed.

**10.** To check the answer to a division problem that has a remainder, multiply the quotient by the divisor. Add the remainder to the product. The result should be the dividend. For example, $16\div5=3$ r1. Check: $(3\times5)+1=16$, the dividend.

**11.** The steps in the Order of Operations Agreement are:

**1.** Do all operations inside parentheses.

**2.** Simplify any number expressions containing exponents.

**3.** Do multiplication and division as they occur from left to right.

**4.** Do addition and subtraction as they occur from left to right.

**12.** A number is a factor of another number if it divides that number evenly (there is no remainder). For example, 7 is a factor of 21 because $21\div7=3$, with a remainder of 0.

**13.** Three is a factor of a number if the sum of the digits of the number is divisible by 3. For the number 285, $2+8+5=15$, which is divisible by 3. Thus 285 is divisible by 3.

## Chapter 1 Review Exercises

**1.** $3\cdot2^3\cdot5^2=3\cdot8\cdot25$
$=24\cdot25=600$

**2.** 10,000 + 300 + 20 + 7

**3.** $18\div1=18$
$18\div2=9$
$18\div3=6$
$18\div6=3$
Factors are 1, 2, 3, 6, 9, and 18.

© 2013 Cengage Learning. All Rights Reserved. May not be scanned, copied or duplicated, or posted to a publicly accessible website, in whole or in part.

**4.**
$$\begin{array}{r} {\scriptstyle 1\,1\,1} \\ 5894 \\ 6301 \\ +\quad 298 \\ \hline 12{,}493 \end{array}$$

**5.**
$$\begin{array}{r} {\scriptstyle 11} \\ {\scriptstyle 8\ \ \not{1}\ \ 16} \\ 4\,\not{9}\,\not{2}\,\not{6} \\ -3\,1\,7\,7 \\ \hline 1\,7\,4\,9 \end{array}$$

**6.**
$$\begin{array}{r} 2{,}135 \\ 7\overline{)14{,}945} \\ -14 \\ \hline 09 \\ -7 \\ \hline 24 \\ -21 \\ \hline 35 \\ -35 \\ \hline 0 \end{array}$$

**7.** $101 > 87$

**8.** $5 \cdot 5 \cdot 7 \cdot 7 \cdot 7 \cdot 7 \cdot 7 = 5^2 \cdot 7^5$

**9.**
$$\begin{array}{r} {\scriptstyle 6} \\ 2019 \\ \times\quad 307 \\ \hline 14133 \\ 60570\phantom{0} \\ \hline 619{,}833 \end{array}$$

**10.**
$$\begin{array}{r} {\scriptstyle 9} \\ {\scriptstyle \not{0}\,10\,11\,2\,14} \\ \not{1}\not{0},\not{1}\not{3}\not{4} \\ -\ 4{,}725 \\ \hline 5{,}409 \end{array}$$

**11.**
$$\begin{array}{r} {\scriptstyle 1\,1} \\ 298 \\ 461 \\ +\quad 322 \\ \hline 1018 \end{array}$$

**12.** $2^3 - 3 \cdot 2 = 8 - 3 \cdot 2 = 8 - 6 = 2$

**13.** 45,700

**14.** Two hundred seventy-six thousand fifty-seven

**15.**
$$\begin{array}{r} 1306 \quad \text{r59} \\ 84\overline{)109{,}763} \\ -84\phantom{{,}763} \\ \hline 257\phantom{63} \\ -252\phantom{63} \\ \hline 56\phantom{3} \\ -0\phantom{3} \\ \hline 563 \\ -504 \\ \hline 59 \end{array}$$

**16.** 2,011,044

**17.**
$$\begin{array}{r} 488 \quad \text{r2} \\ 8\overline{)3906} \\ -32\phantom{06} \\ \hline 70\phantom{6} \\ -64\phantom{6} \\ \hline 66 \\ -64 \\ \hline 2 \end{array}$$

**18.**
$$\begin{aligned} 3^2 + 2^2 \cdot (5-3) &= 3^2 + 2^2 \cdot (2) \\ &= 9 + 4 \cdot 2 \\ &= 9 + 8 = 17 \end{aligned}$$

**19.**
$$\begin{aligned} 8 \cdot (6-2)^2 \div 4 &= 8 \cdot 4^2 \div 4 \\ &= 8 \cdot 16 \div 4 \\ &= 128 \cdot 4 = 32 \end{aligned}$$

**20.**
$$\begin{array}{r|l} \multicolumn{2}{l}{72} \\ 2 & 36 \\ 2 & 18 \\ 2 & 9 \\ 3 & 3 \\ 3 & 1 \end{array}$$

$72 = 2 \cdot 2 \cdot 2 \cdot 3 \cdot 3$

**21.** 2133

**22.**
$$\begin{array}{r} 843 \\ \times\quad 27 \\ \hline 5901 \\ 1686\phantom{0} \\ \hline 22{,}761 \end{array}$$

**23.** **Strategy** To difference in the blood count, subtract the blood count before the operation (6478) from the blood count after the operation (12,789).

© 2013 Cengage Learning. All Rights Reserved. May not be scanned, copied or duplicated, or posted to a publicly accessible website, in whole or in part.

**Solution**

$$\begin{array}{r} 12,789 \\ -6,478 \\ \hline 6,311 \end{array}$$

The difference in the blood count before and after surgery was 6,311 WBC.

**24. Strategy** To find the total pay:

- Multiply the hourly rate ($24) by the number of extra hours worked (20).
- Add the extra wages to the amount for working a 40 hour week ($660).

**Solution**

$$\begin{array}{r} 24 \\ \times 20 \\ \hline 420 \end{array} \text{ additional pay} \qquad \begin{array}{r} 660 \\ +480 \\ \hline 1140 \end{array}$$

The medical transcriptionist's total pay for the week was $1140.

**25. Strategy** To number of patients, divide the total ounces of oil (426) by the number of ounces per client (6).

**Solution**

$$\begin{array}{r} 71 \\ 6\overline{)426} \\ \underline{42} \\ 06 \\ \underline{6} \\ 0 \end{array}$$

The massage therapist had 71 clients.

**26. Strategy** To find the monthly payments:

- Subtract the deposit (2000) from the total amount owed (22,250).
- Divide the amount left by the number of months (50).

**Solution**

$$\begin{array}{r} 22,250 \\ -2000 \\ \hline 20,250 \end{array} \qquad \begin{array}{r} 405 \\ 50\overline{)20,250} \\ \underline{-200} \\ 25 \\ \underline{0} \\ 250 \\ \underline{-250} \\ 0 \end{array}$$

The monthly payment will be $405.

**27. Strategy** To find the total amount deposited, add the two deposits ($3894 and $2985). To find the new checking account balance, add the total amount deposited to the original balance ($5396).

**Solution**

$$\begin{array}{r} 3894 \\ +2985 \\ \hline 6879 \end{array}$$

The total amount deposit is $6879.

$$\begin{array}{r} 5396 \\ +6879 \\ \hline 12,275 \end{array}$$

The new account balance is $12,275

**28. Strategy** To find the total of the car payments over a 12-month period, multiply the amount of each payment ($246) by the number of payments (12).

**Solution**

$$\begin{array}{r} 246 \\ \times 12 \\ \hline 492 \\ 246\phantom{0} \\ \hline 2952 \end{array}$$

The total of the car payment is $2952.

**29. Strategy** To find the difference, subtract the numbers of OTA's (26,600) from the number of PTA's (63,800).

**Solution**

$$\begin{array}{r} 63,800 \\ -26,600 \\ \hline 37,200 \end{array}$$

The difference between the number of OTA's and the number of PTA's is 37,200 people.

**30. Strategy** To find the difference between the number of PTA's, subtract the number of PTA's in 2008 (63,800) from the number in 2018 (85,00).

**Solution**

$$\begin{array}{r} 85,000 \\ -63,800 \\ \hline 21,200 \end{array}$$

The difference between the numbers of PTA's in 2008 and 2018 is 21,200.

© 2013 Cengage Learning. All Rights Reserved. May not be scanned, copied or duplicated, or posted to a publicly accessible website, in whole or in part.

**31. Strategy** To find the average increase per year:

- Subtract the number in 2008 (63,800) from the number in 2018 (85,000).
- Divide the increase by the number of years (10).

**Solution**

$$\begin{array}{r} 85,000 \\ -63,800 \\ \hline 21,200 \end{array}$$

$$21,200 \div 10 = 2,120$$

$$\begin{array}{r} -20 \\ \hline 12 \\ -10 \\ \hline 20 \\ -20 \\ \hline 0 \end{array}$$

The number of PTA's increased an average of 2,120 per year.

**32. Strategy** To find the average increase per year:

- Subtract the number in 2008 (26,600) from the number in 2018 (34,600).
- Divide the increase by the number of years (10).

**Solution**

$$\begin{array}{r} 34,600 \\ -26,600 \\ \hline 8,000 \end{array}$$

$$8,000 \div 10 = 800$$

$$\begin{array}{r} -80 \\ \hline 0 \end{array}$$

The number of OTA's increased an average of 800 per year.

# Chapter 1 Test

**1.** $3^3 \cdot 4^2 = 27 \cdot 16 = 432$

**2.** Two hundred seven thousand sixty-eight

**3.**

$$\begin{array}{r} \overset{0\,17}{\not{1}\not{7}},495 \\ -8,162 \\ \hline 9,333 \end{array}$$

**4.** $20 \div 1 = 20$
$20 \div 2 = 10$
$20 \div 4 = 5$
$20 \div 5 = 4$
Factors are 1, 2, 4, 5, 10, and 20.

**5.**

$$\begin{array}{r} 9736 \\ \times \quad 704 \\ \hline 38,944 \\ 681,520 \\ \hline 6,854,144 \end{array}$$

**6.** $4^2 \cdot (4 - 2) \div 8 + 5 = 4^2 \cdot (2) \div 8 + 5$
$= 16 \cdot (2) \div 8 + 5$
$= 32 \div 8 + 5$
$= 4 + 5 = 9$

**7.** 900,000 + 6000 + 300 + 70 + 8

**8.** 75,000

**9.** $108,764 \div 97 = 1121 \text{ r}27$

$$\begin{array}{r} -97 \\ \hline 117 \\ -97 \\ \hline 206 \\ -194 \\ \hline 124 \\ -97 \\ \hline 27 \end{array}$$

**10.** $3 \cdot 3 \cdot 3 \cdot 7 \cdot 7 = 3^3 \cdot 7^2$

**11.**

$$\begin{array}{r} \scriptstyle 2\ \ 21 \\ 8,756 \\ 9,094 \\ +\ 37,065 \\ \hline 54,915 \end{array}$$

**12.** $84 = 2 \cdot 2 \cdot 3 \cdot 7$

| | 84 |
|---|---|
| 2 | 42 |
| 2 | 21 |
| 3 | 7 |
| 1 | 1 |

© 2013 Cengage Learning. All Rights Reserved. May not be scanned, copied or duplicated, or posted to a publicly accessible website, in whole or in part.

**13.** $16 \div 4 \cdot 2 - (7 - 5)^2 = 16 \div 4 \cdot 2 - 2^2$
$= 16 \div 4 \cdot 2 - 4$
$= 4 \cdot 2 - 4$
$= 8 - 4 = 4$

**14.**
$$\begin{array}{r} {\scriptstyle 6\ \ 5\ 2} \\ 90{,}763 \\ \times \quad\quad 8 \\ \hline 726{,}104 \end{array}$$

**15.** 1,204,006

**16.**
$$\begin{array}{r} 8710 \text{ r2} \\ 7\overline{)60972} \\ -56 \\ \hline 49 \\ -49 \\ \hline 07 \\ -7 \\ \hline 02 \\ -0 \\ \hline 2 \end{array}$$

**17.** 21 > 19

**18.**
$$\begin{array}{r} 703 \\ 8\overline{)5624} \\ -56 \\ \hline 02 \\ -0 \\ \hline 24 \\ -24 \\ \hline 0 \end{array}$$

**19.**
$$\begin{array}{r} 25{,}492 \\ +71{,}306 \\ \hline 96{,}798 \end{array}$$

**20.**
$$\begin{array}{r} {\scriptstyle 1\ 18\ 17} \\ \not{2}\not{9},\not{7}36 \\ -\ 9{,}814 \\ \hline 19{,}922 \end{array}$$

**21. Strategy** To find the difference between the total enrollment in 2016 and 2013:
- Add the numbers in the two columns for 2013 to find the total enrollment for 2013.
- Add the numbers in the two columns for 2016 to find the total enrollment for 2016.
- Subtract the two values to find the difference.

**Solution**
$$\begin{array}{rl} \underline{2013}:\ 41{,}873{,}000 & \text{K}-8 \\ +16{,}000{,}000 & 9-12 \\ \hline 57{,}873{,}000 & \end{array}$$

$$\begin{array}{rl} \underline{2016}:\ 43{,}097{,}000 & \text{K}-8 \\ +16{,}684{,}000 & 9-12 \\ \hline 59{,}781{,}000 & \end{array}$$

$$\begin{array}{rl} 59{,}781{,}000 & 2016 \\ -57{,}873{,}000 & 2013 \\ \hline 1{,}908{,}000 & \end{array}$$

The difference in projected total enrollment between 2016 and 2013 is 1,908,000 students.

**22. Strategy** To find the average enrollment in each of grades 9 through 12 in 2016, divide the total enrollment (16,684,000) in the four grades by 4.

**Solution**
$$\begin{array}{r} 4{,}171{,}000 \\ 4\overline{)16{,}684{,}000} \\ \underline{16}\phantom{,684,000} \\ 06\phantom{84,000} \\ \underline{4}\phantom{84,000} \\ 28\phantom{4,000} \\ \underline{28}\phantom{4,000} \\ 04\phantom{,000} \\ \underline{4}\phantom{,000} \\ 00\phantom{00} \\ \underline{00}\phantom{00} \\ 0\phantom{00} \end{array}$$

The average enrollment in each of grades 9 through 12 in 2016 is projected to be 4,171,000 students.

© 2013 Cengage Learning. All Rights Reserved. May not be scanned, copied or duplicated, or posted to a publicly accessible website, in whole or in part.

**23.** **Strategy** To find how many toothbrushes:

- Find the total number of boxes by multiplying the number of cases (3) by the number of boxes to a case (10).
- Find the total number of toothbrushes by multiplying the total number of boxes by the number of toothbrushes per box (144).

**Solution**

$$\begin{array}{r} 10 \\ \times 3 \\ \hline 30 \end{array} \qquad \begin{array}{r} 144 \\ \times 30 \\ \hline 4320 \end{array}$$

A total of 4,320 toothbrushes were ordered.

**24.** **Strategy** To find the premiums for a year, multiply the amount per month ($237) by the number of months in a year (12).

**Solution**

$$\begin{array}{r} 237 \\ \times\ 12 \\ \hline 474 \\ 237\phantom{0} \\ \hline 2844 \end{array}$$

The insurance costs $2844 per year.

**25a.** **Strategy** To find the total intake, add all of the intakes (120, 210, 90 and 150).

**Solution**

$$\begin{array}{r} 120 \\ 210 \\ 90 \\ +150 \\ \hline 570 \end{array}$$

The total intake was 570 milliliters.

**b.** **Strategy** To find the total output, add all of the outputs (330, 225, and 60).

**Solution**

$$\begin{array}{r} 330 \\ 225 \\ +60 \\ \hline 615 \end{array}$$

The total output is 615 milliliters.

**c.** **Strategy** To find which is greater, compare the total output to the total intake.

$615 > 570$

There was more output than intake.

To find the difference, subtract the total intake (570) from the total output (615).

$$\begin{array}{r} 615 \\ -570 \\ \hline 45 \end{array}$$

Total output was greater by 45 milliliters.

© 2013 Cengage Learning. All Rights Reserved. May not be scanned, copied or duplicated, or posted to a publicly accessible website, in whole or in part.

## Prep Test

**1.** 20

**2.** 120

**3.** 9

**4.** 10

**5.** 7

**6.**
$$\begin{array}{r} 2 \text{ r3} \\ 30\overline{)63} \\ -60 \\ \hline 3 \end{array}$$

**7.** 1, 2, 3, 4, 6, 12

**8.** $8 \cdot 7 + 3 = 56 + 3 = 59$

**9.** 7

**10.** <

## Section 2.1

### Objective A Exercises

**1.**

| | 2 | 5 |
|---|---|---|
| 5 = | | 5 |
| 8 = | 2 · 2 · 2 | |

LCM $= 2 \cdot 2 \cdot 2 \cdot 5 = 40$

**3.**

| | 2 | 3 |
|---|---|---|
| 3 = | | 3 |
| 8 = | 2 · 2 · 2 | |

LCM $= 2 \cdot 2 \cdot 2 \cdot 3 = 24$

**5.**

| | 2 | 3 | 5 |
|---|---|---|---|
| 5 = | | | 5 |
| 6 = | 2 | 3 | |

LCM $= 2 \cdot 3 \cdot 5 = 30$

**7.**

| | 2 | 3 |
|---|---|---|
| 4 = | 2 · 2 | |
| 6 = | 2 | 3 |

LCM $= 2 \cdot 2 \cdot 3 = 12$

**9.**

| | 2 | 3 |
|---|---|---|
| 8 = | 2 · 2 · 2 | |
| 12 = | 2 · 2 | 3 |

LCM $= 2 \cdot 2 \cdot 2 \cdot 3 = 24$

**11.**

| | 2 | 3 | 5 |
|---|---|---|---|
| 5 = | | | 5 |
| 12 = | 2 · 2 | 3 | |

LCM $= 2 \cdot 2 \cdot 3 \cdot 5 = 60$

**13.**

| | 2 | 7 |
|---|---|---|
| 8 = | 2 · 2 · 2 | |
| 14 = | 2 | 7 |

LCM $= 2 \cdot 2 \cdot 2 \cdot 7 = 56$

**15.**

| | 3 |
|---|---|
| 3 = | 3 |
| 9 = | 3 · 3 |

LCM $= 3 \cdot 3 = 9$

**17.**

| | 2 |
|---|---|
| 8 = | 2 · 2 · 2 |
| 32 = | 2 · 2 · 2 · 2 · 2 |

LCM $= 2 \cdot 2 \cdot 2 \cdot 2 \cdot 2 = 32$

**19.**

| | 2 | 3 |
|---|---|---|
| 9 = | | 3 · 3 |
| 36 = | 2 · 2 | 3 · 3 |

LCM $= 2 \cdot 2 \cdot 3 \cdot 3 = 36$

**21.**

| | 2 | 3 | 5 | 11 |
|---|---|---|---|---|
| 44 = | 2 · 2 | | | 11 |
| 60 = | 2 · 2 | 3 | 5 | |

LCM $= 2 \cdot 3 \cdot 5 \cdot 11 = 660$

**23.**

| | 2 | 3 | 17 | 23 |
|---|---|---|---|---|
| 102 = | 2 | 3 | 17 | |
| 184 = | 2 · 2 · 2 | | | 23 |

LCM $= 2 \cdot 2 \cdot 2 \cdot 3 \cdot 17 \cdot 23 = 9384$

**25.**

| | 2 | 3 |
|---|---|---|
| 4 = | 2 · 2 | |
| 8 = | 2 · 2 · 2 | |
| 12 = | 2 · 2 | 3 |

LCM $= 2 \cdot 2 \cdot 2 \cdot 3 = 24$

© 2013 Cengage Learning. All Rights Reserved. May not be scanned, copied or duplicated, or posted to a publicly accessible website, in whole or in part.

**27.**

| | 2 | 3 | 5 |
|---|---|---|---|
| 3 = | | 3 | |
| 5 = | | | 5 |
| 10 = | 2 | | 5 |

LCM $= 2 \cdot 3 \cdot 5 = 30$

**29.**

| | 2 | 3 |
|---|---|---|
| 3 = | | 3 |
| 8 = | 2 · 2 · 2 | |
| 12 = | 2 · 2 | 3 |

LCM $= 2 \cdot 2 \cdot 2 \cdot 3 = 24$

**31.**

| | 2 | 3 |
|---|---|---|
| 9 = | | 3 · 3 |
| 36 = | 2 · 2 | 3 · 3 |
| 64 = | 2 · 2 · 2 · 2 · 2 · 2 | |

LCM $= 2 \cdot 2 \cdot 2 \cdot 2 \cdot 2 \cdot 2 \cdot 3 \cdot 3 = 576$

**33.**

| | 2 | 3 | 5 | 7 |
|---|---|---|---|---|
| 16 = | 2 · 2 · 2 · 2 | | | |
| 30 = | 2 | 3 | 5 | |
| 84 = | 2 · 2 | 3 | | 7 |

LCM $= 2 \cdot 2 \cdot 2 \cdot 2 \cdot 3 \cdot 5 \cdot 7 = 1680$

**35.** True

## Objective B Exercises

**37.**

| | 3 | 5 |
|---|---|---|
| 3 = | 3 | |
| 5 = | | 5 |

GCF = 1

**39.**

| | 2 | 3 |
|---|---|---|
| 6 = | 2 | 3 |
| 9 = | | 3 · 3 |

GCF = 3

**41.**

| | 3 | 5 |
|---|---|---|
| 15 = | 3 | 5 |
| 25 = | | 5 · 5 |

GCF = 5

**43.**

| | 2 | 5 |
|---|---|---|
| 25 = | | 5 · 5 |
| 100 = | 2 · 2 | 5 · 5 |

GCF $= 5 \cdot 5 = 25$

**45.**

| | 2 | 3 | 17 |
|---|---|---|---|
| 32 = | 2 · 2 · 2 · 2 · 2 | | |
| 51 = | | 3 | 17 |

GCF = 1

**47.**

| | 2 | 3 | 5 |
|---|---|---|---|
| 12 = | 2 · 2 | 3 | |
| 80 = | 2 · 2 · 2 · 2 | | 5 |

GCF $= 2 \cdot 2 = 4$

**49.**

| | 2 | 5 | 7 |
|---|---|---|---|
| 16 = | 2 · 2 · 2 · 2 | | |
| 140 = | 2 · 2 | 5 | 7 |

GCF $= 2 \cdot 2 = 4$

**51.**

| | 2 | 3 | 5 |
|---|---|---|---|
| 24 = | 2 · 2 · 2 | 3 | |
| 30 = | 2 | 3 | 5 |

GCF $= 2 \cdot 3 = 6$

**53.**

| | 2 | 3 | 11 |
|---|---|---|---|
| 44 = | 2 · 2 | | 11 |
| 96 = | 2 · 2 · 2 · 2 · 2 | 3 | |

GCF $= 2 \cdot 2 = 4$

**55.**

| | 3 | 5 | 11 |
|---|---|---|---|
| 3 = | 3 | | |
| 5 = | | 5 | |
| 11 = | | | 11 |

GCF = 1

**57.**

| | 2 | 7 |
|---|---|---|
| 7 = | | 7 |
| 14 = | 2 | 7 |
| 49 = | | 7 · 7 |

GCF = 7

**59.**

| | 2 | 3 | 5 |
|---|---|---|---|
| 10 = | 2 | | 5 |
| 15 = | | 3 | 5 |
| 20 = | 2 · 2 | | 5 |

GCF = 5

**61.**

| | 2 | 3 | 5 |
|---|---|---|---|
| 24 = | 2 · 2 · 2 | 3 | |
| 40 = | 2 · 2 · 2 | | 5 |
| 72 = | 2 · 2 · 2 | 3 · 3 | |

GCF $= 2 \cdot 2 \cdot 2 = 8$

© 2013 Cengage Learning. All Rights Reserved. May not be scanned, copied or duplicated, or posted to a publicly accessible website, in whole or in part.

**63.**

| | 3 | 17 | 31 |
|---|---|---|---|
| 17 = | | 17 | |
| 31 = | | | 31 |
| 81 = | $3 \cdot 3 \cdot 3 \cdot 3$ | | |

GCF = 1

**65.**

| | 5 |
|---|---|
| 25 = | $5 \cdot 5$ |
| 125 = | $5 \cdot 5 \cdot 5$ |
| 625 = | $5 \cdot 5 \cdot 5 \cdot 5$ |

GCF = 25

**67.**

| | 2 | 5 | 7 |
|---|---|---|---|
| 28 = | $2 \cdot 2$ | | 7 |
| 35 = | | 5 | 7 |
| 70 = | 2 | 5 | 7 |

GCF = 7

**69.**

| | 2 | 3 | 7 |
|---|---|---|---|
| 32 = | $2 \cdot 2 \cdot 2 \cdot 2 \cdot 2$ | | |
| 56 = | $2 \cdot 2 \cdot 2$ | | 7 |
| 72 = | $2 \cdot 2 \cdot 2$ | $3 \cdot 3$ | |

GCF = $2 \cdot 2 \cdot 2 = 8$

**71.** True

## Applying the Concepts

**73.** The nurse has a 4-day cycle (3 workdays + 1 day off). His friend has a 6-day cycle (5 workdays + 1 day off). The least common multiple of 4 and 6 is 12. After the nurse and his friend have a day off together, they will have another day off together in 12 days.

**75.** The GCF of 3 and 5 is 1. The GCF of 7 and 11 is 1. The GCF of 29 and 43 is 1. Because two prime numbers do not have a common factor other than 1, the GCF of two prime numbers is 1. Because three prime numbers do not have a common factor other than 1, the GCF of three prime numbers is 1.

# Section 2.2

## Objective A Exercises

**1.** Improper fraction

**3.** Proper fraction

**5.** $\frac{3}{4}$

**7.** $\frac{7}{8}$

**9.** $1\frac{1}{2}$

**11.** $2\frac{5}{8}$

**13.** $3\frac{3}{5}$

**15.** $\frac{5}{4}$

**17.** $\frac{8}{3}$

**19.** $\frac{28}{8}$

**21.**

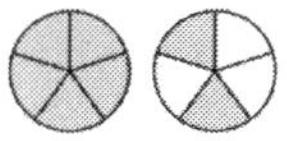

**23.**

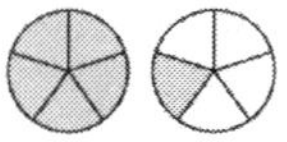

**25.** False

## Objective B Exercises

**27.** $\begin{array}{r} 5 \\ 3\overline{)16} \\ -15 \\ \hline 1 \end{array}$ $\quad \frac{16}{3} = 5\frac{1}{3}$

**29.** $\begin{array}{r} 2 \\ 9\overline{)18} \\ -18 \\ \hline 0 \end{array}$ $\quad \frac{18}{9} = 2$

**31.** $\begin{array}{r} 3 \\ 4\overline{)13} \\ -12 \\ \hline 1 \end{array}$ $\quad \frac{13}{4} = 3\frac{1}{4}$

© 2013 Cengage Learning. All Rights Reserved. May not be scanned, copied or duplicated, or posted to a publicly accessible website, in whole or in part.

**33.** $$\begin{array}{r} 14 \\ 2\overline{)29} \\ \underline{-2} \\ 09 \\ \underline{-8} \\ 1 \end{array} \qquad \frac{29}{2} = 14\frac{1}{2}$$

**35.** $$\begin{array}{r} 17 \\ 3\overline{)51} \\ \underline{-3} \\ 21 \\ \underline{-21} \\ 0 \end{array} \qquad \frac{51}{3} = 17$$

**37.** $$\begin{array}{r} 1 \\ 9\overline{)16} \\ \underline{-9} \\ 7 \end{array} \qquad \frac{16}{9} = 1\frac{7}{9}$$

**39.** $$\begin{array}{r} 1 \\ 5\overline{)9} \\ \underline{-5} \\ 4 \end{array} \qquad \frac{9}{5} = 1\frac{4}{5}$$

**41.** $$\begin{array}{r} 23 \\ 1\overline{)23} \\ \underline{-2} \\ 03 \\ \underline{-3} \\ 0 \end{array} \qquad \frac{23}{1} = 23$$

**43.** $$\begin{array}{r} 1 \\ 16\overline{)31} \\ \underline{-16} \\ 15 \end{array} \qquad \frac{31}{16} = 1\frac{15}{16}$$

**45.** $$\begin{array}{r} 6 \\ 3\overline{)19} \\ \underline{-18} \\ 1 \end{array} \qquad \frac{19}{3} = 6\frac{1}{3}$$

**47.** $$\begin{array}{r} 5 \\ 8\overline{)40} \\ \underline{-40} \\ 0 \end{array} \qquad \frac{40}{8} = 5$$

**49.** $$\begin{array}{r} 1 \\ 3\overline{)3} \\ \underline{-3} \\ 0 \end{array} \qquad \frac{3}{3} = 1$$

**51.** $4\frac{2}{3} = \frac{12+2}{3} = \frac{14}{3}$

**53.** $8\frac{2}{3} = \frac{24+2}{3} = \frac{26}{3}$

**55.** $7\frac{3}{8} = \frac{56+3}{8} = \frac{59}{8}$

**57.** $6\frac{1}{4} = \frac{24+1}{4} = \frac{25}{4}$

**59.** $15\frac{1}{8} = \frac{120+1}{8} = \frac{121}{8}$

**61.** $3\frac{5}{12} = \frac{36+5}{12} = \frac{41}{12}$

**63.** $3\frac{7}{9} = \frac{27+7}{9} = \frac{34}{9}$

**65.** $12\frac{2}{3} = \frac{36+2}{3} = \frac{38}{3}$

**67.** $5\frac{3}{7} = \frac{35+3}{7} = \frac{38}{7}$

**69.** $12\frac{3}{5} = \frac{60+3}{5} = \frac{63}{5}$

**71.** $4\frac{5}{9} = \frac{36+5}{9} = \frac{41}{9}$

**73.** $8\frac{5}{14} = \frac{112+5}{14} = \frac{117}{14}$

## Applying the Concepts

**75.** Students might mention any of the following: fractional parts of an hour, as in three-quarters of an hour; lengths of nails, as in $\frac{3}{4}$-inch nail; lengths of fabric, as in $1\frac{5}{8}$ yards of material; lengths of lumber, as in $2\frac{1}{2}$ feet of pine; ingredients in a recipe, as in $1\frac{1}{2}$ cups sugar; or innings pitched, as in four and two-thirds innings.

© 2013 Cengage Learning. All Rights Reserved. May not be scanned, copied or duplicated, or posted to a publicly accessible website, in whole or in part.

## Section 2.3

### Objective A Exercises

**1.** $10 \div 2 = 5; \frac{1 \cdot 5}{2 \cdot 5} = \frac{5}{10}$

**3.** $48 \div 16 = 3; \frac{3 \cdot 3}{16 \cdot 3} = \frac{9}{48}$

**5.** $32 \div 8 = 4; \frac{3 \cdot 4}{8 \cdot 4} = \frac{12}{32}$

**7.** $51 \div 17 = 3; \frac{3 \cdot 3}{17 \cdot 3} = \frac{9}{51}$

**9.** $16 \div 4 = 4; \frac{3 \cdot 4}{4 \cdot 4} = \frac{12}{16}$

**11.** $9 \div 1 = 9; \frac{3 \cdot 9}{1 \cdot 9} = \frac{27}{9}$

**13.** $60 \div 3 = 20; \frac{1 \cdot 20}{3 \cdot 20} = \frac{20}{60}$

**15.** $60 \div 15 = 4; \frac{11 \cdot 4}{15 \cdot 4} = \frac{44}{60}$

**17.** $18 \div 3 = 6; \frac{2 \cdot 6}{3 \cdot 6} = \frac{12}{18}$

**19.** $49 \div 7 = 7; \frac{5 \cdot 7}{7 \cdot 7} = \frac{35}{49}$

**21.** $18 \div 9 = 2; \frac{5 \cdot 2}{9 \cdot 2} = \frac{10}{18}$

**23.** $3 \div 1 = 3; \frac{7 \cdot 3}{1 \cdot 3} = \frac{21}{3}$

**25.** $45 \div 9 = 5; \frac{7 \cdot 5}{9 \cdot 5} = \frac{35}{45}$

**27.** $64 \div 16 = 4; \frac{15 \cdot 4}{16 \cdot 4} = \frac{60}{64}$

**29.** $98 \div 14 = 7; \frac{3 \cdot 7}{14 \cdot 7} = \frac{21}{98}$

**31.** $48 \div 8 = 6; \frac{5 \cdot 6}{8 \cdot 6} = \frac{30}{48}$

**33.** $42 \div 14 = 3; \frac{5 \cdot 3}{14 \cdot 3} = \frac{15}{42}$

**35.** $144 \div 24 = 6; \frac{17 \cdot 6}{24 \cdot 6} = \frac{102}{144}$

### Objective B Exercises

**37.** $\frac{4}{12} = \frac{\overset{1}{\cancel{2}} \cdot \overset{1}{\cancel{2}}}{\underset{1}{\cancel{2}} \cdot \underset{1}{\cancel{2}} \cdot 3} = \frac{1}{3}$

**39.** $\frac{22}{44} = \frac{\overset{1}{\cancel{2}} \cdot \overset{1}{\cancel{11}}}{\underset{1}{\cancel{2}} \cdot 2 \cdot \underset{1}{\cancel{11}}} = \frac{1}{2}$

**41.** $\frac{2}{12} = \frac{\overset{1}{\cancel{2}}}{\underset{1}{\cancel{2}} \cdot 2 \cdot 3} = \frac{1}{6}$

**43.** $\frac{40}{36} = \frac{\overset{1}{\cancel{2}} \cdot \overset{1}{\cancel{2}} \cdot 2 \cdot 5}{\underset{1}{\cancel{2}} \cdot \underset{1}{\cancel{2}} \cdot 3 \cdot 3} = \frac{10}{9} = 1\frac{1}{9}$

**45.** $\frac{0}{30} = 0$

**47.** $\frac{9}{22} = \frac{3 \cdot 3}{2 \cdot 11} = \frac{9}{22}$

**49.** $\frac{75}{25} = \frac{3 \cdot \overset{1}{\cancel{5}} \cdot \overset{1}{\cancel{5}}}{\underset{1}{\cancel{5}} \cdot \underset{1}{\cancel{5}}} = 3$

**51.** $\frac{16}{84} = \frac{\overset{1}{\cancel{2}} \cdot \overset{1}{\cancel{2}} \cdot 2 \cdot 2}{\underset{1}{\cancel{2}} \cdot \underset{1}{\cancel{2}} \cdot 3 \cdot 7} = \frac{4}{21}$

**53.** $\frac{12}{35} = \frac{2 \cdot 2 \cdot 3}{5 \cdot 7} = \frac{12}{35}$

**55.** $\frac{28}{44} = \frac{\overset{1}{\cancel{2}} \cdot \overset{1}{\cancel{2}} \cdot 7}{\underset{1}{\cancel{2}} \cdot \underset{1}{\cancel{2}} \cdot 11} = \frac{7}{11}$

© 2013 Cengage Learning. All Rights Reserved. May not be scanned, copied or duplicated, or posted to a publicly accessible website, in whole or in part.

**57.** $\frac{16}{12} = \frac{\overset{1}{\cancel{2}} \cdot \overset{1}{\cancel{2}} \cdot 2 \cdot 2}{\underset{1}{\cancel{2}} \cdot \underset{1}{\cancel{2}} \cdot 3} = \frac{4}{3} = 1\frac{1}{3}$

**59.** $\frac{24}{40} = \frac{\overset{1}{\cancel{2}} \cdot \overset{1}{\cancel{2}} \cdot \overset{1}{\cancel{2}} \cdot 3}{\underset{1}{\cancel{2}} \cdot \underset{1}{\cancel{2}} \cdot \underset{1}{\cancel{2}} \cdot 5} = \frac{3}{5}$

**61.** $\frac{8}{88} = \frac{\overset{1}{\cancel{2}} \cdot \overset{1}{\cancel{2}} \cdot \overset{1}{\cancel{2}}}{\underset{1}{\cancel{2}} \cdot \underset{1}{\cancel{2}} \cdot \underset{1}{\cancel{2}} \cdot 11} = \frac{1}{11}$

**63.** $\frac{144}{36} = \frac{\overset{1}{\cancel{2}} \cdot \overset{1}{\cancel{2}} \cdot 2 \cdot 2 \cdot \overset{1}{\cancel{3}} \cdot \overset{1}{\cancel{3}}}{\underset{1}{\cancel{2}} \cdot \underset{1}{\cancel{2}} \cdot \underset{1}{\cancel{3}} \cdot \underset{1}{\cancel{3}}} = 4$

**65.** $\frac{48}{144} = \frac{\overset{1}{\cancel{2}} \cdot \overset{1}{\cancel{2}} \cdot \overset{1}{\cancel{2}} \cdot \overset{1}{\cancel{2}} \cdot \overset{1}{\cancel{3}}}{\underset{1}{\cancel{2}} \cdot \underset{1}{\cancel{2}} \cdot \underset{1}{\cancel{2}} \cdot \underset{1}{\cancel{2}} \cdot \underset{1}{\cancel{3}} \cdot 3} = \frac{1}{3}$

**67.** $\frac{60}{100} = \frac{\overset{1}{\cancel{2}} \cdot \overset{1}{\cancel{2}} \cdot 3 \cdot \overset{1}{\cancel{5}}}{\underset{1}{\cancel{2}} \cdot \underset{1}{\cancel{2}} \cdot 5 \cdot \underset{1}{\cancel{5}}} = \frac{3}{5}$

**69.** $\frac{36}{16} = \frac{\overset{1}{\cancel{2}} \cdot \overset{1}{\cancel{2}} \cdot 3 \cdot 3}{\underset{1}{\cancel{2}} \cdot \underset{1}{\cancel{2}} \cdot 2 \cdot 2} = \frac{9}{4} = 2\frac{1}{4}$

**71.** $\frac{32}{160} = \frac{\overset{1}{\cancel{2}} \cdot \overset{1}{\cancel{2}} \cdot \overset{1}{\cancel{2}} \cdot \overset{1}{\cancel{2}} \cdot \overset{1}{\cancel{2}}}{\underset{1}{\cancel{2}} \cdot \underset{1}{\cancel{2}} \cdot \underset{1}{\cancel{2}} \cdot \underset{1}{\cancel{2}} \cdot \underset{1}{\cancel{2}} \cdot 5} = \frac{1}{5}$

## Applying the Concepts

**73.** $\frac{4}{6}, \frac{6}{9}, \frac{8}{12}, \frac{10}{15}$, and $\frac{12}{18}$ are fractions that are equal to $\frac{2}{3}$.

$\frac{15}{24}$ (brace over columns 1–5)

| | | | | | | | |
|---|---|---|---|---|---|---|---|
| 1 | 2 | 3 | 4 | 5 | | | |
| 6 | 7 | 8 | 9 | 10 | | | |
| 11 | 12 | 13 | 14 | 15 | | | |

$\frac{5}{8}$ (brace under columns 1–5)

**75a. Strategy** To find fraction that were boys, write the number of boys (255) over the total number (500) and reduce.

**Solution** $\frac{255}{500} = \frac{51}{100}$

$\frac{51}{100}$ of the children were boys.

**b. Strategy** To find fraction that were girls,

- Find the number of girls by subtracting the number of boys (255) from the total number (500).
- Write the number of girls over the total number and reduce.

**Solution** $\begin{array}{r} 500 \\ -255 \\ \hline 245 \end{array}$ $\quad \frac{245}{500} = \frac{49}{100}$

$\frac{49}{100}$ of the children were girls.

# Section 2.4

## Objective A Exercises

**1.** $\begin{array}{r} \frac{2}{7} \\ +\frac{1}{7} \\ \hline \frac{3}{7} \end{array}$

**3.** $\begin{array}{r} \frac{1}{2} \\ +\frac{1}{2} \\ \hline \frac{2}{2} \end{array} = 1$

**5.** $\begin{array}{r} \frac{8}{11} \\ +\frac{7}{11} \\ \hline \frac{15}{11} \end{array} = 1\frac{4}{11}$

© 2013 Cengage Learning. All Rights Reserved. May not be scanned, copied or duplicated, or posted to a publicly accessible website, in whole or in part.

**7.** $$\begin{array}{r} \frac{8}{5} \\ \frac{9}{5} \\ +\frac{9}{5} \\ \hline \frac{17}{5} = 3\frac{2}{5} \end{array}$$

**9.** $$\begin{array}{r} \frac{3}{5} \\ \frac{8}{5} \\ +\frac{3}{5} \\ \hline \frac{14}{5} = 2\frac{4}{5} \end{array}$$

**11.** $$\begin{array}{r} \frac{3}{4} \\ \frac{1}{4} \\ +\frac{5}{4} \\ \hline \frac{9}{4} = 2\frac{1}{4} \end{array}$$

**13.** $$\begin{array}{r} \frac{3}{8} \\ \frac{7}{8} \\ +\frac{1}{8} \\ \hline \frac{11}{8} = 1\frac{3}{8} \end{array}$$

**15.** $$\begin{array}{r} \frac{4}{15} \\ \frac{7}{15} \\ +\frac{11}{15} \\ \hline \frac{22}{15} = 1\frac{7}{15} \end{array}$$

**17.** $\frac{5}{12} + \frac{1}{12} + \frac{11}{12} = \frac{17}{12} = 1\frac{5}{12}$

**19.** A whole number other than 1

**21.** The number 1

## Objective B Exercises

**23.** $$\begin{array}{r} \frac{1}{2} = \frac{3}{6} \\ +\frac{2}{3} = \frac{4}{6} \\ \hline \frac{7}{6} = 1\frac{1}{6} \end{array}$$

**25.** $$\begin{array}{r} \frac{3}{14} = \frac{3}{14} \\ +\frac{5}{7} = \frac{10}{14} \\ \hline \frac{13}{14} \end{array}$$

**27.** $$\begin{array}{r} \frac{8}{15} = \frac{32}{60} \\ +\frac{7}{20} = \frac{21}{60} \\ \hline \frac{53}{60} \end{array}$$

**29.** $$\begin{array}{r} \frac{3}{8} = \frac{21}{56} \\ +\frac{9}{14} = \frac{36}{56} \\ \hline \frac{57}{56} = 1\frac{1}{56} \end{array}$$

**31.** $$\begin{array}{r} \frac{3}{20} = \frac{9}{60} \\ +\frac{7}{30} = \frac{14}{60} \\ \hline \frac{23}{60} \end{array}$$

**33.** $$\begin{array}{r} \frac{1}{3} = \frac{6}{18} \\ \frac{5}{6} = \frac{15}{18} \\ +\frac{7}{9} = \frac{14}{18} \\ \hline \frac{35}{18} = 1\frac{17}{18} \end{array}$$

© 2013 Cengage Learning. All Rights Reserved. May not be scanned, copied or duplicated, or posted to a publicly accessible website, in whole or in part.

**35.**
$$\begin{array}{r} \frac{5}{6}=\frac{40}{48} \\ \frac{1}{12}=\frac{4}{48} \\ +\frac{5}{16}=\frac{15}{48} \\ \hline \frac{59}{48}=1\frac{11}{48} \end{array}$$

**37.**
$$\begin{array}{r} \frac{2}{3}=\frac{40}{60} \\ \frac{1}{5}=\frac{12}{60} \\ +\frac{7}{12}=\frac{35}{60} \\ \hline \frac{87}{60}=1\frac{27}{60}=1\frac{9}{20} \end{array}$$

**39.**
$$\begin{array}{r} \frac{2}{3}=\frac{80}{120} \\ \frac{3}{5}=\frac{72}{120} \\ +\frac{7}{8}=\frac{105}{120} \\ \hline \frac{257}{120}=2\frac{17}{120} \end{array}$$

**41.**
$$\begin{array}{r} \frac{2}{3}=\frac{48}{72} \\ \frac{5}{8}=\frac{45}{72} \\ +\frac{7}{9}=\frac{56}{72} \\ \hline \frac{149}{72}=2\frac{5}{72} \end{array}$$

**43.**
$$\begin{array}{r} \frac{3}{8}=\frac{15}{40} \\ +\frac{3}{5}=\frac{24}{40} \\ \hline \frac{39}{40} \end{array}$$

**45.**
$$\begin{array}{r} \frac{3}{8}=\frac{9}{24} \\ \frac{5}{6}=\frac{20}{24} \\ +\frac{7}{12}=\frac{14}{24} \\ \hline \frac{43}{24}=1\frac{19}{24} \end{array}$$

**47.** (ii)

## Objective C Exercises

**49.**
$$\begin{array}{r} 4\frac{1}{2}=4\frac{6}{12} \\ +5\frac{7}{12}=5\frac{7}{12} \\ \hline 9\frac{13}{12}=10\frac{1}{12} \end{array}$$

**51.**
$$\begin{array}{r} 4 \\ +5\frac{2}{7} \\ \hline 9\frac{2}{7} \end{array}$$

**53.**
$$\begin{array}{r} 7\frac{5}{12}=7\frac{20}{48} \\ +2\frac{9}{16}=2\frac{27}{48} \\ \hline 9\frac{47}{48} \end{array}$$

**55.**
$$\begin{array}{r} 6 \\ +2\frac{3}{13} \\ \hline 8\frac{3}{13} \end{array}$$

**57.**
$$\begin{array}{r} 8\frac{29}{30}=8\frac{116}{120} \\ +7\frac{11}{40}=7\frac{33}{120} \\ \hline 15\frac{149}{120}=16\frac{29}{120} \end{array}$$

**59.**
$$\begin{array}{r} 17\frac{3}{8}=17\frac{15}{40} \\ +7\frac{7}{20}=7\frac{14}{40} \\ \hline 24\frac{29}{40} \end{array}$$

**61.**
$$\begin{array}{r} 5\frac{7}{8}=5\frac{21}{24} \\ +27\frac{5}{12}=27\frac{10}{24} \\ \hline 32\frac{31}{24}=33\frac{7}{24} \end{array}$$

© 2013 Cengage Learning. All Rights Reserved. May not be scanned, copied or duplicated, or posted to a publicly accessible website, in whole or in part.

**63.**
$$\begin{aligned} 7\frac{5}{9} &= 7\frac{20}{36} \\ +2\frac{7}{12} &= 2\frac{21}{36} \\ \hline & 9\frac{41}{36} = 10\frac{5}{36} \end{aligned}$$

**65.**
$$\begin{aligned} 2\frac{1}{2} &= 2\frac{6}{12} \\ 3\frac{2}{3} &= 3\frac{8}{12} \\ +4\frac{1}{4} &= 4\frac{3}{12} \\ \hline & 9\frac{17}{12} = 10\frac{5}{12} \end{aligned}$$

**67.**
$$\begin{aligned} 3\frac{1}{2} &= 3\frac{45}{90} \\ 3\frac{1}{5} &= 3\frac{18}{90} \\ +8\frac{1}{9} &= 8\frac{10}{90} \\ \hline & 14\frac{73}{90} \end{aligned}$$

**69.**
$$\begin{aligned} 2\frac{3}{8} &= 2\frac{18}{48} \\ 4\frac{7}{12} &= 4\frac{28}{48} \\ +3\frac{5}{16} &= 3\frac{15}{48} \\ \hline & 9\frac{61}{48} = 10\frac{13}{48} \end{aligned}$$

**71.**
$$\begin{aligned} 5\frac{5}{6} &= 5\frac{20}{24} \\ +3\frac{3}{8} &= 3\frac{9}{24} \\ \hline & 8\frac{29}{24} = 9\frac{5}{24} \end{aligned}$$

**73.**
$$\begin{aligned} 4\frac{8}{9} &= 4\frac{16}{18} \\ +9\frac{1}{6} &= 9\frac{3}{18} \\ \hline & 13\frac{19}{18} = 14\frac{1}{18} \end{aligned}$$

**75.**
$$\begin{aligned} 1\frac{5}{8} &= 1\frac{15}{24} \\ 3 &= 3 \\ +7\frac{7}{24} &= 7\frac{7}{24} \\ \hline & 11\frac{22}{24} = 11\frac{11}{12} \end{aligned}$$

**77.** No

## Objective D Exercises

**79.** **Strategy** To find weight at the end of two months add the two gains $\left(1\frac{3}{8} \text{ and } 1\frac{5}{8}\right)$ to the weight at birth $\left(7\frac{1}{4} \text{ pounds}\right)$.

**Solution**
$$\begin{aligned} 1\frac{3}{8} &= 1\frac{3}{8} \\ 1\frac{5}{8} &= 1\frac{5}{8} \\ +7\frac{1}{4} &= 7\frac{2}{8} \\ \hline & 9\frac{10}{8} = 10\frac{2}{8} = 10\frac{1}{4} \end{aligned}$$

The weight at the end of two months was $10\frac{1}{4}$ pounds.

**81.** **Strategy** To find height at the end of two months add the two gains $\left(\frac{7}{16} \text{ and } \frac{3}{4}\right)$ to the height at birth $\left(20\frac{1}{2} \text{ inches}\right)$.

**Solution**
$$\begin{aligned} \frac{7}{16} &= \frac{7}{16} \\ \frac{3}{4} &= \frac{12}{16} \\ +20\frac{1}{2} &= 20\frac{8}{16} \\ \hline & 20\frac{27}{16} = 21\frac{11}{16} \end{aligned}$$

© 2013 Cengage Learning. All Rights Reserved. May not be scanned, copied or duplicated, or posted to a publicly accessible website, in whole or in part.

The height at the end of two months was $21\frac{11}{16}$ inches.

**83. Strategy** To find the earnings,

- Find the total hours worked by adding the three times $\left(6,\ 3\frac{1}{4},\text{and } 7\frac{3}{4}\text{ hours}\right)$.
- Multiply the total hours by the pay per hour ($24).

**Solution**

$$\begin{array}{r} 6 \\ 3\frac{1}{4} \\ +7\frac{3}{4} \\ \hline 16\frac{4}{4}=17 \end{array} \qquad \begin{array}{r} 17 \\ \times\ 24 \\ \hline 68 \\ 34\ \ \\ \hline 408 \end{array}$$

Elizabeth's earnings for the week was $408.

**85. Strategy** To find the total hours in clinical, add the hours for the three days $\left(4\frac{2}{3},\ 2\frac{1}{2},\text{and } 3\frac{3}{4}\text{ hours}\right)$.

**Solution**

$$\begin{array}{r} 4\frac{2}{3}=4\frac{8}{12} \\ 2\frac{1}{2}=2\frac{6}{12} \\ +\ 3\frac{3}{4}=3\frac{9}{12} \\ \hline 9\frac{23}{12}=10\frac{11}{12} \end{array}$$

The total clinical hours was $10\frac{11}{12}$ hours.

**87. Strategy** To total dry ingredients, add the four dry ingredients together $\left(1\frac{1}{4},\ 18\frac{3}{4},9\frac{1}{3},\text{and } \frac{1}{2}\text{ cups}\right)$.

**Solution**

$$\begin{array}{r} 1\frac{1}{4}=\ 1\frac{3}{12} \\ 8\frac{3}{4}=18\frac{9}{12} \\ 9\frac{1}{3}=\ 9\frac{4}{12} \\ +\ \frac{1}{2}=\ \ \frac{6}{12} \\ \hline 28\frac{22}{12}=29\frac{10}{12} \\ =29\frac{5}{6} \end{array}$$

The total dry ingredients are $29\frac{5}{6}$ cups.

## Applying the Concepts

**89.**

$\frac{1}{3}+\frac{1}{6}+\frac{1}{8}+\frac{1}{12}+\frac{2}{5}$

$=\frac{40}{120}+\frac{20}{120}+\frac{15}{120}+\frac{10}{120}+\frac{48}{120}=\frac{133}{120}=1\frac{13}{120}$

No, this is not possible. The total cannot be greater than 1, which represents all the people surveyed.

# Section 2.5

## Objective A Exercises

**1.** $\begin{array}{r} \frac{9}{17} \\ -\frac{7}{17} \\ \hline \frac{2}{17} \end{array}$

**3.** $\begin{array}{r} \frac{11}{12} \\ -\frac{7}{12} \\ \hline \frac{4}{12}=\frac{1}{3} \end{array}$

**5.** $\begin{array}{r} \frac{9}{20} \\ -\frac{7}{20} \\ \hline \frac{2}{20}=\frac{1}{10} \end{array}$

© 2013 Cengage Learning. All Rights Reserved. May not be scanned, copied or duplicated, or posted to a publicly accessible website, in whole or in part.

**7.** $$\begin{array}{r} \frac{42}{65} \\ -\frac{17}{65} \\ \hline \frac{25}{65} = \frac{5}{13} \end{array}$$

**9.** $$\begin{array}{r} \frac{23}{30} \\ -\frac{13}{30} \\ \hline \frac{10}{30} = \frac{1}{3} \end{array}$$

**11.** $$\begin{array}{r} \frac{13}{14} \\ -\frac{5}{14} \\ \hline \frac{8}{14} = \frac{4}{7} \end{array}$$

**13.** $$\begin{array}{r} \frac{17}{24} \\ -\frac{11}{24} \\ \hline \frac{6}{24} = \frac{1}{4} \end{array}$$

**15.** Yes

## Objective B Exercises

**17.** $$\begin{array}{r} \frac{2}{3} = \frac{4}{6} \\ -\frac{1}{6} = \frac{1}{6} \\ \hline \frac{3}{6} = \frac{1}{2} \end{array}$$

**19.** $$\begin{array}{r} \frac{5}{8} = \frac{35}{56} \\ -\frac{2}{7} = \frac{16}{56} \\ \hline \frac{19}{56} \end{array}$$

**21.** $$\begin{array}{r} \frac{5}{7} = \frac{10}{14} \\ -\frac{3}{14} = \frac{3}{14} \\ \hline \frac{7}{14} = \frac{1}{2} \end{array}$$

**23.** $$\begin{array}{r} \frac{8}{15} = \frac{32}{60} \\ -\frac{7}{20} = \frac{21}{60} \\ \hline \frac{11}{60} \end{array}$$

**25.** $$\begin{array}{r} \frac{9}{16} = \frac{18}{32} \\ -\frac{17}{32} = \frac{17}{32} \\ \hline \frac{1}{32} \end{array}$$

**27.** $$\begin{array}{r} \frac{11}{12} = \frac{55}{60} \\ -\frac{3}{5} = \frac{36}{60} \\ \hline \frac{19}{60} \end{array}$$

**29.** $$\begin{array}{r} \frac{11}{24} = \frac{33}{72} \\ -\frac{7}{18} = \frac{28}{72} \\ \hline \frac{5}{72} \end{array}$$

**31.** $$\begin{array}{r} \frac{11}{12} = \frac{55}{60} \\ -\frac{11}{15} = \frac{44}{60} \\ \hline \frac{11}{60} \end{array}$$

**33.** $$\begin{array}{r} \frac{13}{20} = \frac{39}{60} \\ -\frac{1}{6} = \frac{10}{60} \\ \hline \frac{29}{60} \end{array}$$

**35.** (i)

© 2013 Cengage Learning. All Rights Reserved. May not be scanned, copied or duplicated, or posted to a publicly accessible website, in whole or in part.

## Objective C Exercises

**37.**
$$\begin{array}{r} 16\frac{11}{15} \\ -11\frac{8}{15} \\ \hline 5\frac{3}{15} = 5\frac{1}{5} \end{array}$$

**39.**
$$\begin{array}{r} 5\frac{7}{8} \\ -1 \\ \hline 4\frac{7}{8} \end{array}$$

**41.**
$$\begin{array}{rl} 3 & = 2\frac{21}{21} \\ -2\frac{5}{21} & = 2\frac{5}{21} \\ \hline & \frac{16}{21} \end{array}$$

**43.**
$$\begin{array}{rl} 16\frac{3}{8} & = 15\frac{11}{8} \\ -10\frac{7}{8} & = 10\frac{7}{8} \\ \hline & 5\frac{4}{8} = 5\frac{1}{2} \end{array}$$

**45.**
$$\begin{array}{rl} 8\frac{3}{7} & = 7\frac{10}{7} \\ -2\frac{6}{7} & = 2\frac{6}{7} \\ \hline & 5\frac{4}{7} \end{array}$$

**47.**
$$\begin{array}{rl} 23\frac{7}{8} & = 23\frac{21}{24} \\ -16\frac{2}{3} & = 16\frac{16}{24} \\ \hline & 7\frac{5}{24} \end{array}$$

**49.**
$$\begin{array}{rl} 6 & = 5\frac{5}{5} \\ -4\frac{3}{5} & = 4\frac{3}{5} \\ \hline & 1\frac{2}{5} \end{array}$$

**51.**
$$\begin{array}{rll} 23\frac{3}{20} & = 23\frac{3}{20} & = 22\frac{23}{20} \\ -7\frac{3}{5} & = 7\frac{12}{20} & = 7\frac{12}{20} \\ \hline & & 15\frac{11}{20} \end{array}$$

**53.**
$$\begin{array}{rll} 10\frac{5}{9} & = 10\frac{25}{45} & = 9\frac{70}{45} \\ -5\frac{11}{15} & = 5\frac{33}{45} & = 5\frac{33}{45} \\ \hline & & 4\frac{37}{45} \end{array}$$

**55.** No

## Objective D Exercises

**57. Strategy** To find the amount left

- Find the total amount used by adding the three amounts $\left(\frac{1}{4}, 1\frac{1}{2}, \text{ and } 1\frac{3}{4} \text{ cups}\right)$
- Subtract the amount used from the amount at the beginning (12 cups).

**Solution**

$$\begin{array}{rl} \frac{1}{4} & = \frac{1}{4} \\ 1\frac{1}{2} & = 1\frac{2}{4} \\ +1\frac{3}{4} & = 1\frac{3}{4} \\ \hline & 2\frac{6}{4} = 3\frac{1}{2} \end{array} \qquad \begin{array}{rl} 12 & = 11\frac{2}{2} \\ -2\frac{1}{2} & = -3\frac{1}{2} \\ \hline & 8\frac{1}{2} \end{array}$$

There are $8\frac{1}{2}$ cups of sugar left.

**59a. Strategy** To find the distance to the second checkpoint, add the distance to the first checkpoint $\left(2\frac{2}{5} \text{ miles}\right)$ to the distance to the second checkpoint $\left(5\frac{1}{3} \text{ miles}\right)$.

© 2013 Cengage Learning. All Rights Reserved. May not be scanned, copied or duplicated, or posted to a publicly accessible website, in whole or in part.

**Solution**

$$\begin{array}{r} 2\frac{2}{5} = 2\frac{6}{15} \\ +5\frac{1}{3} = 5\frac{5}{15} \\ \hline 7\frac{11}{15} \end{array}$$

The distance from the starting point to the second checkpoint is $7\frac{11}{15}$ miles.

**b. Strategy** To find the distance from the first starting point to the finish line, subtract the distance to the first checkpoint $\left(2\frac{1}{5}\right)$ from the total distance (10 miles).

**Solution**

$$\begin{array}{r} 10 = 9\frac{5}{5} \\ -2\frac{2}{5} = 2\frac{2}{5} \\ \hline 7\frac{3}{5} \end{array}$$

It is $7\frac{3}{5}$ miles from the first checkpoint to the finish line.

**61a. Strategy** To find the distance, add the distance to be traveled the first day $\left(7\frac{3}{8}\text{ miles}\right)$ to the distance to be traveled the second day $\left(10\frac{1}{3}\text{ miles}\right)$.

**Solution**

$$\begin{array}{r} 7\frac{3}{8} = 7\frac{9}{24} \\ +10\frac{1}{3} = 10\frac{8}{24} \\ \hline 17\frac{17}{24} \end{array}$$

The distance to be traveled during the first 2 days is $17\frac{17}{24}$ miles.

**b. Strategy** To find the distance, subtract the miles traveled in the first two days $\left(17\frac{17}{24}\right)$ from the total miles $\left(27\frac{1}{2}\right)$.

**Solution**

$$\begin{array}{r} 27\frac{1}{2} = 27\frac{12}{24} = 26\frac{36}{24} \\ -17\frac{17}{24} = 17\frac{17}{24} = 17\frac{17}{24} \\ \hline 9\frac{19}{24} \end{array}$$

On the third day, $9\frac{19}{24}$ miles remain to be traveled.

**63.** The difference represents how much farther the hikers plan to travel on the second day than on the first day.

**65a.** The patient has lost $5\frac{1}{4}$ pounds the first week and $4\frac{1}{4}$ pounds the second week. Thus the patient has lost more than 9 pounds the first two weeks. Since less than 13 pounds needs to be lost, the patient can attain the weight class by losing less than 4 pounds. Yes, this is less than the $4\frac{1}{4}$ pounds lost in the second week.

**b. Strategy** To find how much weight must be lost to reach the desired weight:

- Add the amounts of weight lost during the first 2 weeks $\left(5\frac{1}{4}\text{ and }4\frac{1}{4}\text{ pounds}\right)$.
- Subtract the total weight lost so far from the amount that is required $\left(12\frac{3}{4}\text{ pounds}\right)$

© 2013 Cengage Learning. All Rights Reserved. May not be scanned, copied or duplicated, or posted to a publicly accessible website, in whole or in part.

**Solution**

$$\begin{array}{r} 5\frac{1}{4} \\ +4\frac{1}{4} \\ \hline 9\frac{2}{4} = 9\frac{1}{2} \end{array} \qquad \begin{array}{r} 12\frac{3}{4} = 12\frac{3}{4} \\ -9\frac{1}{2} = \ 9\frac{2}{4} \\ \hline 3\frac{1}{4} \end{array}$$

The patient needs to lose $3\frac{1}{4}$ pounds to reach the desired weight.

**67.** The nurse's income is 1, that is, 100%.

$$\begin{array}{r} 1 = \frac{15}{15} \\ -\frac{4}{15} = \frac{4}{15} \\ \hline \frac{11}{15} \end{array}$$

$\frac{11}{15}$ of the nurse's income is not spent for housing.

## Applying the Concepts

**69.** To find the missing number, add $1\frac{5}{8}$ and $4\frac{1}{2}$.

$$\begin{array}{r} 1\frac{5}{8} = 1\frac{5}{8} \\ +4\frac{1}{2} = 4\frac{4}{8} \\ \hline 5\frac{9}{8} = 6\frac{1}{8} \end{array}$$

# Section 2.6

## Objective A Exercises

**1.** $\frac{2}{3} \times \frac{7}{8} = \frac{2 \cdot 7}{3 \cdot 8} = \frac{\cancel{2} \cdot 7}{3 \cdot \cancel{2} \cdot 2 \cdot 2} = \frac{7}{12}$

**3.** $\frac{5}{16} \times \frac{7}{15} = \frac{5 \cdot 7}{16 \cdot 15} = \frac{\cancel{5} \cdot 7}{2 \cdot 2 \cdot 2 \cdot 2 \cdot 3 \cdot \cancel{5}} = \frac{7}{48}$

**5.** $\frac{1}{6} \times \frac{1}{8} = \frac{1 \cdot 1}{6 \cdot 8} = \frac{1 \cdot 1}{2 \cdot 3 \cdot 2 \cdot 2 \cdot 2} = \frac{1}{48}$

**7.** $\frac{11}{12} \times \frac{6}{7} = \frac{11 \cdot 6}{12 \cdot 7} = \frac{11 \cdot \cancel{2} \cdot \cancel{3}}{\cancel{2} \cdot 2 \cdot \cancel{3} \cdot 7} = \frac{11}{14}$

**9.** $\frac{8}{9} \times \frac{27}{4} = \frac{8 \cdot 27}{9 \cdot 4} = \frac{\cancel{2} \cdot \cancel{2} \cdot 2 \cdot \cancel{3} \cdot \cancel{3} \cdot 3}{\cancel{3} \cdot \cancel{3} \cdot \cancel{2} \cdot \cancel{2}} = 6$

**11.** $\frac{5}{6} \times \frac{1}{2} = \frac{5 \cdot 1}{6 \cdot 2} = \frac{5 \cdot 1}{2 \cdot 3 \cdot 2} = \frac{5}{12}$

**13.** $\frac{16}{9} \times \frac{27}{8} = \frac{16 \cdot 27}{9 \cdot 8} = \frac{\cancel{2} \cdot \cancel{2} \cdot \cancel{2} \cdot 2 \cdot \cancel{3} \cdot \cancel{3} \cdot 3}{\cancel{3} \cdot \cancel{3} \cdot \cancel{2} \cdot \cancel{2} \cdot \cancel{2}} = 6$

**15.** $\frac{3}{2} \times \frac{4}{9} = \frac{3 \cdot 4}{2 \cdot 9} = \frac{\cancel{3} \cdot \cancel{2} \cdot 2}{\cancel{2} \cdot \cancel{3} \cdot 3} = \frac{2}{3}$

**17.** $\frac{7}{8} \times \frac{3}{14} = \frac{7 \cdot 3}{8 \cdot 14} = \frac{\cancel{7} \cdot 3}{2 \cdot 2 \cdot 2 \cdot 2 \cdot \cancel{7}} = \frac{3}{16}$

**19.** $\frac{1}{10} \times \frac{3}{8} = \frac{1 \cdot 3}{10 \cdot 8} = \frac{3}{2 \cdot 5 \cdot 2 \cdot 2 \cdot 2} = \frac{3}{80}$

**21.** $\frac{15}{8} \times \frac{16}{3} = \frac{15 \cdot 16}{8 \cdot 3} = \frac{\cancel{3} \cdot 5 \cdot \cancel{2} \cdot \cancel{2} \cdot \cancel{2} \cdot 2}{\cancel{2} \cdot \cancel{2} \cdot \cancel{2} \cdot \cancel{3}} = 10$

**23.** $\frac{1}{2} \times \frac{2}{15} = \frac{1 \cdot 2}{2 \cdot 15} = \frac{1 \cdot \cancel{2}}{\cancel{2} \cdot 3 \cdot 5} = \frac{1}{15}$

**25.** $\frac{5}{7} \times \frac{14}{15} = \frac{5 \cdot 14}{7 \cdot 15} = \frac{\cancel{5} \cdot 2 \cdot \cancel{7}}{\cancel{7} \cdot 3 \cdot \cancel{5}} = \frac{2}{3}$

**27.** $\frac{5}{12} \times \frac{42}{65} = \frac{5 \cdot 42}{12 \cdot 65} = \frac{\cancel{5} \cdot \cancel{2} \cdot \cancel{3} \cdot 7}{\cancel{2} \cdot 2 \cdot \cancel{3} \cdot \cancel{5} \cdot 13} = \frac{7}{26}$

**29.** $\frac{12}{5} \times \frac{5}{3} = \frac{12 \cdot 5}{5 \cdot 3} = \frac{2 \cdot 2 \cdot \cancel{3} \cdot \cancel{5}}{\cancel{5} \cdot \cancel{3}} = 4$

© 2013 Cengage Learning. All Rights Reserved. May not be scanned, copied or duplicated, or posted to a publicly accessible website, in whole or in part.

**31.** $\frac{16}{85}\times\frac{125}{84}=\frac{16\cdot125}{85\cdot84}$

$=\frac{\cancel{2}\cdot\cancel{2}\cdot2\cdot2\cdot\cancel{5}\cdot5\cdot5}{\cancel{5}\cdot17\cdot\cancel{2}\cdot\cancel{2}\cdot3\cdot7}=\frac{100}{357}$

**33.** For example, $\frac{3}{4}$ and $\frac{4}{3}$

**35.** $\frac{32}{9}\times\frac{3}{8}=\frac{32\cdot3}{9\cdot8}=\frac{\cancel{2}\cdot\cancel{2}\cdot\cancel{2}\cdot2\cdot2\cdot\cancel{3}}{\cancel{3}\cdot3\cdot\cancel{2}\cdot\cancel{2}\cdot\cancel{2}}=\frac{4}{3}=1\frac{1}{3}$

**37.** $\frac{7}{3}\times\frac{15}{14}=\frac{7\cdot15}{3\cdot14}=\frac{\cancel{7}\cdot\cancel{3}\cdot5}{\cancel{3}\cdot2\cdot\cancel{7}}=\frac{5}{2}=2\frac{1}{2}$

**39.** $\frac{3}{8}\times\frac{12}{17}=\frac{3\cdot12}{8\cdot17}=\frac{3\cdot\cancel{2}\cdot\cancel{2}\cdot3}{\cancel{2}\cdot\cancel{2}\cdot2\cdot17}=\frac{9}{34}$

## Objective B Exercises

**41.** $14\times\frac{5}{7}=\frac{14\cdot5}{1\cdot7}=\frac{2\cdot\cancel{7}\cdot5}{1\cdot\cancel{7}}=10$

**43.** $\frac{5}{12}\times40=\frac{5\cdot40}{12\cdot1}=\frac{5\cdot\cancel{2}\cdot\cancel{2}\cdot2\cdot5}{\cancel{2}\cdot\cancel{2}\cdot3\cdot1}=\frac{50}{3}=16\frac{2}{3}$

**45.** $\frac{2}{5}\times2\frac{1}{2}=\frac{2}{5}\times\frac{5}{2}=\frac{\cancel{2}\cdot\cancel{5}}{\cancel{5}\cdot\cancel{2}}=1$

**47.** $2\frac{1}{5}\times\frac{5}{22}=\frac{11}{5}\times\frac{5}{22}=\frac{\cancel{11}\cdot\cancel{5}}{\cancel{5}\cdot2\cdot\cancel{11}}=\frac{1}{2}$

**49.** $9\times3\frac{1}{3}=\frac{9}{1}\times\frac{10}{3}=\frac{\cancel{3}\cdot3\cdot2\cdot5}{1\cdot\cancel{3}}=30$

**51.** $5\frac{1}{4}\times8=\frac{21}{4}\times\frac{8}{1}=\frac{3\cdot7\cdot\cancel{2}\cdot\cancel{2}\cdot2}{\cancel{2}\cdot\cancel{2}\cdot1}=42$

**53.** $4\frac{2}{9}\times3=\frac{38}{9}\times\frac{3}{1}=\frac{2\cdot19\cdot\cancel{3}}{\cancel{3}\cdot3\cdot1}=\frac{38}{3}=12\frac{2}{3}$

**55.** $\frac{3}{8}\times4\frac{4}{5}=\frac{3}{8}\times\frac{24}{5}=\frac{3\cdot\cancel{2}\cdot\cancel{2}\cdot\cancel{2}\cdot3}{\cancel{2}\cdot\cancel{2}\cdot\cancel{2}\cdot5}=\frac{9}{5}=1\frac{4}{5}$

**57.** $5\frac{1}{3}\times\frac{5}{16}=\frac{16}{3}\times\frac{5}{16}=\frac{\cancel{2}\cdot\cancel{2}\cdot\cancel{2}\cdot\cancel{2}\cdot5}{3\cdot\cancel{2}\cdot\cancel{2}\cdot\cancel{2}\cdot\cancel{2}}=\frac{5}{3}=1\frac{2}{3}$

**59.** $\frac{5}{7}\times2\frac{1}{3}=\frac{5}{7}\times\frac{7}{3}=\frac{5\cdot\cancel{7}}{\cancel{7}\cdot3}=\frac{5}{3}=1\frac{2}{3}$

**61.** $6\frac{1}{8}\times0=\frac{49}{8}\times0=\frac{49\cdot0}{8}=0$

**63.** $5\frac{3}{16}\times5\frac{1}{3}=\frac{83}{16}\times\frac{16}{3}$

$=\frac{83\cdot\cancel{2}\cdot\cancel{2}\cdot\cancel{2}\cdot\cancel{2}}{\cancel{2}\cdot\cancel{2}\cdot\cancel{2}\cdot\cancel{2}\cdot3}=\frac{83}{3}=27\frac{2}{3}$

**65.** $16\frac{5}{8}\times1\frac{1}{16}=\frac{133}{8}\times\frac{17}{16}=\frac{133\cdot17}{2\cdot2\cdot2\cdot2\cdot2\cdot2\cdot2}$

$=\frac{2261}{128}=17\frac{85}{128}$

**67.** $2\frac{2}{3}\times\frac{3}{20}=\frac{8}{3}\times\frac{3}{20}=\frac{\cancel{2}\cdot\cancel{2}\cdot2\cdot\cancel{3}}{\cancel{3}\cdot\cancel{2}\cdot\cancel{2}\cdot5}=\frac{2}{5}$

**69.** $3\frac{3}{4}\times2\frac{3}{20}=\frac{15}{4}\times\frac{43}{20}$

$=\frac{3\cdot\cancel{5}\cdot43}{2\cdot2\cdot2\cdot2\cdot\cancel{5}}=\frac{129}{16}=8\frac{1}{16}$

**71.** $6\frac{1}{2}\times1\frac{3}{13}=\frac{13}{2}\times\frac{16}{13}=\frac{\cancel{13}\cdot\cancel{2}\cdot2\cdot2\cdot2}{\cancel{2}\cdot\cancel{13}}=8$

**73.** $2\frac{1}{2}\times3\frac{3}{5}=\frac{5}{2}\times\frac{18}{5}=\frac{\cancel{5}\cdot\cancel{2}\cdot3\cdot3}{\cancel{2}\cdot\cancel{5}}=9$

© 2013 Cengage Learning. All Rights Reserved. May not be scanned, copied or duplicated, or posted to a publicly accessible website, in whole or in part.

**75.** $2\frac{1}{8}\times\frac{5}{17}=\frac{17}{8}\times\frac{5}{17}=\frac{\overset{1}{\cancel{17}}\cdot 5}{2\cdot 2\cdot 2\cdot \underset{1}{\cancel{17}}}=\frac{5}{8}$

**77.** $1\frac{3}{8}\times 2\frac{1}{5}=\frac{11}{8}\times\frac{11}{5}=\frac{121}{40}=3\frac{1}{40}$

## Objective C Exercises

**79.** Greater than \$400

**81.** **Strategy** To find the cost, multiply the cost per case (\$190), by the number of cases $\left(2\frac{1}{2}\right)$.

**Solution** $2\frac{1}{2}\times 190=\frac{5}{2}\times\frac{190}{1}=\frac{950}{2}=475$

The cost is \$475.

**83.** **Strategy** To number of feet used, multiply the number of feet (225) by the fraction used $\left(\frac{1}{3}\right)$.

**Solution** $\frac{1}{3}\times 225=\frac{1}{3}\times\frac{225}{1}=\frac{1\cdot 225}{3\cdot}$

$=\frac{225}{3}=75$

75 feet have been used.

**Strategy** To number of feet left, subtract the number of feet used (75) from the number of feet in the roll (225).

**Solution**

$$\begin{array}{r} 225 \\ -75 \\ \hline 150 \end{array}$$

There are 150 feet left.

**85.** **Strategy** To find time required, multiply the time per x-ray $\left(\frac{1}{6}\text{ hour}\right)$ by the number of x-rays (27).

**Solution** $\frac{1}{6}\times 27=\frac{1}{6}\times\frac{27}{1}=\frac{1\cdot 27}{6\cdot 1}$

$=\frac{27}{6}=4\frac{3}{6}=4\frac{1}{2}$

It will $4\frac{1}{2}$ take hours to complete 27 x-rays.

**87.** **Strategy** To find the number of cups mashed bananas, multiply the number in the original recipe $\left(1\frac{1}{2}\right)$, by 3 (triple).

**Solution** $3\times 1\frac{1}{2}=\frac{3}{1}\times\frac{3}{2}=\frac{3\cdot 3}{1\cdot 2}=\frac{9}{2}=4\frac{1}{2}$

$4\frac{1}{2}$ cups of mashed bananas are needed.

**89.** **Strategy** To find how times to increase the recipe, divide the total number of slices needed (70) by number of slices in one recipe (14).

**Solution**

$$\begin{array}{r} 5 \\ 14\overline{)70} \\ \underline{70} \\ 0 \end{array}$$

The recipe will need to be multiplied by 5.

**Strategy** To find how cups of shortening are needed, multiply the number of cups in one recipe $\left(\frac{1}{4}\right)$, by 5.

**Solution** $\frac{1}{4}\times 5=\frac{1}{4}\times\frac{5}{1}=\frac{5}{4}=1\frac{1}{4}$

$1\frac{1}{4}$ cups of shortening are needed.

© 2013 Cengage Learning. All Rights Reserved. May not be scanned, copied or duplicated, or posted to a publicly accessible website, in whole or in part.

**91.** **Strategy** To find the total pay, multiply the number of days $\left(5\frac{1}{2}\text{ days}\right)$ by the pay per day ($168).

**Solution**

$$5\frac{1}{2}\times168=\frac{11}{2}\times\frac{168}{1}=\frac{11\times\overset{84}{\cancel{168}}}{\underset{1}{\cancel{2}}}=11\times84=924$$

The total pay is $924.

## Applying the Concepts

**93.** $\frac{1}{2}$; Any number multiplied by 1 is the number.

**95.** A. The product of any two positive rational numbers, each less than 1, is less than either of the two numbers.

# Section 2.7

## Objective A Exercises

**1.** $\frac{1}{3}\div\frac{2}{5}=\frac{1}{3}\times\frac{5}{2}=\frac{1\cdot5}{3\cdot2}=\frac{5}{6}$

**3.** $\frac{3}{7}\div\frac{3}{7}=\frac{3}{7}\times\frac{7}{3}=\frac{\overset{1}{\cancel{3}}\cdot\overset{1}{\cancel{7}}}{\underset{1}{\cancel{7}}\cdot\underset{1}{\cancel{3}}}=1$

**5.** $0\div\frac{3}{4}=0\times\frac{4}{3}=0$

**7.** $\frac{5}{24}\div\frac{15}{36}=\frac{5}{24}\times\frac{36}{15}=\frac{\overset{1}{\cancel{5}}\cdot\overset{1}{\cancel{2}}\cdot\overset{1}{\cancel{2}}\cdot\overset{1}{\cancel{3}}\cdot\overset{1}{\cancel{3}}}{\underset{1}{\cancel{2}}\cdot\underset{1}{\cancel{2}}\cdot2\cdot\underset{1}{\cancel{3}}\cdot\underset{1}{\cancel{3}}\cdot\underset{1}{\cancel{5}}}=\frac{1}{2}$

**9.** $\frac{1}{9}\div\frac{2}{3}=\frac{1}{9}\times\frac{3}{2}=\frac{\overset{1}{\cancel{3}}}{\underset{1}{\cancel{3}}\cdot3\cdot2}=\frac{1}{6}$

**11.** $\frac{2}{5}\div\frac{4}{7}=\frac{2}{5}\times\frac{7}{4}=\frac{\overset{1}{\cancel{2}}\cdot7}{5\cdot\underset{1}{\cancel{2}}\cdot2}=\frac{7}{10}$

**13.** $\frac{1}{2}\div\frac{1}{4}=\frac{1}{2}\times\frac{4}{1}=\frac{\overset{1}{\cancel{2}}\cdot2}{\underset{1}{\cancel{2}}}=2$

**15.** $\frac{1}{5}\div\frac{1}{10}=\frac{1}{5}\times\frac{10}{1}=\frac{2\cdot\overset{1}{\cancel{5}}}{\underset{1}{\cancel{5}}}=2$

**17.** $\frac{7}{15}\div\frac{14}{5}=\frac{7}{15}\times\frac{5}{14}=\frac{\overset{1}{\cancel{7}}\cdot\overset{1}{\cancel{5}}}{3\cdot\underset{1}{\cancel{5}}\cdot2\cdot\underset{1}{\cancel{7}}}=\frac{1}{6}$

**19.** $\frac{14}{3}\div\frac{7}{9}=\frac{14}{3}\times\frac{9}{7}=\frac{2\cdot\overset{1}{\cancel{7}}\cdot\overset{1}{\cancel{3}}\cdot3}{\underset{1}{\cancel{3}}\cdot\underset{1}{\cancel{7}}}=6$

**21.** $\frac{5}{9}\div\frac{25}{3}=\frac{5}{9}\times\frac{3}{25}=\frac{\overset{1}{\cancel{5}}\cdot\overset{1}{\cancel{3}}}{\underset{1}{\cancel{3}}\cdot3\cdot\underset{1}{\cancel{5}}\cdot5}=\frac{1}{15}$

**23.** $\frac{2}{3}\div\frac{1}{3}=\frac{2}{3}\times\frac{3}{1}=\frac{2\cdot\overset{1}{\cancel{3}}}{\underset{1}{\cancel{3}}}=2$

**25.** $\frac{5}{7}\div\frac{2}{7}=\frac{5}{7}\times\frac{7}{2}=\frac{5\cdot\overset{1}{\cancel{7}}}{\underset{1}{\cancel{7}}\cdot2}=\frac{5}{2}=2\frac{1}{2}$

**27.** $\frac{2}{3}\div\frac{2}{9}=\frac{2}{3}\times\frac{9}{2}=\frac{\overset{1}{\cancel{2}}\cdot\overset{1}{\cancel{3}}\cdot3}{\underset{1}{\cancel{3}}\cdot\underset{1}{\cancel{2}}}=3$

**29.** $\frac{7}{8}\div\frac{3}{4}=\frac{7}{8}\times\frac{4}{3}=\frac{7\cdot\overset{1}{\cancel{2}}\cdot\overset{1}{\cancel{2}}}{\underset{1}{\cancel{2}}\cdot\underset{1}{\cancel{2}}\cdot2\cdot3}=\frac{7}{6}=1\frac{1}{6}$

**31.** $\frac{5}{7}\div\frac{3}{14}=\frac{5}{7}\times\frac{14}{3}=\frac{5\cdot2\cdot\overset{1}{\cancel{7}}}{\underset{1}{\cancel{7}}\cdot3}=\frac{10}{3}=3\frac{1}{3}$

**33.** True

## Objective B Exercises

**35.** $4\div\frac{2}{3}=\frac{4}{1}\times\frac{3}{2}=\frac{\overset{1}{\cancel{2}}\cdot2\cdot3}{\underset{1}{\cancel{2}}}=6$

© 2013 Cengage Learning. All Rights Reserved. May not be scanned, copied or duplicated, or posted to a publicly accessible website, in whole or in part.

**37.** $$\frac{3}{2} \div 3 = \frac{3}{2} \times \frac{1}{3} = \frac{\cancel{3}}{2 \cdot \cancel{3}} = \frac{1}{2}$$

**39.** $$\frac{5}{6} \div 25 = \frac{5}{6} \times \frac{1}{25} = \frac{\cancel{5}}{2 \cdot 3 \cdot \cancel{5} \cdot 5} = \frac{1}{30}$$

**41.** $$6 \div 3\frac{1}{3} = \frac{6}{1} \div \frac{10}{3} = \frac{6}{1} \times \frac{3}{10} = \frac{\cancel{2} \cdot 3 \cdot 3}{\cancel{2} \cdot 5} = \frac{9}{5} = 1\frac{4}{5}$$

**43.** $$6\frac{1}{2} \div \frac{1}{2} = \frac{13}{2} \div \frac{1}{2} = \frac{13}{2} \times \frac{2}{1} = \frac{13 \cdot \cancel{2}}{\cancel{2}} = 13$$

**45.** $$8\frac{1}{4} \div 2\frac{3}{4} = \frac{33}{4} \div \frac{11}{4} = \frac{33}{4} \times \frac{4}{11} = \frac{3 \cdot \cancel{11} \cdot \cancel{2} \cdot \cancel{2}}{\cancel{2} \cdot \cancel{2} \cdot \cancel{11}} = 3$$

**47.** $$4\frac{1}{5} \div 21 = \frac{21}{5} \div \frac{21}{1} = \frac{21}{5} \times \frac{1}{21} = \frac{\cancel{3} \cdot \cancel{7}}{5 \cdot \cancel{3} \cdot \cancel{7}} = \frac{1}{5}$$

**49.** $$\frac{11}{12} \div 2\frac{1}{3} = \frac{11}{12} \div \frac{7}{3} = \frac{11}{12} \times \frac{3}{7} = \frac{11 \cdot \cancel{3}}{2 \cdot 2 \cdot \cancel{3} \cdot 7} = \frac{11}{28}$$

**51.** $$35 \div \frac{7}{24} = \frac{35}{1} \times \frac{24}{7} = \frac{5 \cdot \cancel{7} \cdot 2 \cdot 2 \cdot 2 \cdot 3}{\cancel{7}} = 120$$

**53.** $$\frac{11}{18} \div 2\frac{2}{9} = \frac{11}{18} \div \frac{20}{9} = \frac{11}{18} \times \frac{9}{20}$$
$$= \frac{11 \cdot \cancel{3} \cdot \cancel{3}}{2 \cdot \cancel{3} \cdot \cancel{3} \cdot 2 \cdot 2 \cdot 5} = \frac{11}{40}$$

**55.** $$2\frac{1}{16} \div 2\frac{1}{2} = \frac{33}{16} \div \frac{5}{2} = \frac{33}{16} \times \frac{2}{5}$$
$$= \frac{3 \cdot 11 \cdot \cancel{2}}{\cancel{2} \cdot 2 \cdot 2 \cdot 2 \cdot 5} = \frac{33}{40}$$

**57.** $$1\frac{2}{3} \div \frac{3}{8} = \frac{5}{3} \div \frac{3}{8} = \frac{5}{3} \times \frac{8}{3}$$
$$= \frac{5 \cdot 2 \cdot 2 \cdot 2}{3 \cdot 3} = \frac{40}{9} = 4\frac{4}{9}$$

**59.** $$1\frac{5}{8} \div 4 = \frac{13}{8} \div \frac{4}{1} = \frac{13}{8} \times \frac{1}{4} = \frac{13}{2 \cdot 2 \cdot 2 \cdot 2 \cdot 2} = \frac{13}{32}$$

**61.** $$16 \div 1\frac{1}{2} = 16 \div \frac{3}{2} = \frac{16}{1} \times \frac{2}{3}$$
$$= \frac{2 \cdot 2 \cdot 2 \cdot 2 \cdot 2}{3} = \frac{32}{3} = 10\frac{2}{3}$$

**63.** $$1\frac{1}{3} \div 5\frac{8}{9} = \frac{4}{3} \div \frac{53}{9} = \frac{4}{3} \times \frac{9}{53} = \frac{2 \cdot 2 \cdot \cancel{3} \cdot 3}{\cancel{3} \cdot 53} = \frac{12}{53}$$

**65.** $$82\frac{3}{5} \div 19\frac{1}{10} = \frac{413}{5} \div \frac{191}{10} = \frac{413}{5} \times \frac{10}{191}$$
$$= \frac{7 \cdot 59 \cdot 2 \cdot \cancel{5}}{\cancel{5} \cdot 191} = \frac{826}{191} = 4\frac{62}{191}$$

**67.** $$102 \div 1\frac{1}{2} = \frac{102}{1} \div \frac{3}{2} = \frac{102}{1} \times \frac{2}{3}$$
$$= \frac{2 \cdot \cancel{3} \cdot 17 \cdot 2}{\cancel{3}} = 68$$

**69.** $$8\frac{2}{7} \div 1 = \frac{58}{7} \div 1 = \frac{58}{7} \times 1 = \frac{58}{7} = 8\frac{2}{7}$$

**71.** $$8\frac{8}{9} \div 2\frac{13}{18} = \frac{80}{9} \div \frac{49}{18} = \frac{80}{9} \times \frac{18}{49}$$
$$= \frac{2 \cdot 2 \cdot 2 \cdot 2 \cdot 5 \cdot 2 \cdot \cancel{3} \cdot \cancel{3}}{\cancel{3} \cdot \cancel{3} \cdot 7 \cdot 7}$$
$$= \frac{160}{49} = 3\frac{13}{49}$$

**73.** $$7\frac{3}{8} \div 1\frac{27}{32} = \frac{59}{8} \div \frac{59}{32} = \frac{59}{8} \times \frac{32}{59}$$
$$= \frac{\cancel{59} \cdot \cancel{2} \cdot \cancel{2} \cdot \cancel{2} \cdot 2 \cdot 2}{\cancel{2} \cdot \cancel{2} \cdot \cancel{2} \cdot \cancel{59}} = 4$$

**75.** $$2\frac{3}{4} \div 1\frac{23}{32} = \frac{11}{4} \div \frac{55}{32} = \frac{11}{4} \times \frac{32}{35}$$
$$= \frac{\cancel{11} \cdot \cancel{2} \cdot \cancel{2} \cdot 2 \cdot 2}{\cancel{2} \cdot \cancel{2} \cdot 5 \cdot \cancel{11}} = \frac{8}{5} = 1\frac{3}{5}$$

© 2013 Cengage Learning. All Rights Reserved. May not be scanned, copied or duplicated, or posted to a publicly accessible website, in whole or in part.

**77.** $\frac{14}{77} \div 3\frac{1}{9} = \frac{14}{77} \div \frac{28}{9} = \frac{14}{17} \times \frac{9}{28}$

$= \frac{\overset{1}{\cancel{2}} \cdot \overset{1}{\cancel{7}} \cdot 3 \cdot 3}{17 \cdot \underset{1}{\cancel{2}} \cdot 2 \cdot \underset{1}{\cancel{7}}} = \frac{9}{34}$

**79.** False

## Objective C Exercises

**81.** Less than 16, because $1\frac{1}{3} > 1$

**83.** **Strategy** To find the number of servings in 16 ounces of cereal, divide 16 by the amount in each serving $\left(1\frac{1}{3} \text{ ounces}\right)$.

**Solution**

$16 \div 1\frac{1}{3} = 16 \div \frac{4}{3}$

$= 16 \times \frac{3}{4} = \frac{16 \cdot 3}{4}$

$= 12$

There are 12 servings in 16 ounces of cereal.

**85.** **Strategy** To find the unit price, divide the price ($21) by the number of ounces $\left(1\frac{1}{2}\right)$.

**Solution**

$21 \div 1\frac{1}{2} = 21 \div \frac{3}{2}$

$= \frac{21}{1} \times \frac{2}{3}$

$= \frac{\overset{7}{\cancel{21}} \cdot 2}{\underset{1}{\cancel{3}}}$

$= 14$

The cost per ounce is $14.

**87.** **Strategy** To find the number of miles for one gallon, divide the number of miles (357) by the number of gallons $\left(25\frac{1}{2} \text{ gallons}\right)$.

**Solution**

$357 \div 25\frac{1}{2} = \frac{357}{1} \div \frac{51}{2}$

$= \frac{357}{1} \times \frac{2}{51}$

$= \frac{\overset{1}{\cancel{17}} \cdot 7 \cdot \overset{1}{\cancel{3}} \cdot 2}{\underset{1}{\cancel{3}} \cdot \underset{1}{\cancel{17}}}$

$= 14$

The car can travel 14 miles.

**89a.** **Strategy** To find the total weight of the fat and bone, subtract the weight after trimming $\left(9\frac{1}{3} \text{ pounds}\right)$ from the original weight $\left(10\frac{3}{4} \text{ pounds}\right)$.

**Solution**

$$\begin{array}{rcr} 10\frac{3}{4} & = & 10\frac{9}{12} \\ -9\frac{1}{3} & = & 9\frac{4}{12} \\ \hline & & 1\frac{5}{12} \end{array}$$

The total weight of the fat and bone was $1\frac{5}{12}$ pounds.

**b.** **Strategy** To find the number of servings, divide the weight after trimming $\left(9\frac{1}{3} \text{ pounds}\right)$ by the weight of one serving $\left(\frac{1}{3} \text{ pound}\right)$.

**Solution**

$9\frac{1}{3} \div \frac{1}{3} = \frac{28}{3} \div \frac{1}{3} = \frac{28}{3} \times \frac{3}{1}$

$= \frac{28 \cdot \overset{1}{\cancel{3}}}{\underset{1}{\cancel{3}} \cdot 1} = 28$

The hospital chef can cut 28 servings from the roast.

**91.** **Strategy** To find the number of doses in a bottle, divide the number of

© 2013 Cengage Learning. All Rights Reserved. May not be scanned, copied or duplicated, or posted to a publicly accessible website, in whole or in part.

ounces in a bottle $\left(10\frac{1}{2}\right)$ by the number on ounces in a dose $\left(\frac{1}{2}\right)$.

**Solution** $10\frac{1}{2} \div \frac{1}{2} = \frac{21}{2} \times \frac{2}{1} = \frac{21 \cdot \overset{1}{\not{2}}}{\underset{1}{\not{2}}} = 21$

There are 21 doses in a bottle.

## Applying the Concepts

**93. Strategy** To find the fractional part of money borrowed that is spent on office renovation and equipment purchase, add the fraction spent on office renovation $\left(\frac{19}{50}\right)$ and the fraction spent on equipment $\left(\frac{6}{25}\right)$.

**Solution** $\frac{19}{50} + \frac{6}{25} = \frac{19}{50} + \frac{12}{50} = \frac{31}{50}$

$\frac{31}{50}$ of the money borrowed is spent on office renovation and office equipment.

**95. Strategy** To find the fraction of the bill left to be paid

- Add the fraction paid by insurance $\left(\frac{1}{2}\right)$ to the fraction you already paid $\left(\frac{1}{6}\right)$.
- Subtract the part paid from 1.

**Solution** $\frac{1}{2} + \frac{1}{6} = \frac{3}{6} + \frac{1}{6} = \frac{4}{6} = \frac{2}{3}$

$1 - \frac{2}{3} = \frac{3}{3} - \frac{2}{3} = \frac{1}{3}$

$\frac{1}{3}$ of the bill is left to be paid.

**97. Strategy** To find the fraction that require a low sodium diet

- Add (40, 25, 30, and 50) to find the total number of residences.
- Divde the number on low sodium diet (40) by the total number and reduce the fraction.

**Solution** $\begin{array}{r} 40 \\ 25 \\ 30 \\ +50 \\ \hline 145 \end{array}$ $\quad \frac{40}{145} = \frac{\overset{1}{\not{5}} \cdot 2 \cdot 2 \cdot 2}{\underset{1}{\not{5}} \cdot 29} = \frac{8}{29}$

$\frac{8}{29}$ of the patients require a low sodium diet.

**99. Strategy** To find the fraction that require a some type of restrictions

- Aadd (40, 25, 30, and 50) to find the total number of residences.
- Add the number of patients with some restrictions (40, 25 and 30).
- Divde the number with some restriction by the total number and reduce the fraction.

**Solution** $\begin{array}{r} 40 \\ 25 \\ 30 \\ +50 \\ \hline 145 \end{array}$ $\quad \begin{array}{r} 40 \\ 25 \\ +30 \\ \hline 95 \end{array}$

$\frac{95}{145} = \frac{\overset{1}{\not{5}} \cdot 19}{\underset{1}{\not{5}} \cdot 29} = \frac{19}{29}$

$\frac{19}{29}$ of the patients have some restrictions.

© 2013 Cengage Learning. All Rights Reserved. May not be scanned, copied or duplicated, or posted to a publicly accessible website, in whole or in part.

**101. Strategy** To find how many more cans of soda per week the average teenage boy drinks than the average teenage girl:

- Subtract the daily consumption for the teenage girls $\left(2\frac{1}{3}\text{ cans}\right)$ from the daily consumption for the teenage boys $\left(3\frac{1}{3}\text{ cans}\right)$.
- Multiply the difference by 7.

**Solution** $3\frac{1}{3} - 2\frac{1}{3} = 1$ more can per day

$1 \times 7 = 7 = 7$ more cans per week

The average teenage boy drinks 7 more cans of soda per week than the average teenage girl.

**103a.** $\frac{1}{2} \div \frac{3}{4} = \frac{1}{2} \times \frac{4}{3} = \frac{2}{3}$

Factor · factor = product

In order to find a factor, divide the product by the known factor.

**b.** $1\frac{3}{4} \div \frac{2}{3} = \frac{7}{4} \times \frac{3}{2} = \frac{21}{8} = 2\frac{5}{8}$

# Section 2.8

## Objective A Exercises

**1.** $\frac{11}{40} < \frac{19}{40}$

**3.** $\frac{2}{3} = \frac{14}{21}, \frac{5}{7} = \frac{15}{21}, \frac{2}{3} < \frac{5}{7}$

**5.** $\frac{5}{8} = \frac{15}{24}, \frac{7}{12} = \frac{14}{24}, \frac{5}{8} > \frac{7}{12}$

**7.** $\frac{7}{9} = \frac{28}{36}, \frac{11}{12} = \frac{33}{36}, \frac{7}{9} < \frac{11}{12}$

**9.** $\frac{13}{14} = \frac{39}{42}, \frac{19}{21} = \frac{38}{42}, \frac{13}{14} > \frac{19}{21}$

**11.** $\frac{7}{24} = \frac{35}{120}, \frac{11}{30} = \frac{44}{120}, \frac{7}{24} < \frac{11}{30}$

**13.** $\frac{4}{5}$ is larger.

## Objective B Exercises

**15.** $\left(\frac{5}{12}\right)^2 = \frac{5}{12} \cdot \frac{5}{12} = \frac{25}{144}$

**17.** $\left(\frac{1}{2}\right) \cdot \left(\frac{2}{3}\right)^2 = \left(\frac{1}{2}\right) \cdot \left(\frac{2}{3} \cdot \frac{2}{3}\right) = \frac{\cancel{2} \cdot 2}{\cancel{2} \cdot 3 \cdot 3} = \frac{2}{9}$

**19.** $\left(\frac{1}{3}\right)^2 \cdot \left(\frac{3}{5}\right)^3 = \left(\frac{1}{3} \cdot \frac{1}{3}\right) \cdot \left(\frac{3}{5} \cdot \frac{3}{5} \cdot \frac{3}{5}\right)$

$= \frac{1 \cdot 1 \cdot \cancel{3} \cdot \cancel{3} \cdot 3}{\cancel{3} \cdot \cancel{3} \cdot 5 \cdot 5 \cdot 5} = \frac{3}{125}$

**21.** $\left(\frac{5}{9}\right)^3 \cdot \left(\frac{18}{25}\right)^2 = \left(\frac{5}{9} \cdot \frac{5}{9} \cdot \frac{5}{9}\right) \cdot \left(\frac{18}{25} \cdot \frac{18}{25}\right)$

$= \frac{\cancel{5} \cdot \cancel{5} \cdot \cancel{5} \cdot 2 \cdot \cancel{3} \cdot \cancel{3} \cdot 2 \cdot \cancel{3} \cdot \cancel{3}}{\cancel{3} \cdot \cancel{3} \cdot \cancel{3} \cdot \cancel{3} \cdot 3 \cdot 3 \cdot \cancel{5} \cdot \cancel{5} \cdot \cancel{5} \cdot 5} = \frac{4}{45}$

**23.** $\left(\frac{1}{2}\right)^6 \cdot \left(\frac{32}{35}\right)^2 = \left(\frac{1}{2} \cdot \frac{1}{2} \cdot \frac{1}{2} \cdot \frac{1}{2} \cdot \frac{1}{2} \cdot \frac{1}{2}\right) \cdot \left(\frac{32}{35} \cdot \frac{32}{35}\right)$

$= \frac{\cancel{2} \cdot \cancel{2} \cdot \cancel{2} \cdot \cancel{2} \cdot \cancel{2} \cdot \cancel{2} \cdot 2 \cdot 2 \cdot 2 \cdot 2}{\cancel{2} \cdot \cancel{2} \cdot \cancel{2} \cdot \cancel{2} \cdot \cancel{2} \cdot \cancel{2} \cdot 5 \cdot 7 \cdot 5 \cdot 7} = \frac{16}{1225}$

**25.** $\left(\frac{1}{6}\right) \cdot \left(\frac{6}{7}\right)^2 \cdot \left(\frac{2}{3}\right) = \left(\frac{1}{6}\right) \cdot \left(\frac{6}{7} \cdot \frac{6}{7}\right) \cdot \left(\frac{2}{3}\right)$

$= \frac{\cancel{2} \cdot \cancel{3} \cdot 2 \cdot \cancel{3} \cdot 2}{\cancel{2} \cdot \cancel{3} \cdot 7 \cdot 7 \cdot \cancel{3}} = \frac{4}{49}$

**27.** $3 \cdot \left(\frac{3}{5}\right)^3 \cdot \left(\frac{1}{3}\right)^2 = \left(\frac{3}{1}\right) \cdot \left(\frac{3}{5} \cdot \frac{3}{5} \cdot \frac{3}{5}\right) \cdot \left(\frac{1}{3} \cdot \frac{1}{3}\right)$

$= \frac{\cancel{3} \cdot \cancel{3} \cdot 3 \cdot 3}{5 \cdot 5 \cdot 5 \cdot \cancel{3} \cdot \cancel{3}} = \frac{9}{125}$

© 2013 Cengage Learning. All Rights Reserved. May not be scanned, copied or duplicated, or posted to a publicly accessible website, in whole or in part.

**29.** $$11\cdot\left(\frac{3}{8}\right)^3\cdot\left(\frac{8}{11}\right)^2=\left(\frac{11}{1}\right)\cdot\left(\frac{3}{8}\cdot\frac{3}{8}\cdot\frac{3}{8}\right)\cdot\left(\frac{8}{11}\cdot\frac{8}{11}\right)$$
$$=\frac{\overset{1}{\cancel{11}}\cdot3\cdot3\cdot3\cdot\overset{1}{\cancel{2}}\cdot\overset{1}{\cancel{2}}\cdot\overset{1}{\cancel{2}}\cdot\overset{1}{\cancel{2}}\cdot\overset{1}{\cancel{2}}\cdot\overset{1}{\cancel{2}}}{\underset{1}{\cancel{2}}\cdot\underset{1}{\cancel{2}}\cdot\underset{1}{\cancel{2}}\cdot\underset{1}{\cancel{2}}\cdot\underset{1}{\cancel{2}}\cdot\underset{1}{\cancel{2}}\cdot2\cdot2\cdot2\cdot\underset{1}{\cancel{11}}\cdot11}=\frac{27}{88}$$

## Objective C Exercises

**31.** $$\frac{1}{2}-\frac{1}{3}+\frac{2}{3}=\frac{3}{6}-\frac{2}{6}+\frac{2}{3}$$
$$=\frac{1}{6}+\frac{2}{3}$$
$$=\frac{1}{6}+\frac{4}{6}$$
$$=\frac{5}{6}$$

**33.** $$\frac{1}{3}\div\frac{1}{2}+\frac{3}{4}=\frac{1}{3}\cdot\frac{2}{1}+\frac{3}{4}$$
$$=\frac{2}{3}+\frac{3}{4}$$
$$=\frac{8}{12}+\frac{9}{12}$$
$$=\frac{17}{12}=1\frac{5}{12}$$

**35.** $$\left(\frac{3}{4}\right)^2-\frac{5}{12}=\frac{9}{16}-\frac{5}{12}$$
$$=\frac{27}{48}-\frac{20}{48}$$
$$=\frac{7}{48}$$

**37.** $$\frac{5}{6}\cdot\left(\frac{2}{3}-\frac{1}{6}\right)+\frac{7}{18}=\frac{5}{6}\cdot\left(\frac{4}{6}-\frac{1}{6}\right)+\frac{7}{18}$$
$$=\frac{5}{6}\cdot\frac{3}{6}+\frac{7}{18}$$
$$=\frac{5}{12}+\frac{7}{18}$$
$$=\frac{15}{36}+\frac{14}{36}$$
$$=\frac{29}{36}$$

**39.** $$\frac{7}{12}-\left(\frac{2}{3}\right)^2+\frac{5}{8}=\frac{7}{12}-\frac{4}{9}+\frac{5}{8}$$
$$=\frac{42}{72}-\frac{32}{72}+\frac{45}{72}$$
$$=\frac{55}{72}$$

**41.** $$\frac{3}{4}\cdot\left(\frac{4}{9}\right)^2+\frac{1}{2}=\frac{3}{4}\cdot\frac{16}{81}+\frac{1}{2}$$
$$=\frac{4}{27}+\frac{1}{2}$$
$$=\frac{8}{54}+\frac{27}{54}$$
$$=\frac{35}{54}$$

**43.** $$\left(\frac{1}{2}+\frac{3}{4}\right)\div\frac{5}{8}=\left(\frac{2}{4}+\frac{3}{4}\right)\div\frac{5}{8}$$
$$=\frac{5}{4}\cdot\frac{8}{5}$$
$$=2$$

**45.** $$\frac{3}{8}\div\left(\frac{5}{12}+\frac{3}{8}\right)=\frac{3}{8}\div\left(\frac{10}{24}+\frac{9}{24}\right)$$
$$=\frac{3}{8}\div\frac{19}{24}$$
$$=\frac{3}{8}\cdot\frac{24}{19}$$
$$=\frac{9}{19}$$

**47.** $$\left(\frac{3}{8}\right)^2\div\left(\frac{3}{7}+\frac{3}{14}\right)=\left(\frac{3}{8}\right)^2\div\left(\frac{6}{14}+\frac{3}{14}\right)$$
$$=\left(\frac{3}{8}\right)^2\div\frac{9}{14}$$
$$=\frac{9}{64}\cdot\frac{14}{9}$$
$$=\frac{7}{32}$$

**49.** $$\frac{2}{5}\div\frac{3}{8}\cdot\frac{4}{5}=\frac{2}{5}\cdot\frac{8}{3}\cdot\frac{4}{5}$$
$$=\frac{16}{15}\cdot\frac{4}{5}$$
$$=\frac{64}{75}$$

© 2013 Cengage Learning. All Rights Reserved. May not be scanned, copied or duplicated, or posted to a publicly accessible website, in whole or in part.

## Applying the Concepts

**51a.** $\frac{13}{50}=\frac{26}{100}$ Location

$\frac{1}{4}=\frac{25}{100}$ Food Quality

More people choose location.

**b.** $\frac{1}{4}=\frac{25}{100}$ Food Quality

$\frac{13}{50}=\frac{26}{100}$ Location

$\frac{4}{25}=\frac{16}{100}$ Menu

$\frac{2}{25}=\frac{8}{100}$ Price

$\frac{3}{25}=\frac{12}{100}$ Speed

$\frac{3}{100}=\frac{3}{100}$ Other

The criterion that was cited by most people was location.

## Chapter 2 Concept Review

**1.** To find the LCM of 75, 30, and 50, find the prime factorization of each number and write the factorization of each number in a table. Circle the greatest product in each column. The LCM is the product of the circled numbers.

| | 2 | 3 | 5 |
|---|---|---|---|
| 75 = | | (3) | (5 · 5) |
| 30 = | (2) | 3 | 5 |
| 50 = | 2 | | 5 · 5 |

$\text{LCM} = 2\cdot3\cdot5\cdot5 = 150$

**2.** To find the GCF of 42, 14, and 21, find the prime factorization of each number and write the factorization of each number in a table. Circle the least product in each column that does not have a blank. The GCF is the product of the circled numbers.

| | 2 | 3 | 7 |
|---|---|---|---|
| 42 = | 2 | 3 | (7) |
| 14 = | 2 | | 7 |
| 21 = | | 3 | 7 |

GCF = 7

**3.** To write an improper fraction as a mixed number, divide the numerator by the denominator. The quotient without the remainder is the whole number part of the mixed number. To write the fractional part of the mixed number, write the remainder over the divisor.

**4.** A fraction is in simplest form when the numerator and denominator have no common factors other than 1, For example, $\frac{8}{12}$ is not in simplest form because 8 and 12 have a common factor of 4. $\frac{5}{7}$ is in simplest form because 5 and 7 have no common factors other than 1.

**5.** When adding fractions, you have to convert to equivalent fractions with a common denominator. One way to explain this is that you can combine like things, but you cannot combine unlike things. You can combine 3 apples and 4 apples and get 7 apples. You cannot combine 4 apples and 3 oranges and get a sum consisting of just one item. In adding whole numbers, you add like things: ones, tens, hundreds, and so on. In adding fractions, you can combine 2 *ninths* and 5 *ninths* and get 7 *ninths*, but you cannot add 2 *ninths* and 3 *fifths*.

© 2013 Cengage Learning. All Rights Reserved. May not be scanned, copied or duplicated, or posted to a publicly accessible website, in whole or in part.

**6.** To add mixed numbers, add the fractional parts and then add the whole parts. Then reduce the sum to simplest form.

**7.** To subtract mixed numbers, the first step is to subtract the fractional parts. If we are subtracting a mixed number from a whole number, there is no fractional part in the whole number from which to subtract the fractional part of the mixed number. Therefore, we must borrow a 1 from the whole number and write 1 as an equivalent fraction with a denominator equal to the denominator of the fraction in the mixed number. Then we can subtract the fractional parts and then subtract the whole numbers.

**8.** When multiplying two fractions, it is better to eliminate the common factors before multiplying the remaining factors in the numerator and denominator so that (1) we don't end up with very large products and (2) we don't have the added step of simplifying the resulting fraction.

**9.** Let's look at an example, $\frac{1}{2}\times\frac{1}{3}=\frac{1}{6}$. $\frac{1}{2}$ and $\frac{1}{3}$ are fractions less than 1. The product, $\frac{1}{6}$, is less than $\frac{1}{2}$ and less than $\frac{1}{3}$. Therefore, the product is less than the smaller number.

**10.** Reciprocals are used to rewrite division problems as related multiplication problems. Since "divided by" means the same thing as "times the reciprocal of," we can change the division sign to a multiplication sign and change the divisor to its reciprocal. For example, $9\div 3=9\times\frac{1}{3}$.

**11.** When a fraction is divided by a whole number, we write the whole number as a fraction before dividing so that we can easily determine the reciprocal of the whole number.

**12.** When comparing fractions, we must first look at the denominators. If they are not the same, we must rewrite the fractions as equivalent fractions with a common denominator. If the denominators are the same, we must look at the numerators. The fraction that has the smaller numerator is the smaller fraction.

**13.** We must follow the Order of Operations Agreement in simplifying the expression $\left(\frac{5}{6}\right)^2-\left(\frac{3}{4}-\frac{2}{3}\right)\div\frac{1}{2}$. Therefore, we must first simplify the expression $\frac{3}{4}-\frac{2}{3}$ inside the parentheses: $\frac{3}{4}-\frac{2}{3}=\frac{1}{12}$. Then simplify the exponential expression: $\left(\frac{5}{6}\right)^2=\frac{25}{36}$. Then perform the division: $\frac{1}{12}\div\frac{1}{2}=\frac{1}{6}$. Then perform the subtraction: $\frac{25}{36}-\frac{1}{6}=\frac{19}{36}$.

© 2013 Cengage Learning. All Rights Reserved. May not be scanned, copied or duplicated, or posted to a publicly accessible website, in whole or in part.

## Chapter 2 Review Exercises

**1.** $\frac{30}{45}=\frac{2\cdot\cancel{3}\cdot\cancel{5}}{3\cdot\cancel{3}\cdot\cancel{5}}=\frac{2}{3}$

**2.** $\left(\frac{3}{4}\right)^3\cdot\frac{20}{27}=\left(\frac{3}{4}\cdot\frac{3}{4}\cdot\frac{3}{4}\right)\left(\frac{20}{27}\right)$

$=\frac{\cancel{3}\cdot\cancel{3}\cdot\cancel{3}\cdot\cancel{2}\cdot\cancel{2}\cdot 5}{2\cdot 2\cdot 2\cdot 2\cdot\cancel{2}\cdot\cancel{2}\cdot\cancel{3}\cdot\cancel{3}\cdot\cancel{3}}=\frac{5}{16}$

**3.** $\frac{13}{4}$

**4.**
$$\begin{array}{r} \frac{2}{3}=\frac{12}{18}\\ \frac{5}{6}=\frac{15}{18}\\ +\frac{2}{9}=\frac{4}{18}\\ \hline \frac{31}{18}=1\frac{13}{18}\end{array}$$

**5.** $\frac{11}{18}=\frac{44}{72},\frac{17}{24}=\frac{51}{72},\frac{11}{18}<\frac{17}{24}$

**6.**
$$\begin{array}{r} 18\frac{1}{6}=18\frac{7}{42}=17\frac{49}{42}\\ -3\frac{5}{7}=3\frac{30}{42}=3\frac{30}{42}\\ \hline 14\frac{19}{42}\end{array}$$

**7.** $\frac{2}{7}\left(\frac{5}{8}-\frac{1}{3}\right)\div\frac{3}{5}=\frac{2}{7}\left(\frac{15}{24}-\frac{8}{24}\right)\div\frac{3}{5}$

$=\frac{2}{7}\left(\frac{7}{24}\right)\div\frac{3}{5}=\frac{1}{12}\div\frac{3}{5}=\frac{1}{12}\times\frac{5}{3}=\frac{5}{36}$

**8.** $2\frac{1}{3}\times 3\frac{7}{8}=\frac{7}{3}\times\frac{31}{8}=\frac{7\cdot 31}{3\cdot 8}=\frac{217}{24}=9\frac{1}{24}$

**9.** $1\frac{1}{3}\div\frac{2}{3}=\frac{4}{3}\div\frac{2}{3}=\frac{4}{3}\times\frac{3}{2}=\frac{4\cdot 3}{3\cdot 2}=\frac{2\cdot\cancel{2}\cdot\cancel{3}}{\cancel{3}\cdot\cancel{2}}=2$

**10.**
$$\begin{array}{r} \frac{17}{24}=\frac{34}{48}\\ -\frac{3}{16}=\frac{9}{48}\\ \hline \frac{25}{48}\end{array}$$

**11.** $8\frac{2}{3}\div 2\frac{3}{5}=\frac{26}{3}\div\frac{13}{5}=\frac{26}{3}\times\frac{5}{13}$

$=\frac{26\cdot 5}{3\cdot 13}=\frac{2\cdot\cancel{13}\cdot 5}{3\cdot\cancel{13}}$

$=\frac{10}{3}=3\frac{1}{3}$

**12.**

| | 2 | 3 | 5 |
|---|---|---|---|
| 20 = | (2 · 2) | | 5 |
| 48 = | 2 · 2 · 2 · 2 | 3 | |

GCF $=2\cdot 2=4$

**13.** $36\div 12=3;\ \frac{2\cdot 12}{3\cdot 12}=\frac{24}{36}$

**14.** $\frac{15}{28}\div\frac{5}{7}=\frac{15}{28}\times\frac{7}{5}=\frac{15\cdot 7}{28\cdot 5}=\frac{3\cdot\cancel{5}\cdot\cancel{7}}{2\cdot 2\cdot\cancel{7}\cdot\cancel{5}}=\frac{3}{4}$

**15.** $44\div 11=4;\ \frac{8\cdot 4}{11\cdot 4}=\frac{32}{44}$

**16.** $2\frac{1}{4}\times 7\frac{1}{3}=\frac{9}{4}\times\frac{22}{3}=\frac{9\cdot 22}{4\cdot 3}=\frac{3\cdot\cancel{3}\cdot\cancel{2}\cdot 11}{\cancel{2}\cdot 2\cdot\cancel{3}}$

$=\frac{33}{2}=16\frac{1}{2}$

**17.**

| | 2 | 3 |
|---|---|---|
| 18 = | 2 | 3 · 3 |
| 12 = | (2 · 2) | (3 · 3) |

LCM $=2\cdot 2\cdot 3\cdot 3=36$

**18.** $\frac{16}{24}=\frac{\cancel{2}\cdot\cancel{2}\cdot 2\cdot 2}{\cancel{2}\cdot\cancel{2}\cdot 11}=\frac{4}{11}$

© 2013 Cengage Learning. All Rights Reserved. May not be scanned, copied or duplicated, or posted to a publicly accessible website, in whole or in part.

**19.**
$$\begin{array}{r} \frac{3}{8} \\ \frac{5}{8} \\ +\frac{1}{8} \\ \hline \frac{9}{8} = 1\frac{1}{8} \end{array}$$

**20.**
$$\begin{array}{r} 16 = 15\frac{8}{8} \\ -5\frac{7}{8} = 5\frac{7}{8} \\ \hline 10\frac{1}{8} \end{array}$$

**21.**
$$\begin{array}{r} 4\frac{4}{9} = 4\frac{24}{54} \\ 2\frac{1}{6} = 2\frac{9}{54} \\ +11\frac{17}{27} = 11\frac{34}{54} \\ \hline 17\frac{67}{54} = 18\frac{13}{54} \end{array}$$

**22.**

| | 3 | 5 |
|---|---|---|
| 15 = | 3 | (5) |
| 25 = | | 5 · 5 |

GCF = 5

**23.**
$$\begin{array}{r} 3 \\ 5\overline{)17} \\ -15 \\ \hline 2 \end{array} \qquad \frac{17}{5} = 3\frac{2}{5}$$

**24.**
$$\left(\frac{4}{5}-\frac{2}{3}\right)^2 \div \frac{4}{15} = \left(\frac{12}{15}-\frac{10}{15}\right)^2 \div \frac{4}{15}$$
$$= \left(\frac{2}{15}\right)^2 \div \frac{4}{15} = \left(\frac{2}{15}\right)\left(\frac{2}{15}\right) \div \frac{4}{15}$$
$$= \frac{4}{225} \times \frac{15}{4} = \frac{4 \cdot 15}{225 \cdot 4} = \frac{1}{15}$$

**25.**
$$\begin{array}{r} \frac{3}{8} = \frac{9}{24} \\ 1\frac{2}{3} = 1\frac{16}{24} \\ +3\frac{5}{6} = 3\frac{20}{24} \\ \hline 4\frac{45}{24} = 5\frac{21}{24} = 5\frac{7}{8} \end{array}$$

**26.**

| | 2 | 3 |
|---|---|---|
| 18 = | (2) | 3 · 3 |
| 27 = | | (3 · 3 · 3) |

LCM = 2 · 3 · 3 · 3 = 54

**27.**
$$\begin{array}{r} \frac{11}{18} \\ -\frac{5}{18} \\ \hline \frac{6}{18} = \frac{1}{3} \end{array}$$

**28.** $2\frac{5}{7} = \frac{14+5}{7} = \frac{19}{7}$

**29.** $\frac{5}{6} \div \frac{5}{12} = \frac{5}{6} \cdot \frac{12}{5} = \frac{5 \cdot 12}{6 \cdot 5} = \frac{\overset{1}{\cancel{5}} \cdot \overset{1}{\cancel{2}} \cdot 2 \cdot \overset{1}{\cancel{3}}}{\underset{1}{\cancel{2}} \cdot \underset{1}{\cancel{3}} \cdot \underset{1}{\cancel{5}}} = 2$

**30.** $\frac{5}{12} \times \frac{4}{25} = \frac{5 \cdot 4}{12 \cdot 25} = \frac{\overset{1}{\cancel{5}} \cdot \overset{1}{\cancel{2}} \cdot \overset{1}{\cancel{2}}}{\underset{1}{\cancel{2}} \cdot \underset{1}{\cancel{2}} \cdot 3 \cdot \underset{1}{\cancel{5}} \cdot 5} = \frac{1}{15}$

**31.** $\frac{11}{50} \times \frac{25}{44} = \frac{11 \cdot 25}{50 \cdot 44} = \frac{\overset{1}{\cancel{11}} \cdot \overset{1}{\cancel{5}} \cdot \overset{1}{\cancel{5}}}{2 \cdot \underset{1}{\cancel{5}} \cdot \underset{1}{\cancel{5}} \cdot 2 \cdot 2 \cdot \underset{1}{\cancel{11}}} = \frac{1}{8}$

**32.** $1\frac{7}{8}$

© 2013 Cengage Learning. All Rights Reserved. May not be scanned, copied or duplicated, or posted to a publicly accessible website, in whole or in part.

**33. Strategy** To find the total lose for the 3 months, add the amounts losteach month $\left(4\frac{1}{2}, 3\frac{3}{4}, \text{ and } 4\frac{1}{4} \text{ inches}\right)$.

**Solution**

$$\begin{aligned} 4\frac{1}{2} &= 4\frac{2}{4} \\ 3\frac{3}{4} &= 3\frac{3}{4} \\ +4\frac{1}{4} &= 4\frac{1}{4} \\ \hline 11\frac{6}{4} &= 12\frac{1}{2} \end{aligned}$$

The total weight lose for the 3 months was $12\frac{1}{2}$ pounds.

**34. Strategy** To find the cost of each office multiply the total cost ($324,000) by $\frac{1}{8}$.

**Solution**

$$324,000 \times \frac{1}{8} = \frac{324,000}{8} = 40,500$$

The value of each office is $40,500.

**35. Strategy** To find how many miles the second checkpoint is from the finish line:

- Add the distance to the first checkpoint $\left(4\frac{1}{2} \textit{ miles}\right)$ to the distance between the first checkpoint and the second checkpoint $\left(5\frac{3}{4} \textit{ miles}\right)$.
- Subtract the total distance to the second checkpoint from the entire length of the race (15 miles).

**Solution**

$$\begin{aligned} 4\frac{1}{2} &= 4\frac{2}{4} \\ +5\frac{3}{4} &= 5\frac{3}{4} \\ \hline 9\frac{5}{4} &= 10\frac{1}{4} \end{aligned} \qquad \begin{aligned} 15 &= 14\frac{4}{4} \\ -10\frac{1}{4} &= 10\frac{1}{4} \\ \hline &\phantom{=} 4\frac{3}{4} \end{aligned}$$

The second checkpoint is $4\frac{3}{4}$ miles from the finish line.

**36. Strategy** To find how many miles the ambulance can travel, multiply the number of miles the ambulance can travel on 1 gallon (12) by the number of gallons $\left(34\frac{1}{2}\right)$.

**Solution**

$$12 \times 34\frac{1}{2} = 12 \times \frac{69}{2} = \frac{12 \cdot 69}{2} = 414$$

The ambulance can travel 414 miles.

# Chapter 2 Test

**1.** $\frac{9}{11} \times \frac{44}{81} = \frac{9 \cdot 44}{11 \cdot 81} = \frac{\overset{1}{\cancel{3}} \cdot \overset{1}{\cancel{3}} \cdot 2 \cdot 2 \cdot \overset{1}{\cancel{11}}}{\underset{1}{\cancel{11}} \cdot \underset{1}{\cancel{3}} \cdot \underset{1}{\cancel{3}} \cdot 3 \cdot 3} = \frac{4}{9}$

**2.**

| | 2 | 3 | 5 |
|---|---|---|---|
| 24 = | $2 \cdot 2 \cdot 2$ | 3 | |
| 80 = | $2 \cdot 2 \cdot 2 \cdot 2$ | | 5 |

GCF $= 2 \cdot 2 \cdot 2 = 8$

**3.** $\frac{5}{9} \div \frac{7}{18} = \frac{5}{9} \times \frac{18}{7} = \frac{5 \cdot 2 \cdot \overset{1}{\cancel{3}} \cdot \overset{1}{\cancel{3}}}{\underset{1}{\cancel{3}} \cdot \underset{1}{\cancel{3}} \cdot 7} = \frac{10}{7} = 1\frac{3}{7}$

**4.** $\left(\frac{3}{4}\right)^2 \div \left(\frac{2}{3} + \frac{5}{6}\right) - \frac{1}{12} = \left(\frac{3}{4} \cdot \frac{3}{4}\right) \div \left(\frac{4}{6} + \frac{5}{6}\right) - \frac{1}{12}$

© 2013 Cengage Learning. All Rights Reserved. May not be scanned, copied or duplicated, or posted to a publicly accessible website, in whole or in part.

$$= \frac{9}{16} \div \left(\frac{9}{6}\right) - \frac{1}{12}$$
$$= \frac{9}{16} \div \frac{3}{2} - \frac{1}{12}$$
$$= \frac{9}{16} \times \frac{2}{3} - \frac{1}{12}$$
$$\frac{\overset{1}{\cancel{3}} \cdot 3 \cdot \overset{1}{\cancel{2}}}{2 \cdot 2 \cdot 2 \cdot \underset{1}{\cancel{2}} \cdot \underset{1}{\cancel{3}}} - \frac{1}{12} = \frac{3}{8} - \frac{1}{12} = \frac{9}{24} - \frac{2}{24} = \frac{7}{24}$$

**5.** $9\frac{4}{5} = \frac{45+4}{5} = \frac{49}{5}$

**6.** $5\frac{2}{3} \times 1\frac{7}{17} = \frac{17}{3} \times \frac{24}{17} = \frac{17 \cdot 24}{3 \cdot 17}$

$$= \frac{\overset{1}{\cancel{17}} \cdot 2 \cdot 2 \cdot 2 \cdot \overset{1}{\cancel{3}}}{\underset{1}{\cancel{3}} \cdot \underset{1}{\cancel{17}}} = 8$$

**7.** $\frac{40}{64} = \frac{\overset{1}{\cancel{2}} \cdot \overset{1}{\cancel{2}} \cdot \overset{1}{\cancel{2}} \cdot 5}{\underset{1}{\cancel{2}} \cdot \underset{1}{\cancel{2}} \cdot \underset{1}{\cancel{2}} \cdot 2 \cdot 2 \cdot 2} = \frac{5}{8}$

**8.** $\frac{3}{8} = \frac{9}{24}, \frac{5}{12} = \frac{10}{24}, \frac{3}{8} < \frac{5}{12}$

**9.** $\left(\frac{1}{4}\right)^3 \div \left(\frac{1}{8}\right)^2 - \frac{1}{6} = \left(\frac{1}{4} \cdot \frac{1}{4} \cdot \frac{1}{4}\right) \div \left(\frac{1}{8} \cdot \frac{1}{8}\right) - \frac{1}{6}$

$$= \frac{1}{64} \div \frac{1}{64} - \frac{1}{6}$$
$$= \frac{1}{64} \times \frac{64}{1} - \frac{1}{6}$$
$$= 1 - \frac{1}{6}$$
$$= \frac{6}{6} - \frac{1}{6} = \frac{5}{6}$$

**10.**

| | 2 | 3 | 5 |
|---|---|---|---|
| 24 = | (2 · 2 · 2) | (3) | |
| 40 = | 2 · 2 · 2 | | (5) |

LCM = 2 · 2 · 2 · 3 · 5 = 120

**11.**
$$\frac{17}{24} - \frac{11}{24} = \frac{6}{24} = \frac{1}{4}$$

**12.**
$$5\overline{)18} = 3 \text{ R } 3 \quad (18 - 15 = 3)$$
$$\frac{18}{5} = 3\frac{3}{5}$$

**13.** $6\frac{2}{3} \div 3\frac{1}{6} = \frac{20}{3} \div \frac{19}{6} = \frac{20}{3} \times \frac{6}{19}$

$$= \frac{2 \cdot 2 \cdot 5 \cdot 2 \cdot \overset{1}{\cancel{3}}}{\underset{1}{\cancel{3}} \cdot 19} = \frac{40}{19} = 2\frac{2}{19}$$

**14.** $72 \div 8 = 9;\ \frac{5 \cdot 9}{8 \cdot 9} = \frac{45}{72}$

**15.**
$$\frac{5}{6} = \frac{75}{90}$$
$$\frac{7}{9} = \frac{70}{90}$$
$$+\frac{1}{15} = \frac{6}{90}$$
$$\frac{151}{90} = 1\frac{61}{90}$$

**16.**
$$23\frac{1}{8} = 23\frac{11}{88} = 22\frac{99}{88}$$
$$-9\frac{9}{44} = 9\frac{18}{88} = 9\frac{18}{88}$$
$$13\frac{81}{88}$$

**17.**
$$\frac{9}{16} = \frac{27}{48}$$
$$-\frac{5}{12} = \frac{20}{48}$$
$$\frac{7}{48}$$

**18.** $\left(\frac{2}{3}\right)^4 \left(\frac{27}{32}\right) = \left(\frac{2}{3} \cdot \frac{2}{3} \cdot \frac{2}{3} \cdot \frac{2}{3}\right)\left(\frac{27}{32}\right)$

$$= \frac{\overset{1}{\cancel{2}} \cdot \overset{1}{\cancel{2}} \cdot \overset{1}{\cancel{2}} \cdot \overset{1}{\cancel{2}} \cdot \overset{1}{\cancel{3}} \cdot \overset{1}{\cancel{3}} \cdot \overset{1}{\cancel{3}}}{3 \cdot \underset{1}{\cancel{3}} \cdot \underset{1}{\cancel{3}} \cdot \underset{1}{\cancel{3}} \cdot \underset{1}{\cancel{2}} \cdot \underset{1}{\cancel{2}} \cdot \underset{1}{\cancel{2}} \cdot \underset{1}{\cancel{2}} \cdot 2} = \frac{1}{6}$$

© 2013 Cengage Learning. All Rights Reserved. May not be scanned, copied or duplicated, or posted to a publicly accessible website, in whole or in part.

**19.**
$$\begin{array}{r} \frac{7}{12} \\ \frac{11}{12} \\ +\frac{5}{12} \\ \hline \frac{23}{12} = 1\frac{11}{12} \end{array}$$

**20.**
$$\begin{array}{rl} 12\frac{5}{12} = & 12\frac{25}{60} \\ +9\frac{17}{20} = & 9\frac{51}{60} \\ \hline & 21\frac{76}{60} = 22\frac{16}{60} = 22\frac{4}{15} \end{array}$$

**21.** $\frac{11}{4}$

**22. Strategy** To find the radiologist's earnings, multiply daily earnings ($240) by the number of days worked $\left(3\frac{1}{2}\right)$.

**Solution**
$$240 \times 3\frac{1}{2} = 240 \times \frac{7}{2} = \frac{240 \cdot 7}{2} = 840$$

The radiologist earns $840.

**23. Strategy** To find total length used, add the lengths $\left(14\frac{1}{4},\ 12\frac{5}{8},\text{ and } 15\frac{4}{6}\text{ inches}\right)$

**Solution**
$$\begin{array}{rl} 14\frac{1}{4} = & 14\frac{6}{24} \\ 12\frac{5}{8} = & 12\frac{15}{24} \\ +15\frac{4}{6} = & 15\frac{16}{24} \\ \hline & 41\frac{37}{24} = 42\frac{13}{24} \end{array}$$

A total of $42\frac{13}{24}$ inches was used.

**24. Strategy** To determine the sections that can be cut, divide the total length (36 feet) by the feet in each section $\left(\frac{1}{2}\right)$.

**Solution**
$$36 \div \frac{1}{2} = 36 \times \frac{2}{1} = 72$$

72 sections can be cut.

**25. Strategy** To find the weight after two weeks,

- Add the two loses $\left(1\frac{1}{2}\text{ and }\frac{3}{4}\text{ pounds}\right)$.
- Subtract the total lose from the original weight (122 pounds).

**Solution**
$$\begin{array}{rl} 1\frac{1}{2} = & 1\frac{2}{4} \\ +\frac{3}{4} = & \frac{3}{4} \\ \hline & 1\frac{5}{4} = 2\frac{1}{4} \end{array}$$

$$\begin{array}{rl} 122 = & 121\frac{4}{4} \\ -2\frac{1}{4} = & 2\frac{1}{4} \\ \hline & 119\frac{3}{4} \end{array}$$

The weight after two weeks was $119\frac{3}{4}$ pounds .

## Cumulative Review Exercises

**1.** 290,000

**2.**
$$\begin{array}{r} 9 \quad\ \ 9\ 13 \\ 8\,10\ \ 10\ 3\,17 \\ 3\cancel{9}\cancel{0},\cancel{0}\cancel{4}\cancel{7} \\ -\ 98,769 \\ \hline 291,278 \end{array}$$

**3.**
$$\begin{array}{r} 926 \\ \times\ \ 79 \\ \hline 8334 \\ 6482\ \\ \hline 73,154 \end{array}$$

© 2013 Cengage Learning. All Rights Reserved. May not be scanned, copied or duplicated, or posted to a publicly accessible website, in whole or in part.

**4.**

$$\begin{array}{r} 540 \text{ r}12 \\ 57\overline{)30,792} \\ \underline{-285} \\ 229 \\ \underline{-228} \\ 12 \\ \underline{-0} \\ 12 \end{array}$$

**5.** $4\cdot(6-3)\div 6-1 = 4\cdot 3\div 6-1$

$= 12\div 6-1$

$= 2-1$

$= 1$

**6.**

$$\begin{array}{r|l} & 44 \\ 2 & 22 \\ 2 & 11 \\ 11 & 1 \end{array}$$

$44 = 2\cdot 2\cdot 11$

**7.**

| | 2 | 3 | 5 | 7 |
|---|---|---|---|---|
| 30 = | (2) | (3) | (5) | |
| 42 = | 2 | 3 | | (7) |

LCM $= 2\cdot 3\cdot 5\cdot 7 = 210$

**8.**

| | 2 | 3 | 5 |
|---|---|---|---|
| 60 = | (2 · 2) | 3 | (5) |
| 80 = | 2 · 2 · 2 · 2 | | 5 |

GCF $= 2\cdot 2\cdot 5 = 20$

**9.** $7\frac{2}{3} = \frac{21+2}{3} = \frac{23}{3}$

**10.**

$$\begin{array}{r} 6\,r1 \\ 4\overline{)25} \\ \underline{-24} \\ 1 \end{array} \qquad \frac{25}{4} = 6\frac{1}{4}$$

**11.** $48\div 16 = 3;\ \frac{5\cdot 3}{16\cdot 3} = \frac{15}{48}$

**12.** $\frac{24}{60} = \frac{2\cdot\cancel{2}\cdot\cancel{2}\cdot\cancel{3}}{\cancel{2}\cdot\cancel{2}\cdot\cancel{3}\cdot 5} = \frac{2}{5}$

**13.**

$$\begin{array}{rcl} \frac{7}{12} & = & \frac{28}{48} \\ +\frac{9}{16} & = & \frac{27}{48} \\ \hline & & \frac{55}{48} = 1\frac{7}{48} \end{array}$$

**14.**

$$\begin{array}{rcl} 3\frac{7}{8} & = & 3\frac{42}{48} \\ 7\frac{5}{12} & = & 7\frac{20}{48} \\ +2\frac{15}{16} & = & 2\frac{45}{48} \\ \hline & & 12\frac{107}{48} = 14\frac{11}{48} \end{array}$$

**15.**

$$\begin{array}{rcl} \frac{11}{12} & = & \frac{22}{24} \\ -\frac{3}{8} & = & \frac{9}{24} \\ \hline & & \frac{13}{24} \end{array}$$

**16.**

$$\begin{array}{rcccl} 5\frac{1}{6} & = & 5\frac{3}{18} & = & 4\frac{21}{18} \\ -3\frac{7}{18} & = & 3\frac{7}{18} & = & 3\frac{7}{18} \\ \hline & & & & 1\frac{14}{18} = 1\frac{7}{9} \end{array}$$

**17.** $\frac{3}{8}\times\frac{14}{15} = \frac{3\cdot 14}{8\cdot 15} = \frac{\cancel{3}\cdot\cancel{2}\cdot 7}{2\cdot 2\cdot\cancel{2}\cdot\cancel{3}\cdot 5} = \frac{7}{20}$

**18.** $3\frac{1}{8}\times 2\frac{2}{5} = \frac{25}{8}\times\frac{12}{5} = \frac{25\cdot 12}{8\cdot 5}$

$= \frac{5\cdot\cancel{5}\cdot\cancel{2}\cdot\cancel{2}\cdot 3}{2\cdot\cancel{2}\cdot\cancel{2}\cdot\cancel{5}} = \frac{15}{2} = 7\frac{1}{2}$

**19.** $\frac{7}{16}\div\frac{5}{12} = \frac{7}{16}\times\frac{12}{5} = \frac{7\cdot 12}{16\cdot 5}$

$= \frac{7\cdot\cancel{2}\cdot\cancel{2}\cdot 3}{\cancel{2}\cdot\cancel{2}\cdot 2\cdot 2\cdot 5} = \frac{21}{20} = 1\frac{1}{20}$

© 2013 Cengage Learning. All Rights Reserved. May not be scanned, copied or duplicated, or posted to a publicly accessible website, in whole or in part.

**20.** $6\frac{1}{8} \div 2\frac{1}{3} = \frac{49}{8} \div \frac{7}{3} = \frac{49}{8} \times \frac{3}{7} = \frac{49 \cdot 3}{8 \cdot 7}$

$= \frac{7 \cdot \overset{1}{\cancel{7}} \cdot 3}{2 \cdot 2 \cdot 2 \cdot \underset{1}{\cancel{7}}} = \frac{21}{8} = 2\frac{5}{8}$

**21.** $\left(\frac{1}{2}\right)^3 \cdot \frac{8}{9} = \left(\frac{1}{2} \cdot \frac{1}{2} \cdot \frac{1}{2}\right) \cdot \frac{8}{9} = \frac{1}{8} \cdot \frac{8}{9} = \frac{1}{9}$

**22.** $\left(\frac{1}{2} + \frac{1}{3}\right) \div \left(\frac{2}{5}\right)^2 = \left(\frac{3}{6} + \frac{2}{6}\right) \div \left(\frac{2}{5} \cdot \frac{2}{5}\right)$

$= \frac{5}{6} \div \frac{4}{25} = \frac{5}{6} \times \frac{25}{4} = \frac{5 \cdot 25}{6 \cdot 4} = \frac{125}{24} = 5\frac{5}{24}$

**23. Strategy** To find the amount in the checking account:
- Find the total of the checks written by adding the check amounts ($128, $54, and $315).
- Subtract the total of the checks written from the original balance in the checking account ($1359).

**Solution**

$$\begin{array}{r} 128 \\ 54 \\ +315 \\ \hline 497 \end{array} \qquad \begin{array}{r} 1359 \\ -497 \\ \hline 862 \end{array}$$

The amount in the checking account at the end of the week was $862.

**24. Strategy** To find the total cost:
- Find the cost gloves multiplying the price per box ($17) by the number of boxes ordered (10).
- Find the cost of the depressors by multiplying the price per box ($4) by the number of boxes ordered (20).
- Find the total cost of the order by adding the cost of gloves to the cost of depressors.

**Solution**

$$\begin{array}{r} 17 \\ \times\ 10 \\ \hline 170 \end{array} \qquad \begin{array}{r} 20 \\ \times\ 4 \\ \hline 80 \end{array} \qquad \begin{array}{r} 170 \\ +\ 80 \\ \hline 250 \end{array}$$

The total cost of the order was $250.

**25. Strategy** To find the total length,
- Add the three gains $\left(\frac{3}{4}, \frac{5}{8}, \text{ and } \frac{1}{2} \text{ inches}\right)$.
- Add the total gains to the original length $\left(19\frac{7}{8} \text{ inches}\right)$.

**Solution**

$$\begin{array}{r} \frac{3}{4} = \frac{6}{8} \\ \frac{5}{8} = \frac{5}{8} \\ +\frac{1}{2} = \frac{4}{8} \\ \hline \frac{15}{8} = 1\frac{7}{8} \end{array} \qquad \begin{array}{r} 19\frac{7}{8} \\ +1\frac{7}{8} \\ \hline 20\frac{14}{8} = 21\frac{3}{4} \end{array}$$

The total length after two weeks is $21\frac{3}{4}$ inches.

**26. Strategy** To find the amount, multiply the amount (500 milliliters) by the fraction remaining $\left(\frac{2}{5}\right)$.

**Solution**

$$500 \cdot \frac{2}{5} = \frac{500}{1} \cdot \frac{2}{5} = \frac{\overset{100}{\cancel{500}} \cdot 2}{\underset{1}{\cancel{5}}} = 200$$

There are 200 milliliters left.

**27. Strategy** To find pediatric dose, multiply the adult dose $\left(1\frac{1}{2}\right)$ by $\frac{2}{3}$.

**Solution**

$$1\frac{1}{2} \times \frac{2}{3} = \frac{3}{2} \times \frac{2}{3} = \frac{\overset{1}{\cancel{3}} \cdot \overset{1}{\cancel{2}}}{\underset{1}{\cancel{2}} \cdot \underset{1}{\cancel{3}}} = 1$$

© 2013 Cengage Learning. All Rights Reserved. May not be scanned, copied or duplicated, or posted to a publicly accessible website, in whole or in part.

The pediatric dose is 1 ounce every 4 hours.

**28.** **Strategy** To find how many doses are in the bottle, divide the amount in the bottle (12 ounces) by the amount in each dose $\left(\frac{3}{4}\right)$ ounces.

**Solution**

$$12 \div \frac{3}{4} = \frac{12}{1} \cdot \frac{4}{3} = \frac{\overset{4}{\cancel{12}} \cdot 4}{\underset{1}{\cancel{3}}} = 16$$

There are 16 doses in 1 bottle.

© 2013 Cengage Learning. All Rights Reserved. May not be scanned, copied or duplicated, or posted to a publicly accessible website, in whole or in part.

# Chapter 3: Decimals

## Prep Test

**1.** $\frac{3}{10}$

**2.** 36,900

**3.** Four thousand seven hundred ninety-one

**4.** 6842

**5.** 9394

**6.** 1638

**7.**
$$\begin{array}{r} 844 \\ \times\ 91 \\ \hline 844 \\ 7596\phantom{0} \\ \hline 76,804 \end{array}$$

**8.**
$$\begin{array}{r} 278 \text{ r}18 \\ 23\overline{)6412} \\ -46\phantom{12} \\ \hline 181\phantom{2} \\ -161\phantom{2} \\ \hline 202 \\ -184 \\ \hline 18 \end{array}$$

## Section 3.1

### Objective A Exercises

**1.** The digit 5 is in the thousandths place.

**3.** The digit 5 is in the ten-thousandths place.

**5.** The digit 5 is in the hundredths place.

**7.** $\frac{3}{10} = 0.3$ (three tenths)

**9.** $\frac{21}{100} = 0.21$ (twenty-one hundredths)

**11.**

$\frac{461}{1000} = 0.461$ (four hundred sixty-one thousandths)

**13.** $0.1 = \frac{1}{10}$ (one-tenth)

**15.** $0.47 = \frac{47}{100}$ (forty-seven-hundredths)

**17.**

$0.289 = \frac{289}{1000}$ (two hundredth eighty-nine-thousandths)

**19.** Thirty-seven-hundredths

**21.** Nine and four-tenths

**23.** Fifty-three-ten-thousandths

**25.** Forty-five-thousandths

**27.** Twenty-six and four-hundredths

**29.** 3.0806

**31.** 407.03

**33.** 246.024

**35.** 73.02684

### Objective B Exercises

**37.**
┌ *Given place value*
6.249
└ $4 < 5$
6.249 rounded to the nearest tenth is 6.2.

**39.**
┌ *Given place value*
21.007
└ $0 < 5$
21.007 rounded to the nearest tenth is 21.0.

**41.**
┌ *Given place value*
18.40937
└ $9 > 5$
18.40937 rounded to the nearest hundredth is 18.41.

**43.**
┌ *Given place value*
72.4983
└ $8 > 5$
72.4983 rounded to the nearest hundredth is 72.50.

© 2013 Cengage Learning. All Rights Reserved. May not be scanned, copied or duplicated, or posted to a publicly accessible website, in whole or in part.

**45.**

Given place value
936.2905
5 = 5
936.2905 rounded to the nearest thousandth is 936.291.

**47.**

Given place value
47.3192
3 < 5
47.3192 rounded to the nearest whole number is 47.

**49.**

Given place value
7014.96
9 > 5
7014.96 rounded to the nearest whole number is 7015.

**51.**

Given place value
2.975268
8 > 5
2.975268 rounded to the nearest hundred-thousandth is 2.97527.

**53.** 6.1 rounded to the nearest whole number is 6. The length of the small intestine to the nearest whole number is 6 meters.

**55.** For example, 0.2701

## Applying the Concepts

**57a.** Answers will vary. For example, 0.11, 0.12, 0.13, 0.14, 0.15, 0.16, 0.17, 0.18, and 0.19 are numbers between 0.1 and 0.2. But any number of digits can be attached to 0.1, and the number will be between 0.1 and 0.2. For example, 0.123456789 is a number between 0.1 and 0.2.

**b.** Answers will vary. For example, 1.01, 1.02, 1.03, 1.04, 1.05, 1.06, 1.07, 1.08, and 1.09 are numbers between 1 and 1.1. But any number of digits can be attached to 1.0, and the number will be between 1 and 1.1. For example, 1.0123456789 is a number between 1 and 1.1.

**c.** Answers will vary. For example, 0.001, 0.002, 0.003 and 0.004 are numbers between 0 and 0.005. But any number of digits can be attached to 0.001, 0.002, 0.003, or 0.004, and the number will be between 0 and 0.005. For example, 0.00123456789 is a number between 0 and 0.005.

# Section 3.2

## Objective A Exercises

**1.**
$$\begin{array}{r} {}^{1}\ \ {}^{1}{}^{1} \\ 16.008 \\ 2.0385 \\ +\ 132.06 \\ \hline 150.1065 \end{array}$$

**3.**
$$\begin{array}{r} {}^{1}\ {}^{1} \\ 1.792 \\ 67. \\ +\ 27.0526 \\ \hline 95.8446 \end{array}$$

**5.**
$$\begin{array}{r} {}^{1} \\ 3.02 \\ 62.7 \\ +\ 3.924 \\ \hline 69.644 \end{array}$$

**7.**
$$\begin{array}{r} {}^{1}{}^{1}\ {}^{1} \\ 82.006 \\ 9.95 \\ +\ 0.927 \\ \hline 92.883 \end{array}$$

**9.**
$$\begin{array}{r} {}^{2}{}^{1}\ {}^{1}{}^{1} \\ 4.307 \\ 99.82 \\ +\ 9.078 \\ \hline 113.205 \end{array}$$

**11.**
$$\begin{array}{r} 0.29 \\ +0.4 \\ \hline 0.69 \end{array}$$

© 2013 Cengage Learning. All Rights Reserved. May not be scanned, copied or duplicated, or posted to a publicly accessible website, in whole or in part.

**13.**
$$\begin{array}{r} 7.3 \\ +\ 9.005 \\ \hline 16.305 \end{array}$$

**15.**
$$\begin{array}{r} {}^{2\,1\ \ 1} \\ 8.72 \\ 99.073 \\ +\ \ 2.9736 \\ \hline 110.7666 \end{array}$$

**17.**
$$\begin{array}{r} {}^{2} \\ 8. \\ 89.43 \\ +\ 7.0659 \\ \hline 104.4959 \end{array}$$

**19.**
$$\begin{array}{rcr} 219.9 & \approx & 220 \\ 0.872 & \approx & 1 \\ +\ 13.42 & \approx & +\ \ 13 \\ \hline \text{Cal.: } 234.192 & & \text{Est.: } 234 \end{array}$$

**21.**
$$\begin{array}{rcr} 678.92 & \approx & 679 \\ 97.6 & \approx & 98 \\ +\ \ 5.423 & \approx & +\ \ \ 5 \\ \hline \text{Cal.: } 781.943 & & \text{Est.: } 782 \end{array}$$

**23.** Yes

## Objective B Exercises

**25.** **Strategy** To find the number of viewers, add the three numbers (1.2, 0.8, and 1.4 million).

**Solution**
$$\begin{array}{r} 1.2 \\ 0.8 \\ +1.4 \\ \hline 3.4 \end{array}$$

There were 3.4 million viewers.

**27.** **Strategy** To find length of the large intestines, add the lengths of the four sections (20.32, 45.72, 30.48, and 45.72 centimeters).

**Solution**
$$\begin{array}{r} 20.32 \\ 45.72 \\ 30.48 \\ +45.72 \\ \hline 142.24 \end{array}$$

The approximate total length of the large intestine is 142.24 centimeters.

**29.** **Strategy** To find the weight, add the two gains (1.5 and 0.8 kilograms) to the original weight (15.9 kilograms).

**Solution**
$$\begin{array}{r} 1.5 \\ 0.8 \\ +15.9 \\ \hline 18.2 \end{array}$$

The child now weighs 18.2 kilograms.

**31.** **Strategy**

- To find the total fiber add the fiber for, ½ cup of bran cereal (10.4 grams), ½ cup green beans (2.1 grams), 1 medium apple (3.5 grams), and ½ cup pinto beans (18.8 grams).
- Compare the total to 28 grams to see if John has consumed enough fiber.

**Solution**
$$\begin{array}{r} 10.4 \\ 2.1 \\ 3.5 \\ +18.8 \\ \hline 34.8 \end{array}$$

$34.8 > 28$

John has consumed more than 28 grams of fiber. Yes, he has met his requirement.

© 2013 Cengage Learning. All Rights Reserved. May not be scanned, copied or duplicated, or posted to a publicly accessible website, in whole or in part.

## Applying the Concepts

**33**. Three possible answers are bread, butter, and mayonnaise; raisin bran, butter, and bread; and potatoes, cola, and mayonnaise. Other answers are possible.

# Section 3.3

## Objective A Exercises

**1.**
13
1 3 10
24.037
−18.41
5.627

**3.**
12 9
1 2 10 6 10 10
123.0700
− 9.4273
113.6427

**5.**
15 14 9 9
0 5 4 10 10 10 10
16.5000
− 9.7902
6.7098

**7.**
18
6 8 10
235.790
− 20.093
215.697

**9.**
12 9 9 14
5 2 10 10 4 10
63.0050
− 9.1274
53.8776

**11.**
11 9 9 9
8 1 10 10 10 10
92.0000
− 19.2909
72.7091

**13.**
9
1 10 10
0.3200
−0.0058
0.3142

**15.**
9
2 10 10
3.005
−1.982
1.023

**17.**
10 15
2 15 1 0 5 10
352.160
− 90.994
261.166

**19.**
11
6 1 14
724.32
− 69.
655.32

**21.**
11 13
5 1 13 8 3 10
362.3940
− 19.4672
342.9268

**23.**
9 9
8 10 10 10
19.000
10.372
8.628

**25.** 7.01 − 2.325

**27.** 19.35 − 8.967

**29.**

| | | | |
|---|---|---|---|
| | 3.7529 | ≈ | 4 |
| | −1.00784 | ≈ | −1 |
| Cal.: | 2.74506 | Est.: | 3 |

**31.**

| | | | |
|---|---|---|---|
| | 9.07325 | ≈ | 9 |
| | −1.924 | ≈ | −2 |
| Cal.: | 7.14925 | Est.: | 7 |

© 2013 Cengage Learning. All Rights Reserved. May not be scanned, copied or duplicated, or posted to a publicly accessible website, in whole or in part.

## Objective B Exercises

**33.** **Strategy** To find the remaining balance,

- to find the total debits, add all the debits ($89.65, $6.73, and $134.22).
- subtract the total debits from the original amount ($350).

**Solution**

$$\begin{array}{r} 89.65 \\ 6.73 \\ +134.22 \\ \hline 230.60 \end{array} \qquad \begin{array}{r} 350.00 \\ -230.60 \\ \hline 119.40 \end{array}$$

The remaining balance is $119.40.

**35.** **Strategy** To find additional grams of fiber,

- add the number of grams consumed (5.5, 5.2, and 10.4 grams).
- subtract the grams consumed from 25.

**Solution**

$$\begin{array}{r} 5.5 \\ 4.2 \\ +10.4 \\ \hline 20.1 \end{array} \qquad \begin{array}{r} 25.0 \\ -20.1 \\ \hline 3.9 \end{array}$$

Sheila needs to consume 3.9 more grams of fiber.

**37.** **Strategy** To find the temperature after two hours,

- add the two amounts that the temperature was lowered (1.4° and 0.8°).
- subtract the total lowered from the original temperature (102.1°).

**Solution**

$$\begin{array}{r} 1.4 \\ +0.8 \\ \hline 2.2 \end{array} \qquad \begin{array}{r} 102.1 \\ -2.2 \\ \hline 99.9 \end{array}$$

The temperature after two hours was 99.9°.

## Applying the Concepts

**39a.** Rounding to tenths, the largest difference between a decimal and the decimal rounded to tenths is 0.05. Example: For numbers between 3.7 and 3.8,

(1) Any number between 3.7 and 3.75 (not including 3.75) is rounded to 3.7, so the largest difference is *less than* 0.05.

(2) Any number between 3.75 and 3.8 (including 3.75) is rounded to 3.8, so the largest difference is *equal to* 0.05.

Therefore, rounding to tenths, the largest amount by which the estimate of the sum of two decimals could differ from the exact sum is the sum of the largest differences for each decimal. 0.05 + 0.05 = 0.1.

**b.** For hundredths,

0.005 + 0.005 = 0.01.

**c.** For thousandths,

0.0005 + 0.0005 = 0.001.

# Section 3.4

## Objective A Exercises

**1.**
$$\begin{array}{r} 0.9 \\ \times\ 0.4 \\ \hline 0.36 \end{array}$$

**3.**
$$\begin{array}{r} 0.5 \\ \times\ 0.5 \\ \hline 0.25 \end{array}$$

**5.**
$$\begin{array}{r} 7.7 \\ \times\ 0.9 \\ \hline 6.93 \end{array}$$

© 2013 Cengage Learning. All Rights Reserved. May not be scanned, copied or duplicated, or posted to a publicly accessible website, in whole or in part.

**7.**
$$\begin{array}{r} 9.2 \\ \times\ 0.2 \\ \hline 1.84 \end{array}$$

**9.**
$$\begin{array}{r} 7.4 \\ \times\ 0.1 \\ \hline 0.74 \end{array}$$

**11.**
$$\begin{array}{r} 7.9 \\ \times\quad 5 \\ \hline 39.5 \end{array}$$

**13.**
$$\begin{array}{r} 0.68 \\ \times\quad 4 \\ \hline 2.72 \end{array}$$

**15.**
$$\begin{array}{r} 0.67 \\ \times\ 0.9 \\ \hline 0.603 \end{array}$$

**17.**
$$\begin{array}{r} 2.5 \\ \times\ 5.4 \\ \hline 13.50 \end{array}$$

**19.**
$$\begin{array}{r} 0.83 \\ \times\ 5.2 \\ \hline 166 \\ 415\phantom{0} \\ \hline 4.316 \end{array}$$

**21.**
$$\begin{array}{r} 1.47 \\ \times\ 0.09 \\ \hline 0.1323 \end{array}$$

**23.**
$$\begin{array}{r} 8.92 \\ \times\ 0.004 \\ \hline 0.03568 \end{array}$$

**25.**
$$\begin{array}{r} 0.49 \\ \times\ 0.16 \\ \hline 294 \\ 49\phantom{0} \\ \hline 0.0784 \end{array}$$

**27.**
$$\begin{array}{r} 7.6 \\ \times\ 0.01 \\ \hline 0.076 \end{array}$$

**29.**
$$\begin{array}{r} 8.62 \\ \times\quad 4 \\ \hline 34.48 \end{array}$$

**31.**
$$\begin{array}{r} 64.5 \\ \times\quad 9 \\ \hline 580.5 \end{array}$$

**33.**
$$\begin{array}{r} 2.19 \\ \times\ 9.2 \\ \hline 438 \\ 1971\phantom{0} \\ \hline 20.148 \end{array}$$

**35.**
$$\begin{array}{r} 1.85 \\ \times\ 0.023 \\ \hline 555 \\ 370\phantom{0} \\ \hline 0.04255 \end{array}$$

**37.**
$$\begin{array}{r} 0.478 \\ \times\ 0.37 \\ \hline 3346 \\ 1434\phantom{0} \\ \hline 0.17686 \end{array}$$

**39.**
$$\begin{array}{r} 48.3 \\ \times\ 0.0041 \\ \hline 483 \\ 1932\phantom{0} \\ \hline 0.19803 \end{array}$$

**41.**
$$\begin{array}{r} 0.413 \\ \times\ 0.0016 \\ \hline 2478 \\ 413\phantom{0} \\ \hline 0.0006608 \end{array}$$

**43.**
$$\begin{array}{r} 8.005 \\ \times\ 0.067 \\ \hline 56035 \\ 48030\phantom{0} \\ \hline 0.536335 \end{array}$$

**45.**
$$\begin{array}{r} 4.29 \\ \times\ 0.1 \\ \hline 0.429 \end{array}$$

© 2013 Cengage Learning. All Rights Reserved. May not be scanned, copied or duplicated, or posted to a publicly accessible website, in whole or in part.

**47.** $$\begin{array}{r} 5.29 \\ \underline{\times \quad 0.4} \\ 2.116 \end{array}$$

**49.** $$\begin{array}{r} 0.68 \\ \underline{\times \quad 0.7} \\ 0.476 \end{array}$$

**51.** $$\begin{array}{r} 1.4 \\ \underline{\times 0.73} \\ 42 \\ \underline{98\phantom{0}} \\ 1.022 \end{array}$$

**53.** $$\begin{array}{r} 5.2 \\ \underline{\times \quad 7.3} \\ 156 \\ \underline{364\phantom{0}} \\ 37.96 \end{array}$$

**55.** $$\begin{array}{r} 3.8 \\ \underline{\times \ 0.61} \\ 38 \\ \underline{228\phantom{0}} \\ 2.318 \end{array}$$

**57.** $0.32 \times 10 = 3.2$

**59.** $0.065 \times 100 = 6.5$

**61.** $6.2856 \times 1000 = 6285.6$

**63.** $3.2 \times 1000 = 3200$

**65.** $3.57 \times 10{,}000 = 35{,}700$

**67.** $0.63 \times 10^1 = 6.3$

**69.** $0.039 \times 10^2 = 3.9$

**71.** $4.9 \times 10^4 = 49{,}000$

**73.** $0.067 \times 10^2 = 6.7$

**75.** $$\begin{array}{r} 3.45 \\ \underline{\times \ 0.0035} \\ 1725 \\ \underline{1035\phantom{0}} \\ 0.012075 \end{array}$$

**77.** $$\begin{array}{r} 0.00392 \\ \underline{\times \quad 3.005} \\ 1960 \\ \underline{1176\phantom{000}} \\ 0.01177960 \\ \text{or } 0.0117796 \end{array}$$

**79.** $$\begin{array}{r} 1.348 \\ \underline{\times \quad 0.23} \\ 4044 \\ \underline{2696\phantom{0}} \\ 0.31004 \end{array}$$

**81.** $$\begin{array}{r} 23.67 \\ \underline{\times \ 0.0035} \\ 11835 \\ \underline{7101\phantom{0}} \\ 0.082845 \end{array}$$

**83.** $$\begin{array}{r} 0.45 \\ \underline{\times 5} \\ 2.25 \end{array} \qquad \begin{array}{r} 2.25 \\ \underline{\times 2.3} \\ 675 \\ \underline{450\phantom{0}} \\ 5.175 \end{array}$$

**85.** $$\begin{array}{rcr} 28.5 & \approx & 30 \\ \underline{\times \ 3.2} & \approx & \underline{\times \ 3} \\ \text{Cal.: } 91.2 & & \text{Est.: } 90 \end{array}$$

**87.** $$\begin{array}{rcr} 2.38 & \approx & 2 \\ \underline{\times \ 0.44} & \approx & \underline{\times \ 0.4} \\ \text{Cal.: } 1.0472 & & \text{Est.: } 0.8 \end{array}$$

**89.** $$\begin{array}{rcr} 0.866 & \approx & 0.9 \\ \underline{\times \quad 4.5} & \approx & \underline{\times \quad 5} \\ \text{Cal.: } 3.897 & & \text{Est.: } 4.5 \end{array}$$

**91.** $$\begin{array}{rcr} 4.34 & \approx & 4 \\ \underline{\times \quad 2.59} & \approx & \underline{\times \ 3} \\ \text{Cal.: } 11.2406 & & \text{Est.: } 12 \end{array}$$

**93.** $$\begin{array}{rcr} 8.434 & \approx & 8 \\ \underline{\times \quad 0.044} & \approx & \underline{\times \ 0.04} \\ \text{Cal.: } 0.371096 & & \text{Est.: } 0.32 \end{array}$$

© 2013 Cengage Learning. All Rights Reserved. May not be scanned, copied or duplicated, or posted to a publicly accessible website, in whole or in part.

**95.**

$$\begin{array}{rcr} 28.44 & \approx & 30 \\ \times \underline{\quad 1.12} & \approx & \underline{\times \ 1} \\ \text{Cal.: } 31.8528 & & \text{Est.: } 30 \end{array}$$

## Objective B Exercises

**97. Strategy** To find the amount used in a week,
- Find the amount of insulin used in one day by multiplying the number of units (48) by the number of milliliters per unit (0.01)
- Multiply the amount used in a day by the number of days in a week (7).

**Solution**

$$\begin{array}{r} 48 \\ \underline{\times 0.01} \\ 0.48 \end{array} \qquad \begin{array}{r} 0.48 \\ \underline{\times 7} \\ 3.36 \end{array}$$

Mariel uses 3.36 milliliters of insulin in a week.

**99. Strategy** To find the amount received for the cans, multiply the weight (18.75 pounds) by the cost per pound ($.75).

**Solution**

$$\begin{array}{r} 18.75 \\ \underline{\times \ 0.75} \\ 9375 \\ \underline{1312.5\phantom{0}} \\ 14.06525 \approx 14.06 \end{array}$$

The amount received for the cans is $14.06.

**101. Strategy** To find the cost, multiply the amount to be destroyed (87 pounds) by the cost per pound ($6.95)

**Solution**

$$\begin{array}{r} 6.95 \\ \underline{\times 87} \\ 4865 \\ \underline{5560\phantom{0}} \\ 604.65 \end{array}$$

The cost will be $604.65.

**103. Strategy** To weight, multiply the weight at birth (7.16 pounds) by three.

**Solution**

$$\begin{array}{r} 7.16 \\ \underline{\times \ 3} \\ 21.48 \end{array}$$

The baby weighs 21.48 pounds.

**105a. Strategy** To find the amount of overtime pay, multiply the overtime rate ($52.35) by the number of hours worked (15).

**Solution**

$$\begin{array}{r} 52.35 \\ \underline{\times \quad 15} \\ 26175 \\ \underline{5235\phantom{0}} \\ 785.25 \end{array}$$

The amount of overtime pay is $785.25.

**b. Strategy** To find the nurse's total income for the week, add the overtime pay ($785.25) to the salary ($1396).

**Solution**

$$\begin{array}{r} 785.25 \\ \underline{+\ 1396.00} \\ 2181.25 \end{array}$$

The nurse's total income is $2181.25.

**107. Strategy** To find total for a week, multiply amount per day (0.025) by the number of days in a week (7).

**Solution**

$$\begin{array}{r} 0.025 \\ \underline{\times \quad 7} \\ 0.175 \end{array}$$

The total for a week is 0.175 grams.

© 2013 Cengage Learning. All Rights Reserved. May not be scanned, copied or duplicated, or posted to a publicly accessible website, in whole or in part.

**109. Strategy** To find the total fiber consumed:

- Find the amount of fiber in 1½ green beans, multiply the number of grams in ½ cup of green beans (2.1 grams) by 3.
- Find the amount of fiber in one cup of bran cereal by multiplying the amount in ½ cup of bran cereal (10.4 grams) by 2.
- Find the total amount consumed by adding the amount in ½ grapefruit (0.9 grams) in 1½ cup green beans, and the amount in one cup of bran cereal.

**Solution**

$$\begin{array}{r} 2.1 \\ \underline{\times 3} \\ 6.3 \end{array} \quad \begin{array}{r} 10.4 \\ \underline{\times 2} \\ 20.8 \end{array} \quad \begin{array}{r} 6.3 \\ 20.8 \\ \underline{+0.9} \\ 28.0 \end{array}$$

The patient has consumed 28.0 grams of fiber.

**111. Strategy** To find the cost, multiply the number of payments (87) by the cost per payment ($0.55).

**Solution**

$$\begin{array}{r} 87 \\ \underline{\times 0.55} \\ 435 \\ \underline{435\phantom{0}} \\ 47.85 \end{array}$$

The cost for 87 payments is $47.85.

**113. Strategy** To find the total pay for the RN's:

- Multiply 40 by the number of RN's (4).
- Multiply the number of hours by the pay per hours ($28.50).

To find the total pay for the LPN's:

- Multiply 40 by the number of LPN's (3).
- Multiply the number of hours by the pay per hours ($16.30).

To find the total pay for the CMA's:

- Multiply 40 by the number of CMA's (5).
- Multiply the number of hours by the pay per hours ($13.80).

Add the total pay for the RN's, LPN's, and CMA's.

RN:

$$\begin{array}{r} 40 \\ \underline{\times 4} \\ 160 \end{array} \quad \begin{array}{r} 28.50 \\ \underline{\times 160} \\ 1710 \\ \underline{28.50} \\ 4560.00 \end{array}$$

LPN:

$$\begin{array}{r} 40 \\ \underline{\times 3} \\ 120 \end{array} \quad \begin{array}{r} 16.30 \\ \underline{\times 120} \\ 3260 \\ \underline{16.30} \\ 1956.00 \end{array}$$

CMA:

$$\begin{array}{r} 40 \\ \underline{\times 5} \\ 200 \end{array} \quad \begin{array}{r} 13.80 \\ \underline{\times 200} \\ 2760.00 \end{array}$$

$$\begin{array}{r} 4560 \\ 1956 \\ \underline{+2760} \\ 9276 \end{array}$$

The weekly payroll is $9276.

© 2013 Cengage Learning. All Rights Reserved. May not be scanned, copied or duplicated, or posted to a publicly accessible website, in whole or in part.

## Applying the Concepts

**115.**

$$1.3 = 1\frac{3}{10}$$

$$2.31 = 2\frac{31}{100}$$

$$1\frac{3}{10} \times 2\frac{31}{100} = \frac{13}{10} \times \frac{231}{100} = \frac{3003}{1000} = 3\frac{3}{1000} = 3.003$$

**117.** When a number is multiplied by 10, 100, 1000, 10,000, etc., the decimal point is moved as many places to the right as there are zeros in the multiple of 10. For example, the decimal point in a number multiplied by 1000 would be moved three places to the right.

# Section 3.5

## Objective A Exercises

**1.**

$$\begin{array}{r} 0.82 \\ 3\overline{)2.46} \\ \underline{-24} \\ 06 \\ \underline{-06} \\ 0 \end{array}$$

**3.**

$$\begin{array}{r} 4.8 \\ 0.8.\overline{)3.8.4} \\ \underline{-32} \\ 64 \\ \underline{-64} \\ 0 \end{array}$$

**5.**

$$\begin{array}{r} 89. \\ 0.7.\overline{)62.3.} \\ \underline{-56} \\ 63 \\ \underline{-63} \\ 0 \end{array}$$

**7.**

$$\begin{array}{r} 60. \\ 0.4.\overline{)24.0.} \\ \underline{-24} \\ 00 \\ \underline{-0} \\ 0 \end{array}$$

**9.**

$$\begin{array}{r} 84.3 \\ 0.7.\overline{)59.0.1} \\ \underline{-56} \\ 30 \\ \underline{-28} \\ 21 \\ \underline{-21} \\ 0 \end{array}$$

**11.**

$$\begin{array}{r} 32.3 \\ 0.5.\overline{)16.1.5} \\ \underline{-15} \\ 11 \\ \underline{-10} \\ 15 \\ \underline{-15} \\ 0 \end{array}$$

**13.**

$$\begin{array}{r} 5.06 \\ 0.7.\overline{)3.5.42} \\ \underline{-35} \\ 04 \\ \underline{-0} \\ 42 \\ \underline{-42} \\ 0 \end{array}$$

**15.**

$$\begin{array}{r} 1.3 \\ 6.3.\overline{)8.1.9} \\ \underline{-63} \\ 189 \\ \underline{-189} \\ 0 \end{array}$$

**17.**

$$\begin{array}{r} 0.11 \\ 3.6.\overline{)0.3.96} \\ \underline{-36} \\ 36 \\ \underline{-36} \\ 0 \end{array}$$

**19.**

$$\begin{array}{r} 3.8 \\ 6.9.\overline{)26.2.2} \\ \underline{-207} \\ 552 \\ \underline{-552} \\ 0 \end{array}$$

© 2013 Cengage Learning. All Rights Reserved. May not be scanned, copied or duplicated, or posted to a publicly accessible website, in whole or in part.

**21.**

$6.32 \approx 6.3$

$8.8.\overline{)55.6.20}$
−528
282
−264
180
−176
4

**23.**

$0.57 \approx 0.6$

$9.5.\overline{)5.4.27}$
−475
677
−665
12

**25.**

$2.52 \approx 2.5$

$7.3.\overline{)18.4.00}$
−146
380
−365
150
−146
4

**27.**

$1.07 \approx 1.1$

$0.17.\overline{)0.18.30}$
−17
13
− 0
130
−119
11

**29.**

$130.64 \approx 130.6$

$0.053.\overline{)6.924.00}$
−53
162
−159
34
−0
340
−318
220
−212
8

**31.**

$0.808 \approx 0.81$

$8\overline{)6.467}$
−64
06
− 0
67
−64
3

**33.**

$0.089 \approx 0.09$

$0.72.\overline{)0.06.470}$
− 576
710
− 648
62

**35.**

$40.70$

$0.95.\overline{)38.66.5}$
−380
66
− 0
665
−665
0

**37.**

$0.456 \approx 0.46$

$60.8.\overline{)27.7.380}$
− 2432
3418
−3040
3780
−3648
132

**39.**

$0.0190 \approx 0.019$

$54\overline{)1.0280}$
− 54
488
−486
20
− 0
0

**41.**

$0.0874 \approx 0.087$

$0.5.\overline{)0.0.4370}$
− 40
37
−35
20
−20
0

**43.**

$0.3600 \approx 0.360$

$95.3.\overline{)34.3.1000}$
−2859
5720
−5718
20
− 0
200
− 0
200

© 2013 Cengage Learning. All Rights Reserved. May not be scanned, copied or duplicated, or posted to a publicly accessible website, in whole or in part.

**45.**
$$\begin{array}{r} 0.1031 \approx 0.103 \\ 4.72\overline{)0.48.7100} \\ -472 \\ \hline 151 \\ -0 \\ \hline 1510 \\ -1416 \\ \hline 940 \\ -472 \\ \hline 468 \end{array}$$

**47.**
$$\begin{array}{r} 0.0086 \approx 0.009 \\ 26.7\overline{)0.2.3070} \\ -2136 \\ \hline 1710 \\ -1602 \\ \hline 108 \end{array}$$

**49.**
$$\begin{array}{r} 0.9 \approx 1 \\ 90\overline{)89.76} \\ -810 \\ \hline 87 \end{array}$$

**51.**
$$\begin{array}{r} 2.5 \approx 3 \\ 0.413.\overline{)1.047.8} \\ -826 \\ \hline 2218 \\ -2065 \\ \hline 153 \end{array}$$

**53.**
$$\begin{array}{r} 1.0 \approx 1 \\ 0.778.\overline{)0.790.0} \\ -778 \\ \hline 120 \end{array}$$

**55.**
$$\begin{array}{r} 56.8 \approx 57 \\ 6.9.\overline{)392.0.0} \\ -345 \\ \hline 470 \\ -414 \\ \hline 560 \\ -552 \\ \hline 8 \end{array}$$

**57.** $4.07 \div 10 = 0.407$

**59.** $42.67 \div 10 = 4.267$

**61.** $1.037 \div 100 = 0.01037$

**63.** $8.295 \div 1000 = 0.008295$

**65.** $825.37 \div 1000 = 0.82537$

**67.** $0.32 \div 10^1 = 0.032$

**69.** $23.627 \div 10^2 = 0.23627$

**71.** $0.0053 \div 10^2 = 0.000053$

**73.** $1.8932 \div 10^3 = 0.0018932$

**75.**
$$\begin{array}{r} 18.42 \\ 2.4.\overline{)44.2.08} \\ -24 \\ \hline 202 \\ -192 \\ \hline 100 \\ -96 \\ \hline 48 \\ -48 \\ \hline 0 \end{array}$$

**77.**
$$\begin{array}{r} 16.07 \\ 45\overline{)723.15} \\ -45 \\ \hline 273 \\ -270 \\ \hline 31 \\ -0 \\ \hline 315 \\ -315 \\ \hline 0 \end{array}$$

**79.** $13.5 \div 10^3 = 0.0135$

**81.** $23.678 \div 1000 = 0.023678$

**83.**
$$\begin{array}{r} 0.112 \\ 0.05.\overline{)0.00.560} \\ -5 \\ \hline 06 \\ -5 \\ \hline 10 \\ -10 \\ \hline 0 \end{array}$$

**85.** Cal.: $42.42 \div 3.8 = 11.1632$
Est.: $40 \div 4 = 10$

**87.** Cal.: $389 \div 0.44 = 884.0909$
Est.: $400 \div 0.4 = 1000$

**89.** Cal.: $6.394 \div 3.5 = 1.8269$
Est.: $6 \div 4 = 1.5$

**91.** Cal.: $1.235 \div 0.021 = 58.8095$
Est.: $1 \div 0.02 = 50$

**93.** Cal.: $95.443 \div 1.32 = 72.3053$
Est.: $100 \div 1 = 100$

© 2013 Cengage Learning. All Rights Reserved. May not be scanned, copied or duplicated, or posted to a publicly accessible website, in whole or in part.

## Objective B Exercises

**95a.** Division

**b.** Multiplication

**97.** **Strategy** To find the cost per gown, divide the total cost ($21.35) by the number of gowns (50).

**Solution**

$$\begin{array}{r} 0.427 \approx 0.43 \\ 50\overline{)21.350} \\ \underline{-200} \\ 135 \\ \underline{-100} \\ 350 \\ \underline{-350} \\ 0 \end{array}$$

The cost per gown is $0.43.

**99.** **Strategy** To find the monthly amount, divide total amount (49.8 pounds) by the number of months in a year (12).

**Solution**

$$\begin{array}{r} 4.15 \\ 12\overline{)49.80} \\ \underline{-48} \\ 18 \\ \underline{-12} \\ 60 \\ \underline{-60} \\ 0 \end{array}$$

The patient must lose 4.15 pounds per month.

**101.** **Strategy** To find the number of tablets, divide the dose (0.3 gram) by the tablet strength (0.15 grams).

**Solution**

$$\begin{array}{r} 2 \\ 0.15.\overline{)0.30.} \\ \underline{-30} \\ 0 \end{array}$$

The dose is 2 tablets.

**103.** **Strategy** To find the dividend for each share, divide the total dividends ($6,090,990,120) by the number of shares (3,541,221,500).

**Solution** $6,090,990,120 \div 3,541,221,500 = 1.72$

The dividend for each share is $1.72.

**105.** **Strategy** To find the mileage per gallon:

- Subtract 17,814.2 from 18,130.4 to find the number of miles driven.
- Divide the number of miles driven by the amount of gas used (12.4 gallons).

**Solution**

$$\begin{array}{r} 18,130.4 \\ \underline{-17,814.2} \\ 316.2 \end{array}$$

$$\begin{array}{r} 25.5 \\ 12.4.\overline{)316.2.0} \\ \underline{-248} \\ 682 \\ \underline{-620} \\ 620 \\ \underline{-620} \\ 0 \end{array}$$

The car can travel 25.5 miles on 1 gallon of gasoline.

**107.** **Strategy** To find the average hemoglobin count:

- Add the readings for the past six months (10.9, 11.5, 12.1, 11.8, 13.1, and 11.0)
- Divide by 6.

© 2013 Cengage Learning. All Rights Reserved. May not be scanned, copied or duplicated, or posted to a publicly accessible website, in whole or in part.

**Solution**

$$\begin{array}{r} 10.9 \\ 11.5 \\ 12.1 \\ 11.8 \\ 13.1 \\ +11.0 \\ \hline 70.4 \end{array} \qquad \begin{array}{r} 11.73 \\ 6\overline{)70.40} \\ \underline{-6} \\ 10 \\ \underline{-6} \\ 44 \\ \underline{42} \\ 20 \\ \underline{18} \\ 2 \end{array}$$

The average hemoglobin count is 11.7 grams.

## Applying the Concepts

**109. Strategy** To find how many more women than men were enrolled at institutions of higher learning, subtract the number of men (7.46 million) from the expected number of women (10.03 million).

**Solution**

$$\begin{array}{rl} 10.03 & \text{million} \\ -\ 7.46 & \text{million} \\ \hline 2.57 & \text{million} \end{array}$$

2.57 million more women were enrolled at institutions of higher learning.

**111. Strategy** To find how many times greater, divide the number under 18 ($75.40 thousand) by number over 65 ($38.61 thousand).

**Solution** $75.04 \div 29.31 \approx 2.56$

There are 2.56 times more Americans under 18 that are uninsured than between 18 and 24.

**113. Strategy** To find how many times greater the population of 85 and over is expected to be in 2030 than in 2000, divide the expected population in 2030 (8.9 million) by the population in 2000 (4.2 million).

**Solution** $8.9 \div 4.2 \approx 2.1$

The population of this segment is expected to be 2.1 times greater in 2030 than in 2000.

**115**. To calculate a grade point average, multiply each A times a 4 GP and times 3 hours. Multiply each B times a 3 GP and times 3 hours. Multiply each C by a 2 GP and times 3 hours. Total the products and divide by the total number of hours (4 courses times 3 hours is 12 total hours).

$$\begin{array}{l} 4\times1\times3=12 \\ 3\times1\times3=9 \\ 2\times2\times3=12 \end{array} \qquad \begin{array}{r} 12 \\ 9 \\ +12 \\ \hline 33 \end{array} \qquad \begin{array}{r} 2.75 \\ 12\overline{)33.00} \\ \underline{24} \\ 90 \\ \underline{84} \\ 60 \\ \underline{60} \\ 0 \end{array}$$

The GPA is 2.75.

**117.** $3.45 \div 0.5 = 6.9$

**119.** $6.009 - 4.68 = 1.329$

**121.** $9.876 + 23.12 = 32.996$

**123.** 5.217

**125.** 0.025

# Section 3.6

## Objective A Exercises

**1.** $\begin{array}{r} 0.625 \\ 8\overline{)5.000} \end{array}$

© 2013 Cengage Learning. All Rights Reserved. May not be scanned, copied or duplicated, or posted to a publicly accessible website, in whole or in part.

**3.** $\begin{array}{l} \phantom{3)}0.6666 \approx 0.667 \\ 3\overline{)2.0000} \end{array}$

**5.** $\begin{array}{l} \phantom{6)}\overline{0.1666} \approx 0.167 \\ 6\overline{)1.0000} \end{array}$

**7.** $\begin{array}{l} \phantom{12)}\overline{0.4166} \approx 0.417 \\ 12\overline{)5.0000} \end{array}$

**9.** $\begin{array}{r} 1.750 \\ 4\overline{)7.000} \end{array}$

**11.** $1\frac{1}{2} = \frac{3}{2}$; $\begin{array}{r} 1.500 \\ 2\overline{)3.000} \end{array}$

**13.** $\begin{array}{r} 4.000 \\ 4\overline{)16.000} \end{array}$

**15.** $\begin{array}{r} 0.003 \\ 1000\overline{)3.000} \end{array}$

**17.** $7\frac{2}{25} = \frac{177}{25}$; $\begin{array}{r} 7.080 \\ 25\overline{)177.000} \end{array}$

**19.** $37\frac{1}{2} = \frac{75}{2}$; $\begin{array}{r} 37.500 \\ 2\overline{)75.000} \end{array}$

**21.** $\begin{array}{r} 0.160 \\ 25\overline{)4.000} \end{array}$

**23.** $8\frac{2}{5} = \frac{42}{5}$; $\begin{array}{r} 8.400 \\ 5\overline{)42.000} \end{array}$

**25.** Less than 1, because $54 < 57$

**27.** Greater than 1, because $88 > 80$

## Objective B Exercises

**29.** $0.8 = \frac{8}{10} = \frac{4}{5}$

**31.** $0.32 = \frac{32}{100} = \frac{8}{25}$

**33.** $0.125 = \frac{125}{1000} = \frac{1}{8}$

**35.** $1.25 = 1\frac{25}{100} = 1\frac{1}{4}$

**37.** $16.9 = 16\frac{9}{10}$

**39.** $8.4 = 8\frac{4}{10} = 8\frac{2}{5}$

**41.** $8.437 = 8\frac{437}{1000}$

**43.** $2.25 = 2\frac{25}{100} = 2\frac{1}{4}$

**45.** $0.15\frac{1}{3} = \frac{15\frac{1}{3}}{100} = 15\frac{1}{3} \div 100 = \frac{46}{3} \times \frac{1}{100}$
$= \frac{46}{300} = \frac{23}{150}$

**47.** $0.87\frac{7}{8} = \frac{87\frac{7}{8}}{100} = 87\frac{7}{8} \div 100 = \frac{703}{8} \times \frac{1}{100} = \frac{703}{800}$

**49.** $7.38 = 7\frac{38}{100} = 7\frac{19}{50}$

**51.** $0.57 = \frac{57}{100}$

**53.** $0.66\frac{2}{3} = \frac{66\frac{2}{3}}{100} = 66\frac{2}{3} \div 100 = \frac{200}{3} \times \frac{1}{100} = \frac{2}{3}$

## Objective C Exercises

**55.** $0.15 < 0.50$; $0.15 < 0.5$

**57.** $6.65 > 6.56$

**59.** $2.504 > 2.054$

**61.** $\frac{3}{8} = 0.375$

$0.375 > 0.365$

$\frac{3}{8} > 0.365$

© 2013 Cengage Learning. All Rights Reserved. May not be scanned, copied or duplicated, or posted to a publicly accessible website, in whole or in part.

**63.** $\frac{2}{3} \approx 0.67$

$0.67 > 0.65$

$\frac{2}{3} > 0.65$

**65.** $\frac{5}{9} \approx 0.556$

$0.556 > 0.550$

$0.556 > 0.55$

$\frac{5}{9} > 0.55$

**67.** $\frac{7}{15} \approx 0.467$

$0.620 > 0.467$

$0.62 > 0.467$

$0.62 > \frac{7}{15}$

**69.** $\frac{1}{7} \approx 0.14$

$0.161 > 0.140$

$0.161 > 0.14$

$0.161 > \frac{1}{7}$

**71.** $0.860 > 0.855$; $0.86 > 0.855$

**73.** $1.005 > 0.500$; $1.005 > 0.5$

**75.** $0.172 < 17.2$

## Applying the Concepts

**77.** Car 1 $\frac{360}{367{,}921} < 0.001$

Car 2 $\frac{420}{401{,}346} > 0.001$

Car 3 $\frac{210}{298{,}773} < 0.001$

Car 4 $\frac{320}{330{,}045} < 0.001$

Car 5 $\frac{450}{432{,}989} > 0.001$

Cars 2 and 5 would fail the test.

## Chapter 3 Concept Review

**1.** To round a decimal to the nearest tenth, look at the digit in the hundredths place. If the digit in the hundredths place is less than 5, that digit and all digits to the right are dropped. If the digit in the hundredths place is greater than or equal to 5, increase the digit in the tenths place by 1 and drop all digits to its right.

**2.** The decimal 0.37 is read 37 hundredths. To write the decimal as a fraction, put 37 in the numerator and 100 in the denominator: $\frac{37}{100}$.

**3.** The fraction $\frac{173}{10{,}000}$ is read 173 ten-thousandths. To write the fraction as a decimal, insert one 0 after the decimal point so that the 3 is in the ten-thousandths place: 0.0173.

**4.** When adding decimals of different place values, write the numbers so that the decimal points are on a vertical line.

**5.** Write the decimal point in the product of two decimals so that the number of decimal places in the product is the sum of the decimal places in the factors.

**6.** To estimate the product of two decimals, round each number so that it contains one nonzero digit. Then multiply. For example, to estimate the product of 0.068 and 0.0052, round the two numbers to 0.07 and 0.005; then multiply $0.07 \times 0.005 = 0.00035$.

© 2013 Cengage Learning. All Rights Reserved. May not be scanned, copied or duplicated, or posted to a publicly accessible website, in whole or in part.

**7.** When dividing decimals, move the decimal point in the divisor to the right to make the divisor a whole number. Move the decimal point in the dividend the same number of places to the right. Place the decimal point in the quotient directly over the decimal point in the dividend, and then divide as with whole numbers.

**8.** First convert the fraction to a decimal: The fraction $\frac{5}{8}$ is equal to 0.625. Now compare the decimals: $0.63 > 0.625$. In the inequality $0.63 > 0.625$, replace the decimal 0.625 with the fraction $\frac{5}{8}$: $0.63 > \frac{5}{8}$. The answer is that the decimal 0.63 is greater than the fraction $\frac{5}{8}$.

**9.** When dividing 0.763 by 0.6, the decimal points will be moved one place to the right: $7.63 \div 6$. The decimal 7.63 has digits in the tenths and hundredths places. We need to write a zero in the thousandths place in order to determine the digit in the thousandths place of the quotient so that we can round the quotient to the nearest hundredth.

**10.** To subtract a decimal from a whole number that has no decimal point, write a decimal point in the whole number to the right of the ones place. Then write as many zeros to the right of that decimal point as there are places in the decimal being subtracted from the whole number. For example, the subtraction $5-3.578$ would be written $5.000-3.578$.

## Chapter 3 Review Exercises

**1.**

$$\begin{array}{r} 54.5 \\ 0.067.\overline{)3.651.5} \\ -335 \\ \hline 301 \\ -268 \\ \hline 335 \\ -335 \\ \hline 0 \end{array}$$

**2.**

$$\begin{array}{r} {}^{2\,3\,1\;\;1} \\ 369.41 \\ 88.3 \\ 9.774 \\ +366.474 \\ \hline 833.958 \end{array}$$

**3.** $0.055 < 0.100$; $0.055 < 0.1$

**4.** Twenty-two and ninety-two ten-thousandths

**5.**

0.05678235 (Given place value: 8; $2 < 5$)

0.05678

**6.** $2\frac{1}{3} = \frac{7}{3}$; $3\overline{)7.000}$ = 2.333 ≈ 2.33

**7.** $0.375 = \frac{375}{1000} = \frac{3}{8}$

**8.**

$$\begin{array}{r} {}^{1\;1} \\ 3.42 \\ 0.794 \\ +\;32.5 \\ \hline 36.714 \end{array}$$

**9.** 34.025

**10.** $\frac{5}{8} = 0.625$

$0.625 > 0.620$

$\frac{5}{8} > 0.62$

© 2013 Cengage Learning. All Rights Reserved. May not be scanned, copied or duplicated, or posted to a publicly accessible website, in whole or in part.

**11.** $9\overline{)7.0000}$ = $0.7777 \approx 0.778$

**12.** $0.66 = \dfrac{66}{100} = \dfrac{33}{50}$

**13.**
$$\begin{array}{r} 27.3100 \\ -\ 4.4465 \\ \hline 22.8635 \end{array}$$

**14.**
7.93704 — Given place value; 7 > 5

7.94

**15.**
$$\begin{array}{r} 3.08 \\ \times\ 2.9 \\ \hline 2772 \\ 616\phantom{0} \\ \hline 8.932 \end{array}$$

**16.** Three hundred forty-two and thirty-seven hundredths

**17.** 3.06753

**18.**
$$\begin{array}{r} 34.79 \\ \times\ 0.74 \\ \hline 13916 \\ 24353\phantom{0} \\ \hline 25.7446 \end{array}$$

**19.**
$$\begin{array}{r} 6.594 \\ 0.053.\overline{)0.349.482} \\ -318\phantom{.482} \\ \hline 314\phantom{82} \\ -265\phantom{82} \\ \hline 498\phantom{2} \\ -477\phantom{2} \\ \hline 212 \\ -212 \\ \hline 0 \end{array}$$

**20.**
$$\begin{array}{r} 7.7960 \\ -\ 2.9175 \\ \hline 4.8785 \end{array}$$

**21. Strategy** To find the new balance in your checking account:

- Find the total amount of the checks by adding the check amounts ($145.72 and $88.45).
- Subtract the total check amounts from the original balance ($895.68).

**Solution**
$$\begin{array}{r} 145.72 \\ +\ 88.45 \\ \hline 234.17 \end{array} \qquad \begin{array}{r} 895.68 \\ -\ 234.17 \\ \hline 661.51 \end{array}$$

The new balance in your account is $661.51.

**22. Strategy** To find the cost per mile, divide the total cost ($118) by the number of miles (760 miles).

**Solution**
$$\begin{array}{r} 0.155 \\ 760\overline{)118.000} \\ 760\phantom{00} \\ \hline 4200\phantom{0} \\ 3800\phantom{0} \\ \hline 4000 \\ 3800 \\ \hline \end{array} \qquad 0.155 \approx 0.16$$

The cost is $0.16 per mile.

**23. Strategy** To find hourly wage, divide the yearly wage ($40,040) by the number of hours per year (2080 hours).

**Solution**
$$\begin{array}{r} 19.25 \\ 2080\overline{)40040.00} \\ -2080\phantom{0.00} \\ \hline 19240\phantom{.00} \\ -18720\phantom{.00} \\ \hline 5200\phantom{0} \\ -4160\phantom{0} \\ \hline 10400 \\ -10400 \\ \hline 0 \end{array}$$

The hourly wage is $19.25.

© 2013 Cengage Learning. All Rights Reserved. May not be scanned, copied or duplicated, or posted to a publicly accessible website, in whole or in part.

**24.** **Strategy** To find the additional fiber Mario needs:

- add the fiber he has consumed (3.1 grams, 5.2 grams, and 13.2 grams).
- subtract the total he has consumed from the amount he needs (30 grams).

**Solution**

$$\begin{array}{r} 3.1 \\ 5.2 \\ +13.2 \\ \hline 21.5 \end{array} \qquad \begin{array}{r} 30.0 \\ -21.5 \\ \hline 8.5 \end{array}$$

Mario needs 8.5 more grams of fiber.

**25.** **Strategy** To find the amount of milk served during a 5-day school week, multiply the amount of milk served daily (1.9 million gallons) by 5 days.

**Solution**

$$\begin{array}{r} 1.9 \\ \times\ 5 \\ \hline 9.5 \end{array}$$

During a 5-day school week, 9.5 million gallons of milk are served.

## Chapter 3 Test

**1.** $0.66 < 0.666$

**2.**

$$\begin{array}{r} 13.027 \\ -\ 8.940 \\ \hline 4.087 \end{array}$$

**3.** Forty-five and three hundred two ten-thousandths

**4.** $\frac{9}{13} = 13\overline{)9.0000}$ $0.6923 \approx 0.692$

**5.** $0.825 = \frac{825}{1000} = \frac{33}{40}$

**6.**

*Given place value*

0.07395

5 = 5

0.0740

**7.**

$1.5378 \approx 1.538$

$0.037.\overline{)0.056.9000}$

−37
199
−185
140
−111
290
−259
310
−296
14

**8.**

$$\begin{array}{r} 37.00300 \\ -\ 9.23674 \\ \hline 27.76626 \end{array}$$

**9.**

*Given place value*

7.0954625

4 < 5

7.095

**10.**

232.

$0.006.\overline{)1.392.}$

−12
19
−18
12
−12
0

**11.**

$$\begin{array}{r} 270.93 \\ 97. \\ 1.976 \\ +\ 88.675 \\ \hline 458.581 \end{array}$$

**12.** **Strategy** To find change, subtract the amount of the purchase ($12.43) from $20.

**Solution**

$$\begin{array}{r} 20.00 \\ -\ 12.43 \\ \hline 7.57 \end{array}$$

The change will be $7.57.

© 2013 Cengage Learning. All Rights Reserved. May not be scanned, copied or duplicated, or posted to a publicly accessible website, in whole or in part.

**13.**

$$\begin{array}{r} 1.37 \\ \times\ 0.004 \\ \hline 0.00548 \end{array}$$

**14.**

$$\begin{array}{r} \overset{11}{6}2.3\phantom{00} \\ 4.007 \\ +189.65\phantom{0} \\ \hline 255.957 \end{array}$$

**15.** 209.07086

**16. Strategy** To find the amount of each payment:

- Find the total amount to be paid by subtracting the down payment ($2500) from the cost of the car ($16,734.40).
- Divide the amount remaining to be paid by the number of payments (36).

**Solution**

$$\begin{array}{r} 16,734.40 \\ -\ \ 2,500.00 \\ \hline 14,234.40 \end{array}$$

$$\begin{array}{r} 395.40 \\ 36\overline{)14,234.40} \\ \underline{-108}\phantom{,234.40} \\ 343\phantom{34.40} \\ \underline{-324}\phantom{34.40} \\ 194\phantom{4.40} \\ \underline{-180}\phantom{4.40} \\ 144\phantom{.40} \\ \underline{-144}\phantom{.40} \\ 00 \\ \underline{-\ 0} \\ 0 \end{array}$$

Each payment is $395.40.

**17. Strategy** To find the number of times more the rate is in Mexico, divide the rate in Mexico (17.84) by the rate in the United States (6.14).

**Solution**

$$\begin{array}{r} 2.90 \\ 6.14\overline{)17.84.00} \\ \underline{12.28}\phantom{00} \\ 5560 \\ \underline{5526} \\ 340 \\ \underline{0} \end{array}$$

The infant mortality rate is 2.9 more in Mexico than in the United States.

**18. Strategy** To find total distance walked:

- multiply the number of miles per day for each week by 5 times a week.
- add the totals for each week.

**Solution**

$$\begin{array}{r} 0.25 \\ \underline{\times 5} \\ 1.25 \end{array} \quad \begin{array}{r} 0.5 \\ \underline{\times 5} \\ 2.5 \end{array} \quad \begin{array}{r} 0.75 \\ \underline{\times 5} \\ 3.75 \end{array} \quad \begin{array}{r} 1.25 \\ 2.5\phantom{0} \\ \underline{+3.75} \\ 7.50 \end{array}$$

The patient has walked 7.5 miles after 3 weeks.

**19. Strategy** To find average hours per year, multiply the weekly computer use by a 10th-grade student (6.7 hours) by 52 weeks.

**Solution**

$$\begin{array}{r} 6.7 \\ \times\ \ 52 \\ \hline 134 \\ \underline{335\phantom{0}} \\ 348.4 \end{array}$$

The yearly average computer use by a 10th-grade student is 348.4 hours.

**20. Strategy** To find how many more hours a 2nd-grade student uses a computer than a 5th-grade student:

- Subtract the number of hours the 5th-grade student uses the computer (4.2) from the number

© 2013 Cengage Learning. All Rights Reserved. May not be scanned, copied or duplicated, or posted to a publicly accessible website, in whole or in part.

of hours the 2nd-grade student uses the computer (4.9).

• Multiply the difference by 52 weeks.

**Solution**

$$\begin{array}{r} 4.9 \\ -4.2 \\ \hline 0.7 \end{array} \qquad \begin{array}{r} 52 \\ \times\, 0.7 \\ \hline 36.4 \end{array}$$

On average a 2nd-grade student uses the computer 36.4 hours more per year than a 5th-grade student.

## Cumulative Review Exercises

**1.**
$$\begin{array}{r} 235 \text{ r}17 \\ 89\overline{)20932} \\ -178\phantom{00} \\ \hline 313\phantom{0} \\ -267\phantom{0} \\ \hline 462 \\ -445 \\ \hline 17 \end{array}$$

**2.** $2^3 \cdot 4^2 = 8 \cdot 16 = 128$

**3.** $2^2 - (7-3) \div 2 + 1$
$= 4 - 4 \div 2 + 1$
$= 4 - 2 + 1$
$= 3$

**4.**

| | 2 | 3 |
|---|---|---|
| 9 = | | (3 · 3) |
| 12 = | 2 · 2 | 3 |
| 24 = | (2 · 2 · 2) | 3 |

LCM $= 2 \cdot 2 \cdot 2 \cdot 3 \cdot 3 = 72$

**5.** $\dfrac{22}{5}$ $\quad \begin{array}{r} 4 \text{ r}2 \\ 5\overline{)22} \\ -20 \\ \hline 2 \end{array} \quad \dfrac{22}{5} = 4\dfrac{2}{5}$

**6.** $4\dfrac{5}{8} = \dfrac{32+5}{8} = \dfrac{37}{8}$

**7.** $60 \div 12 = 5;\ \dfrac{5 \cdot 5}{12 \cdot 5} = \dfrac{25}{60}$

**8.**
$$\begin{array}{r} \dfrac{3}{8} = \dfrac{18}{48} \\ \dfrac{5}{12} = \dfrac{20}{48} \\ +\dfrac{9}{12} = \dfrac{27}{48} \\ \hline \dfrac{65}{48} = 1\dfrac{17}{48} \end{array}$$

**9.**
$$\begin{array}{r} 5\dfrac{7}{12} = 5\dfrac{21}{36} \\ +3\dfrac{7}{18} = 3\dfrac{14}{36} \\ \hline 8\dfrac{35}{36} \end{array}$$

**10.**
$$\begin{array}{r} 9\dfrac{5}{9} = 9\dfrac{20}{36} = 8\dfrac{56}{36} \\ -3\dfrac{11}{12} = 3\dfrac{33}{36} = 3\dfrac{33}{36} \\ \hline 5\dfrac{23}{36} \end{array}$$

**11.** $\dfrac{9}{16} \times \dfrac{4}{27} = \dfrac{9 \times 4}{16 \times 27} = \dfrac{\cancel{3} \cdot \cancel{3} \cdot \cancel{2} \cdot \cancel{2}}{\cancel{2} \cdot \cancel{2} \cdot 2 \cdot 2 \cdot \cancel{3} \cdot \cancel{3} \cdot 3} = \dfrac{1}{12}$

**12.** $2\dfrac{1}{8} \times 4\dfrac{5}{17} = \dfrac{17}{8} \times \dfrac{73}{17} = \dfrac{17 \cdot 73}{8 \cdot 17} = \dfrac{73}{8} = 9\dfrac{1}{8}$

**13.** $\dfrac{11}{12} \div \dfrac{3}{4} = \dfrac{11}{12} \times \dfrac{4}{3} = \dfrac{11 \cdot 4}{12 \cdot 3} = \dfrac{11 \cdot \cancel{2} \cdot \cancel{2}}{\cancel{2} \cdot \cancel{2} \cdot 3 \cdot 3} = \dfrac{11}{9} = 1\dfrac{2}{9}$

**14.** $2\dfrac{3}{8} \div 2\dfrac{1}{2} = \dfrac{19}{8} \div \dfrac{5}{2} = \dfrac{19}{8} \times \dfrac{2}{5} = \dfrac{19 \cdot 2}{8 \cdot 5}$

$= \dfrac{19 \cdot \cancel{2}}{2 \cdot 2 \cdot \cancel{2} \cdot 5} = \dfrac{19}{20}$

**15.** $\left(\dfrac{2}{3}\right)^2 \left(\dfrac{3}{4}\right)^3 = \left(\dfrac{2}{3} \cdot \dfrac{2}{3}\right)\left(\dfrac{3}{4} \cdot \dfrac{3}{4} \cdot \dfrac{3}{4}\right)$

$= \dfrac{\cancel{2} \cdot \cancel{2} \cdot \cancel{3} \cdot \cancel{3} \cdot 3}{\cancel{3} \cdot \cancel{3} \cdot \cancel{2} \cdot \cancel{2} \cdot 2 \cdot 2 \cdot 2 \cdot 2} = \dfrac{3}{16}$

© 2013 Cengage Learning. All Rights Reserved. May not be scanned, copied or duplicated, or posted to a publicly accessible website, in whole or in part.

**16.** $\left(\frac{2}{3}\right)^2 - \left(\frac{2}{3} - \frac{1}{2}\right) + 2$

$= \left(\frac{2}{3} \cdot \frac{2}{3}\right) - \left(\frac{4}{6} - \frac{3}{4}\right) + 2$

$= \frac{4}{9} - \frac{1}{6} + 2$

$= \frac{8}{18} - \frac{3}{18} + \frac{36}{18}$

$= \frac{41}{18} = 2\frac{5}{18}$

**17.** Sixty-five and three hundred nine ten-thousandths

**18.**

$$\begin{array}{r} {}^{2\ 3\ 1\ \ 1\ 1\ 1} \\ 379.006\phantom{0} \\ 27.523\phantom{0} \\ 9.8707 \\ +\ 88.2994 \\ \hline 504.6991 \end{array}$$

**19.**

$$\begin{array}{r} {}^{8\ \ 10\ 10\ 4\ 10}_{\phantom{8}\ \ 9\ \ 9\ 14} \\ 2\not{9}.\not{0}\not{0}\not{5}\not{0} \\ -\ 7.9286 \\ \hline 21.0764 \end{array}$$

**20.**

$$\begin{array}{r} 9.074 \\ \times\ \ 6.09 \\ \hline 81666 \\ 544440\phantom{00} \\ \hline 55.26066 \end{array}$$

**21.**

$$\begin{array}{r} 2.1544 \approx 2.154 \\ 8.09.\overline{)17.42.9630} \\ -1618\phantom{0000} \\ \hline 1249\phantom{000} \\ -809\phantom{000} \\ \hline 4406\phantom{00} \\ -4045\phantom{00} \\ \hline 3613\phantom{0} \\ -3236\phantom{0} \\ \hline 3770 \\ -3236 \\ \hline 534 \end{array}$$

**22.** $\frac{11}{15}$ $\quad \begin{array}{r} 0.7333 \approx 0.733 \\ 15\overline{)11.000} \end{array}$

**23.** $0.16\frac{2}{3} = \frac{16\frac{2}{3}}{100} = \frac{\frac{50}{3}}{100} = \frac{50}{3} \div 100 = \frac{50}{3} \times \frac{1}{100}$

$= \frac{50}{300} = \frac{1}{6}$

**24.** $\frac{8}{9} \approx 0.89$

$0.89 < 0.98$

$\frac{8}{9} < 0.98$

**25.** **Strategy** To find how many more calories an active lifestyle burns than an inactive lifestyle, subtract the calories for an inactive lifestyle (2747) from the calories for an active lifestyle (3387).

**Solution**

$$\begin{array}{r} 3387 \\ -2747 \\ \hline 640 \end{array}$$

An active lifestyle burns 640 more calories than an inactive lifestyle.

**26.** **Strategy** To find the loss needed the third month:

- Add the losses for the first two months.
- Subtract this sum from the goal (24 pounds).

**Solution** $9\frac{1}{2} + 6\frac{3}{4} = 9\frac{2}{4} + 6\frac{3}{4}$ pounds

$= 15\frac{5}{4} = 16\frac{1}{4}$

lost first two months

$24 - 16\frac{1}{4} = 23\frac{4}{4} - 16\frac{1}{4} = 7\frac{3}{4}$

pounds

The patient must lose $7\frac{3}{4}$ pounds the third month to achieve the goal.

**27.** **Strategy** To find your balance after you write the checks:

- Find the total of the checks written by adding the amounts of

© 2013 Cengage Learning. All Rights Reserved. May not be scanned, copied or duplicated, or posted to a publicly accessible website, in whole or in part.

the checks ($42.98, $16.43, and $137.56).

• Subtract the total of the checks written from the original balance ($814.35).

**Solution**

$$\begin{array}{r} 42.98 \\ 16.43 \\ +137.56 \\ \hline 196.97 \end{array} \qquad \begin{array}{r} 814.35 \\ -196.97 \\ \hline 617.38 \end{array}$$

Your checking account balance is $617.38.

**28. Strategy** To number of tablets, divide the dosage (1.25 milligrams) by the number of milligrams per tablet (0.5).

**Solution**

$$\begin{array}{r} 2.5 \\ 0.5\overline{)1.25} \\ \underline{10} \\ 25 \\ \underline{25} \\ 0 \end{array}$$

The patient should receive 2½ tablets.

**29. Strategy** To find the amount of income tax you paid:

• Find the amount of tax paid on profit by multiplying the profit ($64,860) by the rate (0.08).

• Add the amount of tax paid on profit to the base tax ($820).

**Solution**

$$\begin{array}{r} 64,860 \\ \times \ \ 0.08 \\ \hline 5188.80 \end{array} \qquad \begin{array}{r} 5188.80 \\ +\ 820.00 \\ \hline 6008.80 \end{array}$$

You paid $6008.80 in income tax last year.

**30. Strategy** To find the number of pounds still left to gain:

• Find the amount already gained by adding the gains $\left(2\frac{1}{2}, 3\frac{3}{4}, 2, \text{ and } 1\frac{3}{4} \text{ pounds}\right)$.

• subtract the total from 10 pounds.

**Solution**

$$\begin{array}{r} 2\frac{1}{2} = 2\frac{2}{4} \\ 3\frac{3}{4} = 3\frac{3}{4} \\ 2 \ \ = 2 \\ +1\frac{3}{4} = 1\frac{3}{4} \\ \hline 8\frac{8}{4} \quad = 10 \end{array}$$

There is no more weight left the gain.

© 2013 Cengage Learning. All Rights Reserved. May not be scanned, copied or duplicated, or posted to a publicly accessible website, in whole or in part.

# Chapter 4: Ratio and Proportion

## Prep Test

**1.** $\frac{8}{10}=\frac{\overset{1}{\not 2}\cdot 2\cdot 2}{\underset{1}{\not 2}\cdot 5}=\frac{4}{5}$

**2.** $\frac{450}{650+250}=\frac{450}{900}=\frac{\overset{1}{\not 4\not 5\not 0}}{2\cdot \underset{1}{\not 4\not 5\not 0}}=\frac{1}{2}$

**3.** $15\overline{)372.0}$ quotient 24.8

**4.** $4\times 33=132$

$62\times 2=124$

$132>124$

$4\times 33$ is greater.

**5.** $5\overline{)20}$ quotient 4 $\quad 4\times 5=20$

## Section 4.1

### Objective A Exercises

**1.** $\frac{3\text{ pints}}{15\text{ pints}}=\frac{3}{15}=\frac{1}{5}$

3 pints: 15 pints = 3 : 15 = 1 : 5

3 pints to 15 pints = 3 to 15 = 1 to 5

**3.** $\frac{\$40}{\$20}=\frac{40}{20}=\frac{2}{1}$

\$40 : \$20 = 40 : 20 = 2 : 1

\$40 to \$20 = 40 to 20 = 2 to 1

**5.** $\frac{3\text{ miles}}{8\text{ miles}}=\frac{3}{8}$

3 miles:8 miles = 3:8

3 miles to 8 miles = 3 to 8

**7.** $\frac{6\text{ minutes}}{6\text{ minutes}}=\frac{6}{6}=\frac{1}{1}$

6 minutes : 6 minutes = 6 : 6 = 1 : 1

6 minutes to 6 minutes = 6 to 6 = 1 to 1

**9.** $\frac{35\text{ cents}}{50\text{ cents}}=\frac{35}{50}=\frac{7}{10}$

35 cents:50 cents = 35 : 50 = 7 : 10

35 cents to 50 cents = 35 to 50 = 7 to 10

**11.** $\frac{30\text{ minutes}}{60\text{ minutes}}=\frac{30}{60}=\frac{1}{2}$

30 minutes : 60 minutes = 30 : 60 = 1 : 2

30 minutes to 60 minutes = 30 to 60 = 1 to 2

**13.** $\frac{32\text{ ounces}}{16\text{ ounces}}=\frac{32}{16}=\frac{2}{1}$

32 ounces:16 ounces = 32 : 16 = 2 : 1

32 ounces to 16 ounces = 32 to 16 = 2 to 1

**15.** $\frac{30\text{ yards}}{12\text{ yards}}=\frac{30}{12}=\frac{5}{2}$

30 yards : 12 yards = 30 : 12 = 5 : 2

30 yards to 12 yards = 30 to 12 = 5 to 2

**17.** $\frac{20\text{ gallons}}{28\text{ gallons}}=\frac{20}{28}=\frac{5}{7}$

20 gallons : 28 gallons = 20 : 28 = 5 : 7

20 gallons to 28 gallons = to 20 to 28 = 5 to 7

**19.** days

### Objective B Exercises

**21.** **Strategy** To find the ratio, write the ratio of housing (\$1600) to total expenses (\$4800) in simplest form.

**Solution** $\frac{\$1600}{\$4800}=\frac{1600}{4800}=\frac{1}{3}$

The ratio is $\frac{1}{3}$.

**23.** **Strategy** To find the ratio, write the ratio of utilities (\$300) to food (\$800) in simplest form.

**Solution** $\frac{\$300}{\$800}=\frac{300}{800}=\frac{3}{8}$

The ratio is $\frac{3}{8}$.

© 2013 Cengage Learning. All Rights Reserved. May not be scanned, copied or duplicated, or posted to a publicly accessible website, in whole or in part.

**25.** **Strategy** To find the ratio, write the ratio of the number of men who participated (65,000) to the number of adult males in the U.S. (50 million) in simplest form.

**Solution** $\frac{65,000}{50,000,000} = \frac{65}{50,000}$
$= \frac{13}{10,000}$

The ratio is $\frac{13}{10,000}$.

**27.** **Strategy** To find the ratio, write the amount of substance being diluted (20 microliters) to the sum of the amount being diluted and amount of water (980 microliters) in simplest terms.

**Solution** $\frac{20}{20+1980} = \frac{20}{2000} = \frac{1}{100}$

The ratio is $\frac{1}{100}$.

**29.** **Strategy** To find the ratio, write in simplest form the in salaries ($1,036,000) over total expenses ($1,850,000).

**Solution** $\frac{1,036,000}{1,850,000} = \frac{14}{25}$

The ratio is $\frac{14}{25}$.

**31.** **Strategy** To find the ratio, write in simplest form, the amount for Internal Medicine ($55,000) over the amount for OB/GYN ($200,000).

**Solution** $\frac{55,000}{200,000} = \frac{11}{40}$

The ratio is $\frac{11}{40}$.

### Applying the Concepts

**33.** No, the value of a ratio is not always less than 1.

For example, a ratio of $8 to $4 is 2 to 1 = $\frac{2}{1}$ = 2

which is greater than 1.

## Section 4.2

### Objective A Exercises

**1.** $\frac{\text{3 pounds}}{\text{4 people}}$

**3.** $\frac{\$80}{\text{12 thermometers}} = \frac{\$20}{\text{3 thermometers}}$

**5.** $\frac{\text{15 patients}}{\text{5 nurses}} = \frac{\text{3 patients}}{\text{1 nurse}}$

**7.** $\frac{\text{16 gallons}}{\text{2 hours}} = \frac{\text{8 gallons}}{\text{1 hour}}$

**9a.** Dollars

**b.** Seconds

### Objective B Exercises

**11.** 15 feet in 1 second

**13.** $\frac{\text{10 feet}}{\text{4 seconds}} = 2.5 \text{ feet / second}$

**15.** $\frac{\$3900}{\text{4 weeks}} = \$975 \text{ / week}$

**17.** $\frac{\text{125 milligrams}}{\text{100 milliliters}} = 1.25 \text{ milligrams/milliliter}$

**19.** $\frac{\$131.88}{\text{7 hours}} = \$18.84 \text{ / hour}$

**21.** $\frac{\text{409.4 miles}}{\text{11.5 gallons}} = 35.6 \text{ miles/gallon}$

© 2013 Cengage Learning. All Rights Reserved. May not be scanned, copied or duplicated, or posted to a publicly accessible website, in whole or in part.

### Objective C Exercises

**23.** **Strategy** To find the number of miles per dollar, divide the total number of miles you get per gallon (26) by the cost per gallon ($3.49).

**Solution**

$$\begin{array}{r} 7.44 \\ 3.49\overline{)26.00} \end{array}$$

You get 7.4 miles per dollar.

**25.** **Strategy** To find the cost per pack for sterile strip closures, divide the total cost ($66) by the number of packs (50).

**Solution**

$$\begin{array}{r} 1.32 \\ 50\overline{)66.00} \end{array}$$

The cost is $1.32 per pack.

**27.** **Strategy** To compare the cost from MediSupp Store to the cost from MedPro:

- Find the cost per closure from MedPro by dividing cost by the total number of gloves per case (24 boxes by 100 gloves per box = 2400).
- Find the cost per closure for MediSupp by dividing the cost ($3.50) by the number of closures per box (100).

**Solution**

MedPro: $\begin{array}{r} 0.0229 \approx .023 \\ 2400\overline{)55.00} \end{array}$

MedSupp: $\begin{array}{r} 0.035 \\ 100\overline{)3.500} \end{array}$

$0.023 < 0.034$

MedPro has the better deal.

**29.** **Strategy** To find number of milligrams per milliliter, divide the number of milligrams (75 milligrams) by the number of milliliters (37.5)

**Solution**

$$\begin{array}{r} 2 \\ 37.5\overline{)75.0} \end{array}$$

There are 2 milligrams/milliliter.

**31.** **Strategy** To find the rate, divide the number of milliliters (1500) by the number of hours (12).

**Solution**

$$\begin{array}{r} 125 \\ 12\overline{)1500} \end{array}$$

The rate is 125 milliliters/hour.

### Applying the Concepts

**33.** The price–earnings ratio of a company's stock is computed by dividing the current price per share of the stock by the annual earnings per share. For example, if the price–earnings ratio of a company's stock is 8.5, the price of the stock is 8.5 times the earnings per share of the stock.

## Section 4.3

### Objective A Exercises

**1.**

$\frac{4}{8} \; \frac{10}{20}$ $\to 8 \times 10 = 80$; $\to 4 \times 20 = 80$

The proportion is true.

**3.**

$\frac{7}{8} \; \frac{11}{12}$ $\to 8 \times 11 = 88$; $\to 7 \times 12 = 84$

The proportion is not true.

**5.**

$\frac{27}{8} \; \frac{9}{4}$ $\to 8 \times 9 = 72$; $\to 27 \times 4 = 108$

The proportion is not true.

**7.**

$\frac{45}{135} \; \frac{3}{9}$ $\to 135 \times 3 = 405$; $\to 45 \times 9 = 405$

The proportion is true.

**9.**

$\frac{50}{2} \; \frac{25}{1}$ $\to 2 \times 25 = 50$; $\to 50 \times 1 = 50$

The proportion is true.

© 2013 Cengage Learning. All Rights Reserved. May not be scanned, copied or duplicated, or posted to a publicly accessible website, in whole or in part.

**11.**

$\frac{6}{5} \times \frac{30}{25}$ $\rightarrow 5 \times 30 = 150$; $\rightarrow 6 \times 25 = 150$

The proportion is true.

**13.**

$\frac{125}{5} \times \frac{250}{10}$ $\rightarrow 5 \times 250 = 1250$; $\rightarrow 125 \times 10 = 1250$

The proportion is true.

**15.**

$\frac{300}{4} \times \frac{450}{7}$ $\rightarrow 4 \times 450 = 1800$; $\rightarrow 300 \times 7 = 2100$

The proportion is not true.

**17.**

$\frac{65}{5} \times \frac{26}{2}$ $\rightarrow 5 \times 26 = 130$; $\rightarrow 65 \times 2 = 130$

The proportion is true.

**19.** Yes

## Objective B Exercises

**21.** Yes

**23.**
$$\begin{aligned} n \times 21 &= 7 \times 9 \\ n \times 21 &= 63 \\ n &= 63 \div 21 \\ n &= 3 \end{aligned}$$

**25.**
$$\begin{aligned} 7 \times n &= 21 \times 35 \\ 7 \times n &= 735 \\ n &= 735 \div 7 \\ n &= 105 \end{aligned}$$

**27.**
$$\begin{aligned} 3 \times 10 &= n \times 15 \\ 30 &= n \times 15 \\ 30 \div 15 &= n \\ 2 &= n \end{aligned}$$

**29.**
$$\begin{aligned} 5 \times 144 &= 12 \times n \\ 720 &= 12 \times n \\ 720 \div 12 &= n \\ 60 &= n \end{aligned}$$

**31.**
$$\begin{aligned} 4 \times 5 &= n \times 9 \\ 20 &= n \times 9 \\ 20 \div 9 &= n \\ 2.22 &\approx n \end{aligned}$$

**33.**
$$\begin{aligned} 36 \times n &= 20 \times 12 \\ 36 \times n &= 240 \\ n &= 240 \div 36 \\ n &\approx 6.67 \end{aligned}$$

**35.**
$$\begin{aligned} 40 \times 8 &= n \times 15 \\ 320 &= n \times 15 \\ 320 \div 15 &= n \\ 21.33 &\approx n \end{aligned}$$

**37.**
$$\begin{aligned} n \times 120 &= 30 \times 65 \\ n \times 120 &= 1950 \\ n &= 1950 \div 120 \\ n &= 16.25 \end{aligned}$$

**39.**
$$\begin{aligned} 1.3 \times 30 &= 16 \times n \\ 39 &= 16 \times n \\ 39 \div 16 &= n \\ 2.44 &\approx n \end{aligned}$$

**41.**
$$\begin{aligned} 1.9 \times n &= 7 \times 13 \\ 1.9 \times n &= 91 \\ n &= 91 \div 1.9 \\ n &\approx 47.89 \end{aligned}$$

## Objective C Exercises

**43.** **Strategy** To find out how many calories are in a 0.5-ounce serving of cereal, write and solve a proportion using $n$ to represent the calories.

**Solution**
$$\frac{6 \text{ ounces}}{600 \text{ calories}} = \frac{0.5 \text{ ounces}}{n \text{ calories}}$$
$$\begin{aligned} 6 \times n &= 600 \times 0.5 \\ 6 \times n &= 300 \\ n &= 300 \div 6 \\ n &= 50 \end{aligned}$$

A 0.5-ounce serving contains 50 calories.

**45.** **Strategy** To find the number of miles a car will travel on 14 gallons of gas, write and solve a proportion using $n$ to represent the number of miles.

© 2013 Cengage Learning. All Rights Reserved. May not be scanned, copied or duplicated, or posted to a publicly accessible website, in whole or in part.

**Solution** $\frac{70.5 \text{ miles}}{3 \text{ gallons}} = \frac{n \text{ miles}}{14 \text{ gallons}}$

$70.5 \times 14 = 3 \times n$

$987 = 3 \times n$

$987 \div 3 = n$

$329 = n$

The car can travel 329 miles on 14 gallons of gas.

**47.** **Strategy** To find out how milliliters of solution are to be prepared, write and solve a proportion using $n$ to represent the milliliters of solution.

**Solution** $\frac{25 \text{ milliliters of alcohol}}{100 \text{ milliliters of solution}} = \frac{175 \text{ milliliters of alchol}}{n \text{ milliliters of solution}}$

$100 \times 175 = 25 \times n$

$17500 = 25n$

$17500 \div 25 = n$

$700 = n$

700 milliliters of solution can be prepared.

**49.** **Strategy** To find out how milliliters of solution are to be prepared, write and solve a proportion using $n$ to represent the milliliters of solution.

**Solution** $\frac{1.5 \text{ grams of sucrose}}{100 \text{ milliliters of solution}} = \frac{3 \text{ grams of sucrose}}{n \text{ milliliters of solution}}$

$100 \times 3 = 1.5 \times n$

$300 = 1.5n$

$300 \div 1.5 = n$

$200 = n$

200 milliliters of solution can be prepared.

**51.** **Strategy** To find the dosage for a person who weighs 150 pounds, write and solve a proportion using $n$ to represent the number of ounces.

**Solution** $\frac{n}{150 \text{ pounds}} = \frac{\frac{1}{3} \text{ ounce}}{40 \text{ pounds}}$

$40 \times n = \frac{1}{3} \times 150$

$40 \times n = 50$

$n = 50 \div 40$

$n = 1.25$

1.25 ounces are required.

**53.** **Strategy** To find amount of acetaminophen:

- Find the total number of tablets taken by multiplying the number of days (3) by the number of times a day (4).
- Write and solve a proportion using $n$ for the amount of acetaminophen.

**Solution** $4 \times 3 = 12$

$\frac{500 \text{ milligrams of acetaminophen}}{1 \text{ tablet}} = \frac{n \text{ milligrams of acetaminophen}}{12 \text{ tablets}}$

$1 \times n = 500 \times 12$

$n = 6000$

The patient has consumed 6000 milligrams of acetaminophen.

**55.** **Strategy** To number of nurse's aides, write and solve a proportion using $n$ to represent the number of nurse's aides.

**Solution** $\frac{1 \text{ nurse's aides}}{12 \text{ residents}} = \frac{n \text{ nurse's aides}}{52 \text{ residents}}$

$12 \times n = 1 \times 52$

$12n = 52$

$n = 4\frac{1}{3}$

Since you cannot have $4\frac{1}{3}$ nurse's aides, you must have 5 nurse's aides.

© 2013 Cengage Learning. All Rights Reserved. May not be scanned, copied or duplicated, or posted to a publicly accessible website, in whole or in part.

**57. Strategy** To find the monthly payment, write and solve a proportion using $n$ to represent the monthly payment.

**Solution**

$$\frac{\$35.35}{\$10,000} = \frac{n}{\$50,000}$$
$$35.35 \times 50,000 = 10,000 \times n$$
$$1,767,500 = 10,000 \times n$$
$$1,767,500 \div 10,000 = n$$
$$176.75 = n$$

The monthly payment is $176.75.

**59. Strategy** To find what dividend Carlos would receive after purchasing additional shares:

- Find the total number of shares owned by adding the original number (50) to the number purchased (300).
- Find the dividend by writing and solving a proportion using $n$ to represent the dividend.

**Solution**

$$\begin{array}{r} 300 \\ +\ 50 \\ \hline 350 \text{ } \textit{shares} \end{array}$$

$$\frac{n}{350 \text{ shares}} = \frac{\$153}{50 \text{ shares}}$$
$$153 \times 350 = n \times 50$$
$$53,550 = n \times 50$$
$$53,550 \div 50 = n$$
$$1071 = n$$

The dividend would be $1071.

**61. Strategy** To find how many grams are in ½ cup of peanut butter, write and solve a proportion using $n$ to represent the grams of carbohydrates.

**Solution**

$$\frac{6.6 \text{ grams}}{2 \text{ tablespoons}} = \frac{n \text{ grams}}{8 \text{ tablespoons}}$$
$$2 \times n = 6.6 \times 8$$
$$2n = 52.8$$
$$n = 52.8 \div 2$$
$$n = 26.4$$

There are 26.4 grams of carbohydrates in 8 tablespoons of peanut butter.

## Applying the Concepts

**63.** The fact that the number of workers per retiree is decreasing means that for each retiree drawing money out of Social Security, there are fewer and fewer workers paying into the Social Security system. In other words, fewer workers are supporting each retiree. Therefore, unless the amount paid into the system by each worker is increased or other radical changes are made, the funds to pay the Social Security benefits will be depleted.

**65.** Answers will vary. Here's an example: One 200-pound bag of fertilizer will cover 5000 square feet of lawn. How many pounds of fertilizer are required for 18,000 square feet of lawn?

# Chapter 4 Concept Review

**1.** If the units in a comparison are different, then the comparison is a rate. For example, the comparison "50 miles in 2 hours" is a rate.

**2.** To find a unit rate, divide the number in the numerator of the rate by the number in the denominator of the rate.

© 2013 Cengage Learning. All Rights Reserved. May not be scanned, copied or duplicated, or posted to a publicly accessible website, in whole or in part.

**3.** To write the ratio $\frac{6}{7}$ using a colon, write the two numbers 6 and 7 separated by a colon: 6 : 7.

**4.** To write the ration 12 : 15 in simplest form, divide both numbers by the GCF of 3: $\frac{12}{3}:\frac{15}{3}=4:5$.

**5.** To write the rate $\frac{342 \text{ miles}}{9.5 \text{ gallons}}$ as a unit rate, divide the number in the numerator by the number in the denominator: $342 \div 9.5 = 36$. $\frac{342 \text{ miles}}{9.5 \text{ gallons}}$ is the rate, 36 miles/gallon is the unit rate.

**6.** A proportion is true if the fractions are equal when written in lowest terms. Another way to describe a true proportion is to say that in a true proportion, the cross products are equal.

**7.** When one of the numbers in a proportion is unknown, we can solve the proportion to find the unknown number. We do this by setting the cross products equal to each other and then solving for the unknown number.

**8.** When setting up a proportion, keep the same units in the numerator and the same units in the denominator.

**9.** To check the solution of a proportion, replace the unknown number in the proportion with the solution. Then find the cross products. If the cross products are equal, the solution is correct. If the cross products are not equal, the solution is not correct.

**10.** To write the ratio 19 : 6 as a fraction, write the first number as the numerator of the fraction and the second number as the denominator: $\frac{19}{6}$.

## Chapter 4 Review Exercises

**1.**
$\frac{2}{9}$ ✕ $\frac{10}{45}$
$10 \rightarrow 9 \times 10 = 90$
$45 \rightarrow 2 \times 45 = 90$
The proportion is true.

**2.** $\frac{\$32}{\$80}=\frac{32}{80}=\frac{2}{5}$
$\$32:\$80 = 32:80 = 2:5$
$32 to $80 = 32 to 80 = 2 to 5

**3.** $\frac{250 \text{ miles}}{4 \text{ hours}} = 62.5 \text{ miles/hour}$

**4.**
$\frac{8}{15}$ ✕ $\frac{32}{60}$
$32 \rightarrow 15 \times 32 = 480$
$60 \rightarrow 8 \times 60 = 480$
The proportion is true.

**5.**
$$\frac{16}{n}=\frac{4}{17}$$
$$16 \times 17 = n \times 4$$
$$272 = n \times 4$$
$$272 \div 4 = n$$
$$68 = n$$

**6.** $\frac{\$500}{40 \text{ hours}} = \$12.50/\text{hour}$

**7.** $\frac{\$8.75}{5 \text{ pounds}} = \$1.75/\text{pound}$

**8.** $\frac{8 \text{ feet}}{28 \text{ feet}}=\frac{8}{28}=\frac{2}{7}$
8 feet:28 feet $= 8:28 = 2:7$
8 feet to 28 feet = 8 to 28 = 2 to 7

© 2013 Cengage Learning. All Rights Reserved. May not be scanned, copied or duplicated, or posted to a publicly accessible website, in whole or in part.

**9.** $\frac{n}{8}=\frac{9}{2}$

$n\times 2=8\times 9$

$n\times 2=72$

$n=72\div 2$

$n=36$

**10.** $\frac{18}{35}=\frac{10}{n}$

$n\times 18=35\times 10$

$n\times 18=350$

$n=350\div 18$

$n\approx 19.44$

**11.** $\frac{6\text{ inches}}{15\text{ inches}}=\frac{6}{15}=\frac{2}{5}$

6 inches:15 inches = 6:15 = 2:5

6 inches to 15 inches = 6 to 15 = 2 to 5

**12.**

$\frac{3}{8}$ ⤫ $\frac{10}{24}$ → $8\times 10=80$, $3\times 24=72$

The proportion is not true.

**13.** $\frac{\$35}{4\text{ hours}}$

**14.** $\frac{326.4\text{ miles}}{12\text{ gallons}}=27.2\text{ miles/gallon}$

**15.** $\frac{12\text{ days}}{12\text{ days}}=\frac{12}{12}=\frac{1}{1}$

12 days:12 days = 12:12 = 1:1

12 days to 12 days = 12 *to* 12 = 1 *to* 1

**16.**

$\frac{5}{7}$ ⤫ $\frac{25}{35}$ → $7\times 25=175$, $5\times 35=175$

The proportion is true.

**17.** $\frac{24}{11}=\frac{n}{30}$

$24\times 30=n\times 11$

$720=n\times 11$

$720\div 11=n$

$65.45\approx n$

**18.** $\frac{250\text{ milligrams}}{5\text{ milliliters}}=\frac{50\text{ milligrams}}{1\text{ milliliter}}$

**19. Strategy** To find the ratio:

- Find the amount of the increase by subtracting the current price ($25) from the original price ($20).
- Write the ratio between the increase and the original price.

**Solution**

$$\begin{array}{r}25\\-20\\\hline 5\end{array}$$

$\frac{\$5}{\$20}=\frac{1}{4}$ The ratio is $\frac{1}{4}$.

**20. Strategy** To find the number of hours needed, write and solve a proportion using *n* for the number of hours.

**Solution** $\frac{3.62\text{ hours}}{1\text{ resident}}=\frac{n}{50\text{ residents}}$

$1\times n=3.62\times 50$

$n=181$

181 nursing staffing hours are needed.

**21. Strategy** To find the ratio, write the ratio of the number of nurses (5) to the number of patients (15). Compare this to the ratio $\frac{1}{4}$.

**Solution** $\frac{5\text{ nurses}}{15\text{ patients}}=\frac{1\text{ nurse}}{3\text{ patient}}$

$\frac{1}{3}\ ?\ \frac{1}{4}$

$\frac{4}{12}>\frac{3}{12}$

The ratio $\frac{1}{3}$ is higher than the rate required.

**22. Strategy** To find the ratio of the hours worked to the total hours in a day:

- Find total number of hours worked by adding the hours from each home (8 and 4).

© 2013 Cengage Learning. All Rights Reserved. May not be scanned, copied or duplicated, or posted to a publicly accessible website, in whole or in part.

• Write in simplest terms the ratio of the hours worked to the total number of hours in a day (24).

**Solution**

$$\begin{array}{r} 8 \\ +4 \\ \hline 12 \end{array}$$

$$\frac{12 \text{ hours worked}}{24 \text{ hours in a day}} = \frac{1}{2}$$

The ratio is $\frac{1}{2}$.

**23. Strategy** To find the ratio, write in the lowest terms the collections to the expenses.

**Solution** $\frac{\$9750}{\$15{,}500} = \frac{39}{62}$

The ratio is $\frac{39}{62}$.

**24. Strategy** To find the cost per ounce, divide the cost ($59.55) by the number of ounces (128).

**Solution** $128\overline{)59.950}$ = 0.468

The cost is $0.47 per ounce.

**25. Strategy** To find the amount per dose:

• Find the total number of doses by multiplying the number of doses per day (4) by the number of days (7).

• Find the amount per dose by dividing the total amount (140 milliliters) by the number of doses.

**Solution**

$$\begin{array}{r} 4 \\ \times 7 \\ \hline 28 \end{array} \qquad 28\overline{)140} = 5$$

There are 5 milliliters in each dose.

**26. Strategy** To find the total amount of medication:

• Find the total number of doses by multiplying the number of tablets (2) by the number of doses per day (3) by the number of days (4).

• Find the total amount of medication by multiplying the number of doses by the amount of medication in each dose (250 milligrams).

**Solution**

$$2 \times 3 \times 4 = 24 \qquad \begin{array}{r} 250 \\ \times 24 \\ \hline 6000 \end{array}$$

The patient took a total of 6000 milligrams of medication.

**27. Strategy** To find the ratio, write the amount of substance being diluted (100 microliters) to the sum of the amount being diluted and amount of diluting agent (4900 microliters) in simplest terms.

**Solution** $\frac{100}{100+4900} = \frac{100}{5000} = \frac{1}{50}$

The ratio is $\frac{1}{50}$.

**28. Strategy** To find the ratio, write the amount of substance being diluted (50 milliliters) to the sum of the amount being diluted and amount of water (100 milliliters) in simplest terms.

**Solution** $\frac{50}{100+50} = \frac{50}{150} = \frac{1}{3}$

The ratio is $\frac{1}{3}$.

© 2013 Cengage Learning. All Rights Reserved. May not be scanned, copied or duplicated, or posted to a publicly accessible website, in whole or in part.

**29.** **Strategy** To find amount of alcohol, write and solve a proportion using $n$ to represent the amount of alcohol.

**Solution**
$$\frac{3}{20}=\frac{n}{250}$$
$$20\times n=3\times 250$$
$$20n=750$$
$$n=750\div 20$$
$$n=37.5$$

37.5 milliliters of alcohol are needed.

**30.** **Strategy** To find amount of solution, write and solve a proportion using $n$ to represent the amount of solution.

**Solution**
$$\frac{1}{100}=\frac{2.5}{n}$$
$$100\times 2.5=1\times n$$
$$250=n$$

250 milliliters of solution can be made.

## Chapter 4 Test

**1.** $\dfrac{\$46{,}036.80}{12\text{ months}}=\$3836.40/\text{month}$

**2.** $\dfrac{40\text{ miles}}{240\text{ miles}}=\dfrac{40}{240}=\dfrac{1}{6}$

40 miles : 240 miles = 40 : 240 = 1 : 6

40 miles to 240 miles = 40 to 240 = 1 to 6

**3.** $\dfrac{125\text{ milligrams}}{5\text{ milliliters}}=\dfrac{25\text{ milligrams}}{1\text{ milliliter}}$

**4.**
$\dfrac{40}{125}$ ⤫ $\dfrac{5}{25}$ $\rightarrow 125\times 5=625$, $\rightarrow 40\times 25=1000$

The proportion is not true.

**5.** $\dfrac{12\text{ days}}{8\text{ days}}=\dfrac{12}{8}=\dfrac{3}{2}$

12 days : 8 days = 12 : 8 = 3 : 2

12 days to 8 days = 12 to 8 = 3 to 2

**6.** $\dfrac{5}{12}=\dfrac{60}{n}$
$$n\times 5=12\times 60$$
$$n\times 5=720$$
$$n=720\div 5$$
$$n=144$$

**7.** $\dfrac{256.2\text{ miles}}{8.4\text{ gallons}}=30.5\text{ miles/gallon}$

**8.** $\dfrac{\$27}{\$81}=\dfrac{27}{81}=\dfrac{1}{3}$

\$27 : \$81 = 27 : 81 = 1 : 3

\$27 to \$81 = 27 to 81 = 1 to 3

**9.**
$\dfrac{5}{14}$ ⤫ $\dfrac{25}{70}$ $\rightarrow 14\times 25=350$, $\rightarrow 5\times 70=350$

The proportion is true.

**10.** $\dfrac{n}{18}=\dfrac{9}{4}$
$$n\times 4=9\times 18$$
$$n\times 4=162$$
$$n=162\div 4$$
$$n=40.5$$

**11.** $\dfrac{\$72}{16\text{ thermometers}}=\dfrac{\$9}{2\text{ thermometers}}$

**12.** $\dfrac{18\text{ feet}}{30\text{ feet}}=\dfrac{18}{30}=\dfrac{3}{5}$

18 feet : 30 feet = 18 : 30 = 3 : 5

18 feet to 30 feet = 18 to 30 = 3 to 5

**13.** **Strategy** To find the dividend on 500 shares of the healthcare stock, write and solve a proportion using $n$ to represent the dividend.

© 2013 Cengage Learning. All Rights Reserved. May not be scanned, copied or duplicated, or posted to a publicly accessible website, in whole or in part.

**Solution** $\frac{n}{500 \text{ shares}} = \frac{\$62.50}{50 \text{ shares}}$

$n \times 50 = 500 \times \$62.50$

$n \times 50 = 31,250$

$n = 31,250 \div 50$

$n = 625$

The dividend is $625.

**14. Strategy** To find the ratio, write the ratio of blood vessels (60,000 miles) to the nerve cells (45 miles) in simplest form.

**Solution** $\frac{60,000 \text{ miles}}{45 \text{ miles}} = \frac{4000}{3}$

The ratio is $\frac{4000}{3}$.

**15.** $\frac{450 \text{ milliliters}}{3 \text{ hours}} = 150 \text{ milliliters/hour}$

The infusion rate is 150 milliliters/hour.

**16. Strategy** To estimate the number of pounds of water in a college student weighing 150 pounds, write and solve a proportion using *n* to represent the number of pounds of water.

**Solution** $\frac{88 \text{ pounds water}}{100 \text{ pounds body weight}} = \frac{n}{150 \text{ pounds body weight}}$

$88 \times 150 = n \times 100$

$13,200 = n \times 100$

$13,200 \div 100 = n$

$132 = n$

The college student's body contains 132 pounds of water.

**17. Strategy** To find how many calories are in 2 cups, write and solve a proportion using *n* to represent the number of calories.

**Solution** $\frac{108 \text{ calories}}{\frac{1}{2} \text{ cup}} = \frac{n \text{ calories}}{2 \text{ cups}}$

$\frac{1}{2} \times n = 108 \times 2$

$\frac{1}{2} n = 216$

$n = 216 \times \frac{2}{1}$

$n = 432$

There are 432 calories in 2 cups of brown rice.

**18. Strategy** To find how many ounces of medication are required for a person who weighs 175 pounds, write and solve a proportion using *n* to represent the ounces of medication.

© 2013 Cengage Learning. All Rights Reserved. May not be scanned, copied or duplicated, or posted to a publicly accessible website, in whole or in part.

**Solution**

$$\frac{\frac{1}{4}\text{ ounce}}{50\text{ pounds}} = \frac{n}{175\text{ pounds}}$$

$$\frac{1}{4} \times 175 = n \times 50$$

$$43.75 = n \times 50$$

$$43.75 \div 50 = n$$

$$0.875 = n$$

The amount of medication required is 0.875 ounce.

**19. Strategy** To find number of milliliters per dose, write and solve a proportion using $n$ to represent the number of milliliters per dose.

**Solution**

$$\frac{100\text{ milligrams}}{5\text{ milliliters}} = \frac{350\text{ milligrams}}{n}$$

$$5 \times 350 = 100 \times n$$

$$1750 = 100n$$

$$1750 \div 100 = n$$

$$17.5 = n$$

There are 17.5 milliliters per dose.

**Strategy** To find the number of milliliters consumed in a day, multiply the number in one dose by the number of doses per day (4).

**Solution**

$$\begin{array}{r} 17.5 \\ \underline{\times 4} \\ 70.0 \end{array}$$

There are 70 milliliters per day.

**20. Strategy** To find the amount of solution, write a solve a proportion using $n$ as the amount of solution.

**Solution**

$$\frac{2.25\text{ grams of salt}}{250\text{ milliliters of distilled water}} = \frac{4.5\text{ grams of salt}}{n\text{ milliliters of distilled water}}$$

$$250 \times 4.5 = 2.25 \times n$$

$$1125 = 2.25n$$

$$1125 \div 2.25 = n$$

$$500 = n$$

500 milliliters of solution can be made.

© 2013 Cengage Learning. All Rights Reserved. May not be scanned, copied or duplicated, or posted to a publicly accessible website, in whole or in part.

## Cumulative Review Exercises

**1.**
$$\begin{array}{r} \overset{1\ 10\ 10\ 8\ 15}{\cancel{2}\cancel{0},\cancel{0}\cancel{9}\cancel{5}} \\ -10{,}937 \\ \hline 9{,}158 \end{array}$$

**2.** $2 \cdot 2 \cdot 2 \cdot 2 \cdot 3 \cdot 3 = 3 = 2^4 \cdot 3^3$

**3.**
$$\begin{aligned} 4-(5-2)^2 \div 3+2 &= 4-(-3)^2 \div 3+2 \\ &= 4-9 \div 3+2 \\ &= 4-3+2 \\ &= 1+2=3 \end{aligned}$$

**4.**
$$\begin{array}{r|l} & 160 \\ \hline 2 & 80 \\ 2 & 40 \\ 2 & 20 \\ 2 & 10 \\ 2 & 5 \\ 5 & 1 \end{array}$$

$160 = 2 \cdot 2 \cdot 2 \cdot 2 \cdot 2 \cdot 5$

**5.**

| | 2 | 3 |
|---|---|---|
| 9 = | | 3 · 3 |
| 12 = | (2 · 2) | 3 |
| 18 = | 2 | (3 · 3) |

LCM $= 2 \cdot 2 \cdot 3 \cdot 3 = 36$

**6.**

| | 2 | 3 | 7 |
|---|---|---|---|
| 28 = | 2 · 2 | | (7) |
| 42 = | (2) | 3 | 7 |

GCF $= 2 \cdot 7 = 14$

**7.** $\dfrac{40}{64} = \dfrac{\cancel{2} \cdot \cancel{2} \cdot \cancel{2} \cdot 5}{\cancel{2} \cdot \cancel{2} \cdot \cancel{2} \cdot 2 \cdot 2 \cdot 2} = \dfrac{5}{8}$

**8.**
$$\begin{array}{r} 3\frac{5}{6} = 3\frac{25}{30} \\ +4\frac{7}{15} = 4\frac{14}{30} \\ \hline 7\frac{39}{30} = 8\frac{9}{30} = 8\frac{3}{10} \end{array}$$

**9.**
$$\begin{array}{r} 10\frac{1}{6} = 10\frac{3}{18} = 9\frac{21}{18} \\ -4\frac{5}{9} = 4\frac{10}{18} = 4\frac{10}{18} \\ \hline 5\frac{11}{18} \end{array}$$

**10.**
$$\begin{aligned} \frac{11}{12} \times 3\frac{1}{11} &= \frac{11}{12} \times \frac{34}{11} \\ &= \frac{11 \times 34}{12 \times 11} \\ &= \frac{\cancel{11} \cdot \cancel{2} \cdot 17}{2 \cdot \cancel{2} \cdot 3 \cdot \cancel{11}} = \frac{17}{6} = 2\frac{5}{6} \end{aligned}$$

**11.**
$$\begin{aligned} 3\frac{1}{3} \div \frac{5}{7} &= \frac{10}{3} \div \frac{5}{7} \\ &= \frac{10}{3} \times \frac{7}{5} \\ &= \frac{10 \cdot 7}{3 \cdot 5} = \frac{2 \cdot \cancel{5} \cdot 7}{3 \cdot \cancel{5}} = \frac{14}{3} = 4\frac{2}{3} \end{aligned}$$

**12.**
$$\begin{aligned} \left(\frac{2}{5} + \frac{3}{4}\right) \div \frac{3}{2} &= \left(\frac{8}{20} + \frac{15}{20}\right) \div \frac{3}{2} \\ &= \frac{23}{20} \times \frac{2}{3} \\ &= \frac{23 \times 2}{20 \times 3} = \frac{23 \cdot \cancel{2}}{2 \cdot \cancel{2} \cdot 5 \cdot 2} = \frac{23}{30} \end{aligned}$$

**13.** Four and seven hundred nine ten-thousandths

**14.** 2.10

2.09762 — *Given place value* (the 9 in the hundredths place); $7 > 5$

**15.**
$$\begin{array}{r} 1.9898 \approx 1.990 \\ 8.09\overline{)16.09.7600} \\ -\ 809 \\ \hline 8007 \\ -7281 \\ \hline 7266 \\ -6472 \\ \hline 7940 \\ -7281 \\ \hline 6590 \\ -6472 \\ \hline 118 \end{array}$$

© 2013 Cengage Learning. All Rights Reserved. May not be scanned, copied or duplicated, or posted to a publicly accessible website, in whole or in part.

**16.**

$$0.06\frac{2}{3} = \frac{6\frac{2}{3}}{100} = 6\frac{2}{3} \div 100 = \frac{20}{3} \div 100$$
$$= \frac{20}{3} \times \frac{1}{100}$$
$$= \frac{20 \cdot 1}{3 \cdot 100} = \frac{1}{15}$$

**17.** $\dfrac{25 \text{ miles}}{200 \text{ miles}} = \dfrac{25}{200} = \dfrac{1}{8}$

**18.** $\dfrac{87¢}{6 \text{ pencils}} = \dfrac{29¢}{2 \text{ pencils}}$

**19.** $\dfrac{250.5 \text{ miles}}{7.5 \text{ gallons of gas}} = 33.4 \text{ miles/gallon}$

**20.**

$$\frac{40}{n} = \frac{160}{17}$$
$$40 \times 17 = n \times 160$$
$$680 = n \times 160$$
$$680 \div 160 = n$$
$$4.25 = n$$

**21.** $\dfrac{457.6 \text{ miles}}{8 \text{ hours}} = 57.2 \text{ miles/hour}$

The car's speed is 57.2 miles/hour.

**22.**

$$\frac{12}{5} = \frac{n}{15}$$
$$12 \times 15 = n \times 5$$
$$180 = n \times 5$$
$$180 \div 5 = n$$
$$36 = n$$

**23. Strategy** To find your new checking account balance:

- Find the total cost of the scrubs by multiplying the number of scrubs (3) by the cost per scrub ($25.95).
- Find the total of the purchases by adding the total cost of the scrubs to the other purchase ($75.45).
- Subtract the total of the purchases from the original balance ($485.80).

**Solution**

| | | |
|---|---|---|
| 25.95 | 77.85 | 485.80 |
| ×3 | +75.45 | −153.30 |
| 77.85 | 153.30 | 332.50 |

The total of the purchases was $153.30. The new balance was $332.50

**24. Strategy** To find the change:

- Find the amount to be paid by adding the two purchases ($89.95 and $205).
- Subtract the amount owed from the amount of money given (two $100 and two $50).

**Solution**

| | |
|---|---|
| 205.00 | $2 \times 100 = 200$ |
| +89.95 | $2 \times 50 = 100$ |
| 294.95 | 300 |

$$\begin{array}{r} 300.00 \\ -294.95 \\ \hline 5.05 \end{array}$$

The change is $5.05.

**25. Strategy** To find which sex has the greater population:

- Find the population for males by adding the populations in the four categories (4,000,000, 10,500,000, 10,200,000, and 9,900,000).
- Find the population for females by adding the populations in the four categories (7,900,000, 10,000,000, 10,200,000, and 10,100,000).
- Compare the two totals.

© 2013 Cengage Learning. All Rights Reserved. May not be scanned, copied or duplicated, or posted to a publicly accessible website, in whole or in part.

**Solution**

| Males | Females |
|---|---|
| 4,000,000 | 7,900,000 |
| 10,500,000 | 10,000,000 |
| 10,200,000 | 10,200,000 |
| +9,900,000 | +10,100,000 |
| 34,600,000 | 38,200,000 |

38,200,000 > 34,600,000

Females has the greatest population.

**26. Strategy** To find difference in the populations:

- Find the population for males by adding the populations in the two categories (4,000,000, and 10,500,000).
- Find the population for females by adding the populations in the two categories (7,900,000, and10,000,000).
- Find the difference between the two totals.

**Solution**

| Males | Females |
|---|---|
| 4,000,000 | 7,900,000 |
| +10,500,000 | +10,000,000 |
| 14,500,000 | 17,900,000 |

$$\begin{array}{r} 17{,}900{,}000 \\ -14{,}500{,}000 \\ \hline 3{,}400{,}000 \end{array}$$

Females have 3,400,000 more.

**27. Strategy** To find the difference, subtract the population for males (9,900,000) from the population for females (10,100,000).

**Solution**

$$\begin{array}{r} 10{,}100{,}000 \\ -9{,}900{,}000 \\ \hline 200{,}000 \end{array}$$

The population for females is 200,000 more.

**28. Strategy** To find the amount left to lose:

- Find the total amount lost by adding the 4 loses $\left(2\frac{1}{2}, 3\frac{3}{4}, 2, \text{ and } 1\frac{3}{4} \text{ pounds}\right)$.
- Subtract the total lost from 20 pounds.

**Solution**

$$\begin{array}{r} 2\frac{1}{2} = 2\frac{2}{4} \\ 3\frac{3}{4} = 3\frac{3}{4} \\ 2 \;\; = 2 \\ +1\frac{3}{4} = 1\frac{3}{4} \\ \hline 8\frac{8}{4} = 10 \end{array} \qquad \begin{array}{r} 20 \\ -10 \\ \hline 10 \end{array}$$

The patient has 10 more pounds to lose.

**29. Strategy** To find the unit rate, divide the number of milliliters (300) by the number of hours (4).

**Solution**

$$4\overline{)300} = 125$$

$$\begin{array}{r} 28 \\ \hline 20 \\ 20 \\ \hline 0 \end{array}$$

The rate is 125 milliliters/hour.

© 2013 Cengage Learning. All Rights Reserved. May not be scanned, copied or duplicated, or posted to a publicly accessible website, in whole or in part.

**30.** **Strategy** To find how many ounces of medication are required for a person who weighs 160 pounds, write and solve a proportion using $n$ to represent the number of ounces.

**Solution**

$$\frac{n}{160} = \frac{\frac{1}{2}\text{ ounce}}{50\text{ pounds}}$$

$$n \times 50 = \frac{1}{2} \times 160$$

$$n \times 50 = 80$$

$$n = 80 \div 50$$

$$n = 1.6$$

1.6 ounces of medication are required.

© 2013 Cengage Learning. All Rights Reserved. May not be scanned, copied or duplicated, or posted to a publicly accessible website, in whole or in part.

# Chapter 5: Percents

## Prep Test

1. $19\times\frac{1}{100}=\frac{19}{100}$

2. $23\times 0.01=0.23$

3. $0.47\times 100=47$

4. $0.06\times 47,500=2850$

5.
$$\begin{array}{r} 4000. \\ 0.015.\overline{)60.000.} \\ -60 \\ \hline 00 \\ -0 \\ \hline 00 \\ -0 \\ \hline 0 \end{array}$$

6. $8\div\frac{1}{4}=\frac{8}{1}\times\frac{4}{1}=32$

7. $\frac{5}{8}\times\frac{100}{1}=\frac{5\cdot \cancel{2}\cdot \cancel{2}\cdot 5\cdot 5}{\cancel{2}\cdot \cancel{2}\cdot 2}=\frac{125}{2}=62\frac{1}{2}=62.5$

8. $\frac{200}{3}=66\frac{2}{3}$

9. $16\overline{)28.00}$ with quotient $1.75$

## Section 5.1

### Objective A Exercises

1. $25\%=25\times\frac{1}{100}=\frac{25}{100}=\frac{1}{4}$
   $25\%=25\times 0.01=0.25$

3. $130\%=130\times\frac{1}{100}=\frac{130}{100}=1\frac{3}{10}$
   $130\%=130\times 0.01=1.30$

5. $100\%=100\times\frac{1}{100}=\frac{100}{100}=1$
   $100\%=100\times 0.01=1.00$

7. $73\%=73\times\frac{1}{100}=\frac{73}{100}$
   $73\%=73\times 0.01=0.73$

9. $383\%=383\times\frac{1}{100}=\frac{383}{100}=3\frac{83}{100}$
   $383\%=383\times 0.01=3.83$

11. $70\%=70\times\frac{1}{100}=\frac{70}{100}=\frac{7}{10}$
    $70\%=70\times 0.01=0.70$

13. $88\%=88\times\frac{1}{100}=\frac{88}{100}=\frac{22}{25}$
    $88\%=88\times 0.01=0.88$

15. $32\%=32\times\frac{1}{100}=\frac{32}{100}=\frac{8}{25}$
    $32\%=32\times 0.01=0.32$

17. $66\frac{2}{3}\%=66\frac{2}{3}\times\frac{1}{100}=\frac{200}{3}\times\frac{1}{100}$
    $=\frac{200}{300}=\frac{2}{3}$

19. $83\frac{1}{3}\%=83\frac{1}{3}\times\frac{1}{100}=\frac{250}{3}\times\frac{1}{100}$
    $=\frac{250}{300}=\frac{5}{6}$

21. $11\frac{1}{9}\%=11\frac{1}{9}\times\frac{1}{100}=\frac{100}{9}\times\frac{1}{100}$
    $=\frac{100}{900}=\frac{1}{9}$

23. $45\frac{5}{11}\%=45\frac{5}{11}\times\frac{1}{100}=\frac{500}{11}\times\frac{1}{100}$
    $=\frac{500}{1100}=\frac{5}{11}$

25. $4\frac{2}{7}\%=4\frac{2}{7}\times\frac{1}{100}=\frac{30}{7}\times\frac{1}{100}$
    $=\frac{30}{700}=\frac{3}{70}$

27. $6\frac{2}{3}\%=6\frac{2}{3}\times\frac{1}{100}=\frac{20}{3}\times\frac{1}{100}=\frac{20}{300}=\frac{1}{15}$

© 2013 Cengage Learning. All Rights Reserved. May not be scanned, copied or duplicated, or posted to a publicly accessible website, in whole or in part.

**29.** $6.5\% = 6.5 \times 0.01 = 0.065$

**31.** $12.3\% = 12.3 \times 0.01 = 0.123$

**33.** $0.55\% = 0.55 \times 0.01 = 0.0055$

**35.** $8.25\% = 8.25 \times 0.01 = 0.0825$

**37.** $5.05\% = 5.05 \times 0.01 = 0.0505$

**39.** $2\% = 2 \times 0.01 = 0.02$

**41.** Greater than

## Objective B Exercises

**43.** $0.73 = 0.73 \times 100\% = 73\%$

**45.** $0.01 = 0.01 \times 100\% = 1\%$

**47.** $2.94 = 2.94 \times 100\% = 294\%$

**49.** $0.006 = 0.006 \times 100\% = 0.6\%$

**51.** $3.106 = 3.106 \times 100\% = 310.6\%$

**53.** $0.70 = 0.70 \times 100\% = 70\%$

**55.** $\frac{37}{100} = \frac{37}{100} \times 100\% = \frac{3700}{100}\% = 37\%$

**57.** $\frac{2}{5} = \frac{2}{5} \times 100\% = \frac{200}{5}\% = 40\%$

**59.** $\frac{1}{8} = \frac{1}{8} \times 100\% = \frac{100}{8}\% = 12.5\%$

**61.** $1\frac{1}{2} = 1\frac{1}{2} \times 100\% = \frac{3}{2} \times 100\% = \frac{300}{2}\% = 150\%$

**63.** $1\frac{2}{3} = 1\frac{2}{3} \times 100\% = \frac{5}{3} \times 100\% = \frac{500}{3}\% \approx 166.7\%$

**65.** $\frac{7}{8} = \frac{7}{8} \times 100\% = \frac{700}{8}\% = 87.5\%$

**67.** $\frac{12}{25} = \frac{12}{25} \times 100\% = \frac{1200}{25}\% = 48\%$

**69.** $\frac{1}{3} = \frac{1}{3} \times 100\% = \frac{100}{3}\% = 33\frac{1}{3}\%$

**70.** $2\frac{3}{8} = 2\frac{3}{8} \times 100\% = \frac{19}{8} \times 100\%$

$= \frac{1900}{8}\% = 237\frac{1}{2}\%$

**71.**

$1\frac{2}{3} = 1\frac{2}{3} \times 100\% = \frac{5}{3} \times 100\% = \frac{500}{3}\% = 166\frac{2}{3}\%$

**73.** $\frac{7}{8} = \frac{7}{8} \times 100\% = \frac{700}{8}\% = 87\frac{1}{2}\%$

**75.** Less than

## Applying the Concepts

**77.** **Strategy** To find the percent of those with AB-:

- Add the percents the other blood types.
- Subtract the sum from 100%.

**Solution**

| | |
|---|---|
| 37% | O+ |
| 8% | O− |
| 33% | A+ |
| 7% | A− |
| 9% | B+ |
| 2% | B− |
| +3% | AB+ |
| 99% | |

$100\% - 99\% = 1\%$

1% have blood type AB–.

**79.** $15\% = \frac{15}{100} = \frac{3}{20}$; the dilution ratio is $\frac{3}{20}$.

90% of the solution is water.

# Section 5.2

## Objective A Exercises

**1.** $0.08 \times 100 = n$

$8 = n$

**3.** $0.27 \times 40 = n$

$10.8 = n$

© 2013 Cengage Learning. All Rights Reserved. May not be scanned, copied or duplicated, or posted to a publicly accessible website, in whole or in part.

**5.** $0.0005 \times 150 = n$
$0.075 = n$

**7.** $1.25 \times 64 = n$
$80 = n$

**9.** $0.107 \times 485 = n$
$51.895 = n$

**11.** $0.0025 \times 3000 = n$
$7.5 = n$

**13.** $0.80 \times 16.25 = n$
$13 = n$

**15.** $0.015 \times 250 = n$
$3.75 = n$

**17.** $\frac{1}{6} \times 120 = n$
$20 = n$

**19.** $0.05 \times 95 = n$ or $0.75 \times 6 = n$
$4.75 = n$ $\quad 4.5 = n$

Because $4.75 > 4.5$, 5% of 95 is larger.

**21.** $0.79 \times 16 = n$ or $0.20 \times 65 = n$
$12.64 = n$ $\quad 13 = n$

Because $12.64 < 13$, 79% of 16 is smaller.

**23.** Less than

## Objective B Exercises

**25.** Less than

**27. Strategy** To find how many were occasional donors Medicine, write and solve the basic percent equation using $n$ to represent the number occasional donors. The percent is 19% and the base is 16 million (16,000,000).

**Solution** $19\% \times 16,000,000 = n$
$0.19 \times 16,000,000 = n$
$3,040,000 = n$

3,040,000 were occasional donors.

**29. Strategy** To find the number of patients who use natural products, write and solve the basic percent equation using n to represent the number of people who use natural products. The percent is 17.7% and the base is 23,393.

**Solution** $17.7\% \times 23,393 = n$
$0.177 \times 23,393 = n$
$4140.561 = n$
$4141 \approx n$

4141 of those surveyed use natural products.

**31. Strategy** To find the number who do not use CAM:

• Find the percent who do use CAM by subtracting the percent who do use CAM (12%) from 100%.

• Write and solve the basic percent equation using $n$ to represent the number of children who do use CAM. The percent is 100% - 12% and the base is 73,000,000.

**Solution**

$$\begin{array}{r} 100\% \\ -12\% \\ \hline 88\% \end{array}$$

$88\% \times 73,000,000 = n$
$0.88 \times 73,000,000 = n$
$64,240,000 = n$

64,240,000 children do not use CAM.

© 2013 Cengage Learning. All Rights Reserved. May not be scanned, copied or duplicated, or posted to a publicly accessible website, in whole or in part.

**33. Strategy** To find the number of ounces of cobalt and chrome:

- Find the number of ounces of cobalt by writing and solving the basic percent equation using $n$ to represent the number of ounces of cobalt. The percent is 34% and the base is 18 ounces.
- Find the number of ounces of chrome by writing and solving the basic percent equation using $n$ to represent the number of ounces of chrome. The percent is 19% and the base is 18 ounces.

**Solution**

| Cobalt: | Chrome: |
|---|---|
| $34\% \times 18 = n$ | $19\% \times 18 = n$ |
| $0.34 \times 18 = n$ | $0.19 \times 18 = n$ |
| $6.12 = n$ | $3.42 = n$ |
| $6.1 \approx n$ | $3.4 \approx n$ |

There are 6.1 ounces of cobalt and 3.4 ounces of chrome.

**35. Strategy** To find new hourly wage:

- Find the amount of the raise by writing and solving the basic percent equation using $n$ to represent the raise. The percent is 6% and the base is \$32.40.
- Add the raise to the original salary.

**Solution**

$2.5\% \times 32.40 = n$

$0.025 \times 32.40 = n$

$0.81 = n$

$$\begin{array}{r} 32.40 \\ \underline{+0.81} \\ 33.21 \end{array}$$

The new hourly wage is \$33.21.

# Section 5.3

## Objective A Exercises

**1.** $n \times 75 = 24$

$n = 24 \div 75$

$n = 0.32$

$n = 32\%$

**3.** $n \times 90 = 15$

$n = 15 \div 90$

$n = 0.16\frac{2}{3}$

$n = 16\frac{2}{3}\%$

**5.** $n \times 12 = 24$

$n = 24 \div 12$

$n = 2$

$n = 200\%$

**7.** $n \times 16 = 6$

$n = 6 \div 16$

$n = 0.375$

$n = 37.5\%$

**9.** $n \times 100 = 18$

$n = 18 \div 100$

$n = 0.18$

$n = 18\%$

**11.** $n \times 2000 = 5$

$n = 5 \div 2000$

$n = 0.0025$

$n = 0.25\%$

**13.** $n \times 6 = 1.2$

$n = 1.2 \div 6$

$n = 0.2$

$n = 20\%$

**15.** $n \times 4.1 = 16.4$

$n = 16.4 \div 4.1$

$n = 4$

$n = 400\%$

© 2013 Cengage Learning. All Rights Reserved. May not be scanned, copied or duplicated, or posted to a publicly accessible website, in whole or in part.

**17.** $n \times 40 = 1$
$n = 1 \div 40$
$n = 0.025$
$n = 2.5\%$

**19.** $n \times 48 = 18$
$n = 18 \div 48$
$n = 0.375$
$n = 37.5\%$

**21.** $n \times 2800 = 7$
$n = 7 \div 2800$
$n = 0.0025$
$n = 0.25\%$

**23.** False

## Objective B Exercises

**25.** **Strategy** To find what percent of the total expenses is salaries, write and solve the basic percent equation using $n$ to represent the unknown percent. The base is \$12,300 and the amount is \$5800.

**Solution** $n \times 12{,}300 = 5800$
$n = 5800 \div 12300$
$n = 0.471$
$n \approx 0.47$

Salaries for technicians are 47% of the total expenses.

**27.** **Strategy** To find what percent of the vegetables was wasted, write and solve the basic percent equation using $n$ to represent the unknown percent. The base is 63 billion and the amount is 16 billion.

**Solution** $n \times 63$ billion $= 16$ billion
$n = 16$ billion $\div 63$ billion
$n \approx 0.254$

Approximately 25.4% of the vegetables were wasted.

**29.** **Strategy** To find the percent of Americans with diabetes that have not been diagnosed:
• Find the total number of Americans with diabetes by adding the number that have been diagnosed (14.6 million) to the number that have not been diagnosed (6.2 million).
• Write and solve the basic percent equation using $n$ to represent the percent of Americans with diabetes that have not been diagnosed. The base is the total number of Americans with diabetes and the amount is 6.2 million.

**Solution** $14.6 + 6.2 = 20.8$
$n \times 20.8 = 6.2$
$n = 6.2 \div 20.8$
$n \approx 0.2981$

Approximately 29.8% of Americans with diabetes have not been diagnosed.

## Applying the Concepts

**31.** **Strategy** To find what percent of the daily amount of total carbohydrates in one serving of cereal, write and solve the basic percent equation using $n$ to represent the percent. The base is total daily amount (300 g) and the amount is 23 g.

© 2013 Cengage Learning. All Rights Reserved. May not be scanned, copied or duplicated, or posted to a publicly accessible website, in whole or in part.

**Solution** $n \times 300 = 23$

$n = 23 \div 300$

$n \approx 0.0733$

One serving of cereal has 7.3% of the total daily recommended amount of carbohydrates.

**33. Strategy** To find what percent of the total calories come from fat, write and solve the basic percent equation using $n$ to represent the percent. The base is total calories (110) and the amount is 15 calories.

**Solution** $n \times 110 = 15$

$n = 15 \div 110$

$n \approx 0.136$

13.6% of the calories are from fat.

**35.** The sum of the percents in the percent column is 113%. In order for the responses to be possible, the sum of the percents must be 100%.

# Section 5.4

## Objective A Exercises

**1.** $0.12 \times n = 9$

$n = 9 \div 0.12$

$n = 75$

**3.** $0.16 \times n = 8$

$n = 8 \div 0.16$

$n = 50$

**5.** $0.10 \times n = 10$

$n = 10 \div 0.10$

$n = 100$

**7.** $0.30 \times n = 25.5$

$n = 25.5 \div 0.30$

$n = 85$

**9.** $0.025 \times n = 30$

$n = 30 \div 0.025$

$n = 1200$

**11.** $1.25 \times n = 24$

$n = 24 \div 1.25$

$n = 19.2$

**13.** $2.4 \times n = 18$

$n = 18 \div 2.4$

$n = 7.5$

**15.** $0.15 \times n = 4.8$

$n = 4.8 \div 0.15$

$n = 32$

**17.** $0.128 \times n = 25.6$

$n = 25.6 \div 0.128$

$n = 200$

**19.** $0.30 \times n = 2.7$

$n = 2.7 \div 0.30$

$n = 9$

**21.** $\frac{1}{6} \times n = 84$

$n = 84 \div \frac{1}{6}$

$n = 504$

**23.** Less than

## Objective B Exercises

**25. Strategy** To find the original cost, write and solve the basic percent equation using $n$ to represent the original cost. The percent is 70% and the amount is 1500.

**Solution** $70\% \times n = 1500$

$0.7 \times n = 1500$

$n = 1500 \div 0.7$

$n \approx 2142.86$

The original cost was $2142.86.

**27. Strategy** To find the total number of

© 2013 Cengage Learning. All Rights Reserved. May not be scanned, copied or duplicated, or posted to a publicly accessible website, in whole or in part.

patients, write and solve the basic percent equation using $n$ to represent the total number of patients. The percent is 17% and the amount is 51 people.

**Solution**

$$17\% \times n = 51$$
$$0.17 \times n = 51$$
$$n = 51 \div 0.17$$
$$n = 300$$

300 patients were treated this month.

**29.** **Strategy** To find the total number of problems, write and solve the basic percent equation using $n$ to represent the total number. The percent is 75% and the amount is 120.

**Solution**

$$75\% \times n = 120$$
$$0.75 \times n = 120$$
$$n = 120 \div 0.75$$
$$n = 160$$

There 160 questions on the exam.

**31a.** **Strategy** To find the number of times checked in a week, write and solve the basic percent equation using $n$ to represent the number times checked. The percent is 15% and the amount is 6.

**Solution**

$$15\% \times n = 6$$
$$0.15 \times n = 6$$
$$n = 6 \div 0.15$$
$$n = 40$$

Tyler checked his blood 40 times that week.

**b.** **Strategy** To find the number of times the blood sugar was in the normal range, subtract the number of times it was out of range (6) from the total number of times checked.

**Solution**

$$\begin{array}{r} 40 \\ \underline{-6} \\ 34 \end{array}$$

Tyler's blood sugar was in the normal range 34 times.

## Applying the Concepts

**33.** $30\% \times n = 0.45$ milligrams

$n = 0.45 \div 0.30$

$n = 1.5$ milligrams

The recommended daily amount of thiamin for an adult is 1.5 milligrams.

# Section 5.5

## Objective A Exercises

**1.**

$$\frac{26}{100} = \frac{n}{250}$$
$$26 \times 250 = n \times 100$$
$$6500 = n \times 100$$
$$6500 \div 100 = n$$
$$65 = n$$

**3.**

$$\frac{n}{100} = \frac{37}{148}$$
$$148 \times n = 37 \times 100$$
$$148 \times n = 3700$$
$$n = 3700 \div 148$$
$$n = 25$$

37 is 25% of 148.

**5.**

$$\frac{68}{100} = \frac{51}{n}$$
$$68 \times n = 100 \times 51$$
$$68 \times n = 5100$$
$$n = 5100 \div 68$$
$$n = 75$$

© 2013 Cengage Learning. All Rights Reserved. May not be scanned, copied or duplicated, or posted to a publicly accessible website, in whole or in part.

**7.** $\frac{n}{100} = \frac{43}{344}$

$n \times 344 = 100 \times 43$

$n \times 344 = 4300$

$n = 4300 \div 344$

$n = 12.5$

12.5% of 344 is 43.

**9.** $\frac{20.5}{100} = \frac{82}{n}$

$n \times 20.5 = 82 \times 100$

$n \times 20.5 = 8200$

$n = 8200 \div 20.5$

$n = 400$

**11.** $\frac{6.5}{100} = \frac{n}{300}$

$300 \times 6.5 = n \times 100$

$1950 = n \times 100$

$1950 \div 100 = n$

$19.5 = n$

**13.** $\frac{n}{100} = \frac{7.4}{50}$

$50 \times n = 7.4 \times 100$

$50 \times n = 740$

$n = 740 \div 50$

$n = 14.8$

7.4 is 14.8% of 50.

**15.** $\frac{50.5}{100} = \frac{n}{124}$

$50.5 \times 124 = n \times 100$

$6262 = n \times 100$

$6262 \div 100 = n$

$62.62 = n$

**17.** $\frac{220}{100} = \frac{33}{n}$

$n \times 220 = 33 \times 100$

$n \times 220 = 3300$

$n = 3300 \div 220$

$n = 15$

**19a.** (ii) and (iii)

**b.** (i) and (iv)

## Objective B Exercises

**21.** **Strategy** To find the length of time the drug will be effective as determined by the testing service, write and solve a proportion using $n$ to represent the length of time determined by the testing service. The percent is 80% and the base is 6 hours.

**Solution** $\frac{80}{100} = \frac{n}{6}$

$100 \times n = 80 \times 6$

$100 \times n = 480$

$n = 480 \div 100$

$n = 4.8$

The length of time that the drug will be effective, as determined by the testing service, is 4.8 hours.

**23.** **Strategy** To find the amount of dextrose, write and solve a proportion using $n$ to represent the amount of dextrose. The percent is 10% and the base is 350 milliliters.

**Solution** $10\% \times 350 = n$

$0.1 \times 350 = n$

$35 = n$

The patient has received 35 grams of dextrose.

**25.** **Strategy** To find the total number of donors, write and solve a proportion using $n$ to represent the number of donors. The percent is 45% and the amount is 18.

**Solution** $45\% \times n = 18$

$0.45 \times n = 18$

$n = 18 \div 0.45$

$n = 40$

© 2013 Cengage Learning. All Rights Reserved. May not be scanned, copied or duplicated, or posted to a publicly accessible website, in whole or in part.

40 donors participated.

**27. Strategy** To find the percent that have some college experience but have not earned a college degree, write and solve a proportion using $n$ to represent the percent of baby boomers living in the United States that have some college experience but have not earned a college degree. The base is 78 million and the amount is 45 million.

**Solution**

$$\frac{n}{100} = \frac{45}{78}$$
$$n \times 78 = 100 \times 45$$
$$n \times 78 = 4500$$
$$n = 4500 \div 78$$
$$n \approx 57.7$$

57.7% of baby boomers living in the United States have some college experience but have not earned a college degree

**29. Strategy** To find the percent of the deaths due to lung cancer:

- Find the total number of deaths.
- Write and solve a proportion using $n$ to represent the percent. The base is the total deaths and the amount is 128,900.

**Solution**

$$\begin{array}{r} 128{,}900 \\ 126{,}000 \\ 92{,}900 \\ 44{,}000 \\ 15{,}900 \\ +35{,}300 \\ \hline 443{,}000 \end{array}$$

$$\frac{n}{100} = \frac{128{,}900}{443{,}000}$$
$$100 \times 128{,}900 = n \times 443{,}000$$
$$12{,}890{,}000 = n \times 443{,}000$$
$$12{,}890{,}000 \div 443{,}000 = n$$
$$0.291 \approx n$$

29.1% of the deaths were due to lung cancer.

## Chapter 5 Concept Review

**1.** To write 197% as a fraction, remove the percent sign and multiply by $\frac{1}{100}$: $197 \times \frac{1}{100} = \frac{197}{100}$.

**2.** To write 6.7% as a decimal, remove the percent sign and multiply by 0.01: $6.7 \times 0.01 = 0.067$.

**3.** To write $\frac{9}{5}$ as a percent, multiply by 100%:

$\frac{9}{5} \times 100\% = 180\%$.

**4.** To write 56.3 as a percent, multiply by 100%:

$56.3 \times 100\% = 5630\%$.

**5.** The basic percent equation is Percent × base = amount.

**6.** To find what percent of 40 is 30, use the basic percent equation: $n \times 40 = 30$. To solve for $n$, we *divide* 30 by 40: $30 \div 40 = 0.75 = 75\%$.

**7.** To find 11.7% of 532, use the basic percent equation and write the percent as a decimal: $0.117 \times 532 = n$. To solve for $n$, we *multiply* 0.117 by 532: $0.117 \times 532 = 62.244$.

**8.** To answer the question "36 is 240% of what number?", use the basic percent equation and write

© 2013 Cengage Learning. All Rights Reserved. May not be scanned, copied or duplicated, or posted to a publicly accessible website, in whole or in part.

the percent as a decimal: $2.4 \times n = 36$ . To solve for $n$, we *divide* 36 by 2.4: $36 \div 2.4 = 15$ .

**9.** To use the proportion method to solve a percent problem, identify the percent, the amount, and the base. Then use the proportion $\frac{\text{percent}}{100} = \frac{\text{amount}}{\text{base}}$ .

Substitute the known values into this proportion and solve for the unknown.

**10.** To answer the question "What percent of 1400 is 763?" by using the proportion method, first identify the base (1400) and the amount (763). The percent is unknown. Substitute 1400 for the base and 763 for the amount in the proportion $\frac{\text{percent}}{100} = \frac{\text{amount}}{\text{base}}$ .

Then solve the proportion $\frac{n}{100} = \frac{763}{1400}$ for $n$.

$n = 54.5$, so 54.5% of 1400 is 763.

## Chapter 5 Review Exercises

**1.** $0.30 \times 200 = n$

$60 = n$

**2.** $n \times 80 = 16$

$n = 16 \div 80$

$n = 0.2$

$n = 20\%$

**3.** $1\frac{3}{4} \times 100\% = 1.75 \times 100\% = 175\%$

**4.** $0.20 \times n = 15$

$n = 15 \div 0.20$

$n = 75$

**5.** $12\% = 12 \times \frac{1}{100} = \frac{12}{100} = \frac{3}{25}$

**6.** $0.22 \times 88 = n$

$19.36 = n$

**7.** $n \times 20 = 30$

$n = 30 \div 20$

$n = 1.5$

$n = 150\%$

**8.** $\frac{1}{6} \times n = 84$

$n = 84 \div \frac{1}{6}$

$n = 84 \times 6$

$n = 504$

**9.** 42% = 42 × 0.01 = 0.42

**10.** $0.075 \times 72 = n$

$5.4 = n$

**11.** $\frac{2}{3} \times n = 105$

$n = 105 \div \frac{2}{3}$

$n = 105 \times \frac{3}{2}$

$n = 157.5$

**12.** 7.6% = 7.6 × 0.01 = 0.076

**13.** $1.25 \times 62 = n$

$77.5 = n$

**14.** $16\frac{2}{3}\% = 16\frac{2}{3} \times \frac{1}{100} = \frac{50}{3} \times \frac{1}{100} = \frac{50}{300} = \frac{1}{6}$

**15.** $\frac{n}{100} = \frac{40}{25}$

$n \times 25 = 40 \times 100$

$n \times 25 = 4000 \div 25$

$n = 160$

160% of 25 is 40.

© 2013 Cengage Learning. All Rights Reserved. May not be scanned, copied or duplicated, or posted to a publicly accessible website, in whole or in part.

**16.** $\frac{20}{100}=\frac{15}{n}$

$20\times n=100\times 15$

$20\times n=1,500$

$n=1,500\div 20$

$n=75$

**17.** $0.38\times 100\%=38\%$

**18.** $0.78\times n=8.5$

$n=8.5\div 0.78$

$n\approx 10.89\approx 10.9$

**19.** $n\times 30=2.2$

$n=2.2\div 30$

$n\approx 0.073$

$n\approx 7.3\%$

**20.** $n\times 15=2.2$

$n=92\div 15$

$n\approx 6.133$

$n\approx 613.3\%$

**21. Strategy** To find the percent of the questions answered correctly:

- Find the number of questions answered correctly by subtracting the number missed (9) from the total number of questions (60).
- Write and solve a proportion using $n$ to represent the percent. The base is 60 and the amount is the number of questions answered correctly.

**Solution** $60-9=51$

$\frac{n}{100}=\frac{51}{60}$

$n\times 60=51\times 100$

$n\times 60=5100$

$n=5100\div 60$

$n=85$

The student answered 85% of the questions correctly.

**22. Strategy** To find maximum number of calories that should come from fat, write and solve the basic percent equation using $n$ to represent the calories from fat. The percent is 35% and the base is 1850 calories.

**Solution** $35\%\times 1850=n$

$0.35\times 1850=n$

$647.5=n$

$648\approx n$

The maximum number of calories from fat is 648.

**23. Strategy** To find what percent of budget used for health care, write and solve a basic percent equations using $n$ as the unknown percent. The base is \$45,000 and the amount is \$2250.

**Solution** $\frac{n}{100}=\frac{2250}{45,000}$

$100\times 2250=n\times 45,000$

$225,000=n\times 45,000$

$225,000\div 45,000=n$

$5=n$

5% of the budget is allocated for healthcare.

**24. Strategy** To find the total cost of the defibrillator:

- Find the amount of the sales tax by writing and solving the basic percent equation using $n$ to represent the sales tax. The percent is 6.5% and the base is \$1850.
- Add the sales tax to the cost of the defibrillator (\$1850).

**Solution** $6.5\%\times 1850=n$

$0.065\times 1850=n$

$120.25=n$

$$\begin{array}{r} 1850.00 \\ +\ 120.25 \\ \hline 1970.25 \end{array}$$

The total cost of the defibrillator is \$1970.25.

© 2013 Cengage Learning. All Rights Reserved. May not be scanned, copied or duplicated, or posted to a publicly accessible website, in whole or in part.

**25. Strategy** To find the percent of women who wore sunscreen often, write and solve the basic percent equation using $n$ to represent the unknown percent. The base is 350 women and the amount is 275 women.

**Solution**
$$n \times 350 = 275$$
$$n = 275 \div 350$$
$$n \approx 0.7857$$
Approximately 78.6% of the women wore sunscreen often.

**26. Strategy** To find the world's population in 2000, write and solve the basic percent equation using $n$ to represent the population in 2000. The percent is 149% and the amount is 9,100,000,000 people.

**Solution**
$$149\% \times n = 9{,}100{,}000{,}000$$
$$1.49 \times n = 9{,}100{,}000{,}000$$
$$n = 9{,}100{,}000{,}000 \div 1.49$$
$$n \approx 6{,}100{,}000{,}000$$
The world's population in 2000 was approximately 6,100,000,000 people.

**27. Strategy** To find the number of women who had colonoscopies, write and solve a proportion using $n$ to represent the number of women. The percent is 60% and the amount is 636,000.

**Solution**
$$60\% \times 636{,}000 = n$$
$$0.6 \times 636{,}000 = n$$
$$318{,}600 = n$$
318,600 women had colonoscopies.

**28. Strategy** To find the total GDP, write and solve a proportion using $n$ to represent the total GDP. The percent is 16.2% and the amount is 2.3 trillion.

**Solution**
$$16.2\% \times n = 2.3$$
$$0.162 \times n = 2.3$$
$$n = 2.3 \div 0.162$$
$$n \approx 14$$
The Gross Domestic Product is \$14 trillion.

## Chapter 5 Test

**1.** $97.3\% \times 97.3 \times 0.01 = 0.973$

**2.** $83\frac{1}{3}\% = 83\frac{1}{3} \times \frac{1}{100} = \frac{250}{3} \times \frac{1}{100} = \frac{250}{3006} = \frac{5}{6}$

**3.** $0.3 \times 100\% = 30\%$

**4.** $1.63 \times 100\% = 163\%$

**5.** $\frac{3}{2} \times 100\% = 1.5 \times 100\% = 150\%$

**6.** $\frac{2}{3} \times 100\% = \frac{200}{3}\% = 66\frac{2}{3}\%$

**7.**
$$77\% \times 65 = n$$
$$0.77 \times 65 = n$$
$$50.05 = n$$

**8.**
$$47.2\% \times 130 = n$$
$$0.472 \times 130 = n$$
$$61.36 = n$$

**9.** $7\%$ of $120 = n$ or $76\%$ of $13 = n$
$$0.07 \times 120 = n \qquad 0.76 \times 13 = n$$
$$8.4 = n \qquad 9.88 = n$$

$9.88 > 8.4$, so 76% of 13 is larger.

**10.** $13\%$ of $200 = n$ or $212\%$ of $12 = n$
$$0.13 \times 200 = n \qquad 2.12 \times 12 = n$$
$$26 = n \qquad 25.44 = n$$

$25.44 < 26$, so 212% of 12 is smaller.

**11. Strategy** To find the amount spent for advertising, write and solve the basic percent equation using $n$

© 2013 Cengage Learning. All Rights Reserved. May not be scanned, copied or duplicated, or posted to a publicly accessible website, in whole or in part.

to represent the amount spent for advertising. The percent is 6% and the base is $750,000.

**Solution**
$$6\% \times 750,000 = n$$
$$0.06 \times 750,000 = n$$
$$45,000 = n$$

The amount spent for advertising is $45,000.

**12. Strategy** To find how many carbohydrates should be in the diet, write and solve a basic percent equation using $n$ to represent the carbohydrate calories. The percent is 45% and the base is 2000 calories.

**Solution**
$$45\% \times 2000 = n$$
$$0.45 \times 2000 = n$$
$$900 = n$$

The minimum number of calories from carbohydrates is 900.

**13. Strategy** To find the percent, write and solve the basic percent equation using $n$ to represent the percent of the daily recommended amount of potassium provided by one serving of cereal with skim milk. The amount is 440 milligrams and the base is 3000 milligrams.

**Solution**
$$n \times 3000 = 440$$
$$n = 440 \div 3000$$
$$n \approx 0.147$$

14.7% of the daily recommended amount of potassium is provided.

**14. Strategy** To find the percent:

- Add the number of calories provided by a serving of cereal with skim milk (180 calories) to the additional number of calories provided using 2% milk (20 calories).
- Write and solve the basic percent equation using $n$ to represent the percent of the daily recommended number of calories provided by one serving of this cereal with 2% milk. The base is the total number of calories recommended per day (2200 calories) and the amount is the total number of calories provided by the single serving of cereal with 2% milk.

**Solution** Total number of calories
$= 180 + 20 = 200$
$$n \times 2200 = 200$$
$$n = 200 \div 2200$$
$$n \approx 0.091$$

9.1% of the daily recommended number of calories is provided.

**15. Strategy** To find what percent did not have complications:

- Find the number who did not have complications by subtracting the number that had complications (18) from the total number of surgeries (540),
- Find the percent who did not have complications by writing and solving a basic percent equation using $n$ to represent the percent. The base is the total number of surgeries (540)

© 2013 Cengage Learning. All Rights Reserved. May not be scanned, copied or duplicated, or posted to a publicly accessible website, in whole or in part.

and the amount is the number who did not have complications.

**Solution**

$$\frac{n}{100} = \frac{522}{540}$$

540 − 18 = 522

$$100 \times 522 = n \times 540$$
$$52{,}200 = n \times 540$$
$$52{,}200 \div 540 = n$$
$$96.7 \approx n$$

96.7% of the patients had no complications after surgery.

**16. Strategy** To find what percent of the questions the student answered correctly:

• Find how many questions the student answered correctly by subtracting the number missed (7) from the total number of questions (80).

• Write and solve the basic percent equation using $n$ to represent the percent of questions answered correctly. The base is 80 and the amount is the number of questions answered correctly.

**Solution**

$$80 - 7 = 73$$
$$n \times 80 = 73$$
$$n = 73 \div 80$$
$$n = 0.9125$$
$$n \approx 91.3$$

The student answered approximately 91.3% of the questions correctly.

**17.** $15\% \times n = 12$

$$0.15 \times n = 12$$
$$n = 12 \div 0.15$$
$$n = 80$$

**18.** $150\% \times n = 42.5$

$$1.5 \times n = 42.5$$
$$n = 42.5 \div 1.5$$
$$n \approx 28.3$$

**19. Strategy** To find the amount of dextrose received, write and solve the basic percent equation using $n$ to represent the amount of dextrose. The percent is 5% and the base is 500.

**Solution**

$$5\% \times 500 = n$$
$$0.05 \times 500 = n$$
$$25 = n$$

The patient has received 25 grams of dextrose.

**20. Strategy** To find what percent the increase is of the original price:

• Find the amount of the increase by subtracting the original value ($285,000) from the price 5 years later ($456,000).

• Write and solve the basic percent equation using $n$ to represent the percent. The base is the original price ($285,000) and the amount is the amount of the increase.

**Solution**

456,000 − 285,000 = 171,000

$$n \times 285{,}000 = 171{,}000$$
$$n = 171{,}000 \div 285{,}000$$
$$n = 0.60$$
$$n = 60\%$$

The increase is 60% of the original price.

© 2013 Cengage Learning. All Rights Reserved. May not be scanned, copied or duplicated, or posted to a publicly accessible website, in whole or in part.

**21.** $\dfrac{86}{100}=\dfrac{123}{n}$

$$86\times n=123\times 100$$
$$86\times n=12{,}300$$
$$n=12{,}300\div 86$$
$$n\approx 143.02$$
$$n\approx 143.0$$

**22.** $\dfrac{n}{100}=\dfrac{120}{12}$

$$12\times n=100\times 120$$
$$12\times n=12{,}000$$
$$n=12{,}000\div 12$$
$$n=1000$$

1000% of 12 is 120.

**23. Strategy** To find the dollar increase in the hourly wage:

- Write and solve a proportion to find the hourly wage last year. Let $n$ represent last year's wage. The amount is \$16.24 and the percent is 112%.
- Subtract last year's wage from this year's wage (\$16.24).

**Solution** $\dfrac{112}{100}=\dfrac{16.24}{n}$

$$112\times n=16.24\times 100$$
$$112\times n=1624$$
$$n=1624\div 112$$
$$n=14.5$$

$$\begin{array}{r}16.24\\-\ 14.50\\\hline 1.74\end{array}$$

The dollar increase is \$1.74.

**24. Strategy** To find what percent the pour daily calories is in the pizza, write and solve a basic percent equation using $n$ as the percent. The base is 1800 calories and the amount is 300 calories.

**Solution** $\dfrac{n}{100}=\dfrac{300}{1800}$

$$100\times 300=n\times 1800$$
$$30{,}000=n\times 1800$$
$$30{,}000\div 1800=n$$
$$16.7\approx n$$

One slice of pizza is 16.7% of your daily calories.

**25. Strategy** To find the original weight, write and solve a basic percent equation using $n$ to represent original weight. The percent is 3.6% and the amount is 9 pounds.

**Solution** $3.6\%\times n=9$

$$0.036\times n=9$$
$$n=9\div 0.036$$
$$n=250$$

Jeanne's original weight was 250 pounds.

## Cumulative Review Exercises

**1.** $18\div(7-4)^2+2=18\div(3)^2+2$

$$=18\div 9+2$$
$$=2+2=4$$

**2.**

| | 2 | 3 | 5 |
|---|---|---|---|
| 16 = | (2·2·2·2) | | |
| 24 = | 2·2·2 | (3) | |
| 30 = | 2 | 3 | (5) |

LCM = $2\cdot 2\cdot 2\cdot 2\cdot 3\cdot 5=240$

**3.** 

$$\begin{array}{rcl}2\frac{1}{3}&=&2\frac{8}{24}\\3\frac{1}{2}&=&3\frac{12}{24}\\+4\frac{5}{8}&=&4\frac{15}{24}\\\hline &&9\frac{35}{24}=10\frac{11}{24}\end{array}$$

© 2013 Cengage Learning. All Rights Reserved. May not be scanned, copied or duplicated, or posted to a publicly accessible website, in whole or in part.

**4.**

$$\begin{array}{rcccc} 27\frac{5}{12} & = & 27\frac{20}{48} & = & 26\frac{68}{48} \\ -14\frac{9}{16} & = & 14\frac{27}{48} & = & 14\frac{27}{48} \\ \hline & & & & 12\frac{41}{48} \end{array}$$

**5.**

$$\begin{aligned} 7\frac{1}{3} \times 1\frac{5}{7} &= \frac{22}{3} \times \frac{12}{7} \\ &= \frac{22 \times 12}{3 \times 7} \\ &= \frac{2 \cdot 11 \cdot 2 \cdot 2 \cdot \overset{1}{\cancel{3}}}{\underset{1}{\cancel{3}} \cdot 7} \\ &= \frac{88}{7} = 12\frac{4}{7} \end{aligned}$$

**6.**

$$\begin{aligned} \frac{14}{27} \div 1\frac{7}{9} &= \frac{14}{27} \div \frac{16}{9} \\ &= \frac{14}{27} \times \frac{9}{16} \\ &= \frac{14 \times 9}{27 \times 16} \\ &= \frac{\overset{1}{\cancel{2}} \cdot 7 \cdot \overset{1}{\cancel{3}} \cdot \overset{1}{\cancel{3}}}{3 \cdot \underset{1}{\cancel{3}} \cdot \underset{1}{\cancel{3}} \cdot \underset{1}{\cancel{2}} \cdot 2 \cdot 2 \cdot 2} \\ &= \frac{7}{24} \end{aligned}$$

**7.**

$$\begin{aligned} \left(\frac{3}{4}\right)^3 \left(\frac{8}{9}\right)^2 &= \left(\frac{3}{4} \cdot \frac{3}{4} \cdot \frac{3}{4}\right) \left(\frac{8}{9} \cdot \frac{8}{9}\right) \\ &= \frac{27}{64} \cdot \frac{64}{81} \\ &= \frac{1}{3} \end{aligned}$$

**8.**

$$\begin{aligned} \left(\frac{2}{3}\right)^2 - \left(\frac{3}{8} - \frac{1}{3}\right) \div \frac{1}{2} &= \frac{4}{9} - \left(\frac{9}{24} - \frac{8}{24}\right) \div \frac{1}{2} \\ &= \frac{4}{9} - \frac{1}{24} \div \frac{1}{2} \\ &= \frac{4}{9} - \left(\frac{1}{24} \times \frac{1}{2}\right) \\ &= \frac{4}{9} - \frac{1}{12} \\ &= \frac{16}{36} - \frac{3}{36} = \frac{13}{36} \end{aligned}$$

**9.**

3.07973 (Given place value: 7; 9 > 5)

3.08

**10.**

$$\begin{array}{r} \scriptstyle 2\ \ 10\ 8\ \overset{9}{10}\ 12 \\ \cancel{3}.\cancel{0}\cancel{9}\cancel{0}\cancel{2} \\ -1.9706 \\ \hline 1.1196 \end{array}$$

**11.**

$$\begin{array}{r} 34.28125 \\ 0.032.\overline{)1.097.00000} \\ -96 \\ \hline 137 \\ -128 \\ \hline 90 \\ -64 \\ \hline 260 \\ -256 \\ \hline 40 \\ -32 \\ \hline 80 \\ -64 \\ \hline 160 \\ -160 \\ \hline 0 \end{array}$$

$34.28125 \approx 34.2813$

**12.** $3\frac{5}{8} = \frac{29}{8}$

$$\begin{array}{r} 3.625 \\ 8\overline{)29.000} \\ -24 \\ \hline 50 \\ -48 \\ \hline 20 \\ -16 \\ \hline 40 \\ -40 \\ \hline 0 \end{array}$$

**13.** $1.75 = \frac{175}{100} = \frac{7}{4} = 1\frac{3}{4}$

**14.** $\frac{3}{8} = 0.375$

$\frac{3}{8} < 0.87$

**15.**

$$\begin{aligned} \frac{3}{8} &= \frac{20}{n} \\ 3 \times n &= 8 \times 20 \\ 3 \times n &= 160 \\ n &= 160 \div 3 \\ n &\approx 53.3 \end{aligned}$$

© 2013 Cengage Learning. All Rights Reserved. May not be scanned, copied or duplicated, or posted to a publicly accessible website, in whole or in part.

**16.** $\dfrac{\$153.60}{8 \text{ hours}} = \$19.20/\text{hour}$

**17.** $18\frac{1}{3}\% = 18\frac{1}{3} \times \frac{1}{100} = \frac{55}{3} \times \frac{1}{100} = \frac{55}{300} = \frac{11}{60}$

**18.** $\frac{5}{6} \times 100\% = \frac{500}{6}\% = 83\frac{1}{3}\%$

**19.** $16.3\% \times 120 = n$

$0.163 \times 120 = n$

$19.56 = n$

**20.** $n \times 18 = 24$

$n = 24 \div 18$

$n = 1.33....$

$n = 133\frac{1}{3}\%$

**21.** $125\% \times n = 12.4$

$1.25 \times n = 12.4$

$n = 12.4 \div 1.25$

$n = 9.92$

**22.** $n \times 35 = 120$

$n = 120 \div 35$

$n \approx 3.4285$

$n \approx 342.9\%$

**23.** **Strategy** To find Sergio's take-home pay:

• Find the amount deducted by multiplying the income (\$740) by $\frac{1}{5}$.

• Subtract the amount deducted from the income.

**Solution** $\frac{1}{5} \times \$740 = \$148$

$\$740 - \$148 = \$592$

Sergio's take-home pay is \$592.

**24.** **Strategy** To find the amount of the monthly payment:

• Find the amount that will be paid by payments by subtracting the down payment (\$2000) from the price of the car (\$12,530).

• Divide the total amount remaining to be paid by the number of payments (36).

**Solution**

$$\begin{array}{r} 12{,}530 \\ -2000 \\ \hline 10{,}530 \end{array} \qquad 36\overline{)10{,}530.00} = 292.50$$

Each monthly payment is \$292.50.

**25.** **Strategy** To find the number of tablets, write and solve a proportion using $n$ to represent the number of tablets.

**Solution** $\dfrac{0.25 \text{ grams of medication}}{1 \text{ tablet}} = \dfrac{0.5 \text{ grams of medication}}{n \text{ tablets}}$

$1 \times 0.5 = 0.25 \times n$

$0.5 = 0.25 \times n$

$0.5 \div 0.25 = n$

$2 = n$

2 tablets are needed to give 0.5 grams of medication.

**26.** **Strategy** To find the property tax on a dental office valued at \$344,000, write and solve a proportion using $n$ to represent the tax.

© 2013 Cengage Learning. All Rights Reserved. May not be scanned, copied or duplicated, or posted to a publicly accessible website, in whole or in part.

**Solution**

$$\frac{6880}{344{,}000} = \frac{n}{500{,}000}$$
$$6880 \times 500{,}000 = 344{,}000 \times n$$
$$3{,}440{,}000{,}000 = 344{,}000 \times n$$
$$3{,}440{,}000{,}000 \div 344{,}000 = n$$
$$10{,}000 = n$$

The property tax is $10,000.

**27. Strategy** To find the number of African-Americans with type A+ blood, write and solve a basic percent equation us $n$ as the number with type A+. The percent is 24% and the base is 37,300,000.

**Solution**

$$24\% \times 37{,}300{,}000 = n$$
$$0.24 \times 37{,}300{,}000 = n$$
$$8{,}952{,}000 = n$$

There are 8,952,000 African-Americans with type A+ blood.

**28. Strategy** To find what percent of the people favored Brand B

• Find the number of people who favored Brand B by subtracting the number of people who favored Brand A (165) from the total surveyed (300).

• Write and solve the basic percent equation using $n$ to represent the percent of people who favored Brand B. The base is 300 and the amount is the number of people favored Brand B.

**Solution**

$$\begin{array}{r} 300 \\ -165 \\ \hline 135 \end{array}$$

$$n \times 300 = 135$$
$$n = 135 \div 300$$
$$n = 0.45$$
$$n = 45\%$$

45% of the people favored Brand B.

**29. Strategy** To find the maximum calories from saturated fat in a week:

- To find the maximum calories in one day, write and solve the basic percent equation using $n$ to represent the calories from saturated fat. The percent is 7% and the base is 2000 calories.
- To find the maximum calories in a week, multiply the maximum number of calories in a day by the number of days in a week (7 days).

**Solution**

$$7\% \times 2000 = n$$
$$0.07 \times 2000 = n$$
$$140 = n$$

$$\begin{array}{r} 140 \\ \times 7 \\ \hline 980 \end{array}$$

The maximum number of calories in one week from saturated fat is 980.

**30. Strategy** To find what percent of the children tested had levels of lead that exceeded federal standards, write and solve a proportion using $n$ to represent the percent who had levels of lead that exceeded federal standards. The base is 5500 and the amount is 990.

© 2013 Cengage Learning. All Rights Reserved. May not be scanned, copied or duplicated, or posted to a publicly accessible website, in whole or in part.

**Solution**

$$\frac{n}{100} = \frac{990}{5500}$$

$$n \times 5500 = 990 \times 100$$

$$n \times 5500 = 99{,}000$$

$$n = 99{,}000 \div 5500$$

$$n = 18$$

18% of the children tested had levels of lead that exceeded federal standards.

© 2013 Cengage Learning. All Rights Reserved. May not be scanned, copied or duplicated, or posted to a publicly accessible website, in whole or in part.

# Chapter 6: Applications for Business and Consumers

## Prep Test

**1.** $3.75 \div 5 = 0.75$

**2.** $3.47 \times 15 = 52.05$

**3.** $874.50 - 369.99 = 504.51$

**4.** $0.065 \times 150{,}000 = 9750$

**5.** $1500 \times 0.06 \times 0.5 = 90 \times 0.5 = 45$

**6.** $1372.47 + 36.91 + 5.00 + 2.86 = 1417.24$

**7.**

$$\begin{array}{r} 3.333 \\ 3\overline{)10.000} \\ \underline{-9\phantom{.000}} \\ 1\,0\phantom{00} \\ \underline{-9\phantom{00}} \\ 10\phantom{0} \\ \underline{-9\phantom{0}} \\ 10 \\ \underline{-9} \\ 1 \end{array} \approx 3.33$$

**8.**

$$\begin{array}{r} 0.6052 \\ 570\overline{)345.0000} \\ \underline{-3420\phantom{000}} \\ 300\phantom{00} \\ \underline{-\phantom{0}0\phantom{00}} \\ 3000\phantom{0} \\ \underline{-2850\phantom{0}} \\ 1500 \\ \underline{-1140} \\ 360 \end{array} \approx 0.605$$

**9.** $0.379 < 0.397$

## Section 6.1

### Objective A Exercises

**1. Strategy** To find the unit cost, divide the total cost ($.99) by the number of units (18).

**Solution** $0.99 \div 18 = 0.055$

The unit cost is $0.055 per ounce.

**3. Strategy** To find the unit cost, divide the total cost ($2.99) by the number of units (8).

**Solution** $2.99 \div 8 \approx 0.3737$

The unit cost is $0.374 per ounce.

**5. Strategy** To find the unit cost, divide the total cost ($3.99) by the number of units (50).

**Solution** $3.99 \div 50 = 0.0798$

The unit cost is $0.080 per tablet.

**7. Strategy** To find the unit cost, divide the total cost ($5.35) by the number of ounces (18).

**Solution** $5.35 \div 18 \approx 0.297$

The unit price is $.297 per ounce.

**9. Strategy** To find the unit cost, divide the total cost ($2.99) by the number of units (15).

**Solution** $2.99 \div 15 \approx 0.1993$

The unit cost is $0.199 per ounce.

**11.** To find the unit cost, divide the price of one pint of ice cream by 2.

### Objective B Exercises

**13. Strategy** To find the more economical purchase, compare the unit costs.

**Solution** Kraft: $3.98 \div 40 = 0.0995$

Springfield:

$3.39 \div 32 \approx 0.1059$

$0.0995 < 0.1059$

The Kraft mayonnaise is the more economical purchase.

© 2013 Cengage Learning. All Rights Reserved. May not be scanned, copied or duplicated, or posted to a publicly accessible website, in whole or in part.

**15.** **Strategy** To find the more economical purchase, compare the unit costs.

**Solution** L'Oréal shampoo:

$4.69 \div 13 \approx 0.3608$

Cortexx shampoo:

$3.99 \div 12 = 0.3325$

$0.3325 < 0.3608$

Cortexx shampoo is the more economical purchase.

**17.** **Strategy** To find the more economical purchase, compare the unit costs.

**Solution** Ultra Mr. Clean:

$2.67 \div 20 = 0.1335$

Ultra Spic and Span:

$2.19 \div 14 \approx 0.1564$

$0.1335 < 0.1564$

Ultra Mr. Clean is the more economical purchase.

**19.** **Strategy** To find the more economical purchase, compare the unit costs.

**Solution** Bertolli: $9.49 \div 34 \approx 0.2791$

Pompeian: $2.39 \div 8 \approx 0.2988$

$0.2791 < 0.2988$

Bertolli olive oil is the more economical purchase.

**21.** **Strategy** To find the more economical purchase, compare the unit costs.

**Solution** Wagner's:

$3.95 \div 1.5 \approx 2.6333$

Durkee: $2.84 \div 1 = 2.84$

$2.6333 < 2.84$

Wagner's vanilla extract is the more economical purchase.

**23.** A box of Tea A contains twice as many bags as a box of Tea B, so a box of Tea B contains half as many bags as a box of Tea A. If a box of Tea B cost half as much as a box of Tea A, then the price per tea bag would be equal. But, because the price of a box of Tea B is greater than half the price of a box of Tea A, the price per tea bag for Tea B is greater than the price per bag for Tea A. A box of Tea A is the more economical purchase.

## Objective C Exercises

**25.** **Strategy** To find the total cost, multiply the unit cost (\$.98) by the number of units (75).

**Solution** $0.98 \times 75 = 73.50$

The total cost is \$73.50.

**27.** **Strategy** To find the total cost, multiply the unit cost (\$4.69) by the number of units (3.6).

**Solution** $4.69 \times 3.6 = 16.884$

The total cost is \$16.88.

**29.** **Strategy** To find the total cost, multiply the unit cost (\$5.99) by the number of units (0.65).

**Solution** $5.99 \times 0.65 \approx 3.893$

The total cost is \$3.89.

**31.** **Strategy** To find the total cost, multiply the unit cost (\$9.49) by the number of units (2.8).

**Solution** $9.49 \times 2.8 = 26.572$

The total cost is \$26.57.

## Applying the Concepts

**33.** Students might explain that unit pricing is used in grocery stores. The unit price of a product is the total price divided by the

© 2013 Cengage Learning. All Rights Reserved. May not be scanned, copied or duplicated, or posted to a publicly accessible website, in whole or in part.

number of units the product contains. Consumers can use this information to determine which size of a product is the more economical purchase.

## Section 6.2

### Objective A Exercises

**1.** **Strategy** To find the percent increase:

• Find the amount of the increase by subtracting the number of bison whose meat was consumed in 2005 (17,674 bison) from the number consumed this year (50,000 bison).

• Write and solve the basic percent equation for percent. The base is 17,674 and the amount is the amount of the increase.

**Solution** 50,000 – 17,674 = 32,326

Percent × base = amount

$n \times 17{,}674 = 32{,}326$

$n = 32{,}326 \div 17{,}674$

$n \approx 1.829$

The percent increase is 182.9%.

**3.** **Strategy** To find the percent increase:

• Subtract the number of stores before the increase (420) from the number of stores after the increase (914).

• Write and solve the basic percent equation for percent. The base is 420 and the amount is the amount of the increase.

**Solution** 914 – 420 = 494

Percent × base = amount

$n \times 420 = 494$

$n = 494 \div 420$

$n \approx 1.176$

The percent increase is 117.6%.

**5.** **Strategy** To find the percent increase:

• Find the amount of the increase by subtracting the cost in 2003 ($9249) from the cost in 2008 ($12,298).

• Write and solve the basic percent equation for percent. The base is $9249 and the amount is the amount of the increase.

**Solution** 12,298 – 9,249 = 3049

Percent × base = amount

$n \times 9249 = 3049$

$n = 3049 \div 9240$

$n = 0.330$

The percent increase is 33.0%.

**7.** **Strategy** To find the percent increase:

• Find the amount of the increase by subtracting the amount Americans spent on pets a decade ago ($17 billion) from the amount spent ten years later ($35.9 billion).

• Write and solve the basic percent equation for percent. The base is 17 billion and the amount is the amount of the increase.

© 2013 Cengage Learning. All Rights Reserved. May not be scanned, copied or duplicated, or posted to a publicly accessible website, in whole or in part.

**Solution** $35.9 - 17 = 18.9$

$$\begin{aligned} \text{Percent} \times \text{base} &= \text{amount} \\ n \times 17 &= 18.9 \\ n &= 18.9 \div 17 \\ n &\approx 1.1117 \end{aligned}$$

The percent increase is 111.2%.

**9.** $\$12 \times 0.10 + \$12 = \$1.20 + \$12 = \$13.20$

$\$12(1.10) = \$13.20$

Yes

## Objective B Exercises

**11.** (3) Markup rate × cost = markup

(2) Cost + markup = selling price

**13. Strategy** To find the markup, solve the basic percent equation for amount. The percent is 40% and the base is \$8.75.

**Solution**

$$\begin{aligned} \text{Percent} \times \text{base} &= \text{amount} \\ 40\% \times 8.75 &= n \\ 0.4 \times 8.75 &= n \\ 3.50 &= n \end{aligned}$$

The markup is \$3.50.

**15. Strategy** To find the markup rate, solve the basic percent equation for percent. The base is \$20 and the amount is \$12.

**Solution**

$$\begin{aligned} \text{Percent} \times \text{base} &= \text{amount} \\ n \times 20 &= 12 \\ n &= 12 \div 20 \\ n &= 0.60 = 60\% \end{aligned}$$

The markup rate is 60%.

**17. Strategy** To find the selling price:

- Solve the basic percent equation for amount to find the markup.
- Add the markup to the cost.

**Solution**

$$\begin{aligned} \text{Percent} \times \text{base} &= \text{amount} \\ 45\% \times 12 &= n \\ 0.45 \times 12 &= n \\ 5.40 &= n \end{aligned}$$

The markup is \$5.40.

$5.40 + 12 = 17.40$

The selling price is \$17.40.

**19. Strategy** To find the selling price:

- Solve the basic percent equation for amount to find the amount of the markup.
- Add the amount of the markup to the cost (\$15).

**Solution**

$$\begin{aligned} \text{Percent} \times \text{base} &= \text{amount} \\ 48\% \times 15 &= n \\ 0.48 \times 15 &= n \\ 7.20 &= n \end{aligned}$$

$7.20 + 15 = 22.20$

The selling price is \$22.20.

## Objective C Exercises

**21. Strategy** To find the percent decrease, solve the basic percent equation for percent. The base is 45 and the amount is 18.

**Solution**

$$\begin{aligned} \text{Percent} \times \text{base} &= \text{amount} \\ n \times 45 &= 18 \\ n &= 18 \div 45 \\ n &= 0.40 = 40\% \end{aligned}$$

The amount represents a decrease of 40%.

**23a. Strategy** To find the percent decrease:

- Find the amount of the decrease by subtracting the population in 2005 (886,671) from the population in 1990 (1,027,974).
- Write and solve the basic percent equation for percent.

© 2013 Cengage Learning. All Rights Reserved. May not be scanned, copied or duplicated, or posted to a publicly accessible website, in whole or in part.

The base is 1,027,974 and the amount is the amount of the decrease.

**Solution** 1,027,974 – 886,671 = 141,303

$$\text{Percent} \times \text{base} = \text{amount}$$
$$n \times 1{,}027{,}974 = 141{,}303$$
$$n = 141{,}303 \div 1{,}027{,}974$$
$$n \approx 0.137 = 13.7\%$$

The amount represents a decrease of 13.7%.

**b. Strategy** To find the percent decrease:

- Find the amount of the decrease by subtracting the population in 2005 (1,463,281) from the population in 1990 (1,585,577).
- Write and solve the basic percent equation for percent. The base is 1,585,577 and the amount is the amount of the decrease.

**Solution** 1,585,577 – 1,463,281 = 122,296

$$\text{Percent} \times \text{base} = \text{amount}$$
$$n \times 1{,}585{,}577 = 122{,}296$$
$$n = 122{,}296 \div 1{,}585{,}577$$
$$n \approx 0.077 = 7.7\%$$

The amount represents a decrease of 7.7%.

**c. Strategy** To find the percent decrease:

- Find the amount of the decrease by subtracting the population in 2005 (2,842,518) from the population in 2000 (2,896,016).
- Write and solve the basic percent equation for percent. The base is 2,896,016 and the amount is the amount of the decrease.

**Solution** 2,896,016 – 2,842,518 = 53,498

$$\text{Percent} \times \text{base} = \text{amount}$$
$$n \times 2{,}896{,}016 = 53{,}498$$
$$n = 53{,}498 \div 2{,}896{,}016$$
$$n \approx 0.018 = 1.8\%$$

The amount represents a decrease of 1.8%.

**25. Strategy** To find how much value the car loses, solve the basic percent equation for amount. The base is $28,200 and the percent is 30%.

**Solution**

$$\text{Percent} \times \text{base} = \text{amount}$$
$$30\% \times 28{,}200 = n$$
$$0.30 \times 28{,}200 = n$$
$$8460 = n$$

The car loses $8460 in value after 1 year.

**27a. Strategy** To find the amount of decrease, solve the basic percent equation for amount. The base is $176 and the percent is 20%.

**Solution**

$$\text{Percent} \times \text{base} = \text{amount}$$
$$20\% \times 176 = n$$
$$0.20 \times 176 = n$$
$$35.2 = n$$

The amount of the decrease was $35.20.

**b. Strategy** To find the average monthly gasoline bill now, subtract the amount of the decrease ($35.20) from the original amount ($76).

© 2013 Cengage Learning. All Rights Reserved. May not be scanned, copied or duplicated, or posted to a publicly accessible website, in whole or in part.

**Solution** $176 - 35.20 = 140.80$

The average monthly gasoline bill now is $140.80.

**29. Strategy** To find the percent decrease:

- Find the amount of the decrease by the number of smokers after the program (36) from the original number (45).
- Solve the basic percent equation for percent. The amount is the amount of the decrease and the base is 45.

**Solution** $45 - 36 = 9$

$$\text{Percent} \times \text{base} = \text{amount}$$
$$n \times 45 = 9$$
$$n = 9 \div 45$$
$$n = 0.2 = 20\%$$

The amount represents a decrease of 20%.

## Objective D Exercises

**31.** (3) Discount rate ×regular price = discount

(2) Regular price – discount = sale price

**33. Strategy** To find the discount rate, solve the basic percent equation for percent. The base is $24 and the amount is $8.

**Solution** Percent × base = amount

$$n \times 24 = 8$$
$$n = 8 \div 24$$
$$n = 0.333\ldots = 33\frac{1}{3}\%$$

The discount rate is $33\frac{1}{3}\%$.

**35. Strategy** To find the discount, solve the basic percent equation for amount. The percent is 20% and the base is $400.

**Solution** Percent × base = amount

$$20\% \times 400 = n$$
$$0.20 \times 400 = n$$
$$80 = n$$

The discount is $80.

**37. Strategy** To find the discount rate, solve the basic percent equation for percent. The base is $60 and the amount is $18.

**Solution** Percent × base = amount

$$n \times 60 = 18$$
$$n = 18 \div 60$$
$$n = 0.30 = 30\%$$

The discount rate is 30%.

**39a. Strategy** To find the discount, solve the basic percent equation for amount. The percent is 20% and the base is $1.25.

**Solution** Percent x base = amount

$$20\% \times 1.25 = n$$
$$0.20 \times 1.25 = n$$
$$0.25 = n$$

The discount is $.25 per pound.

**b. Strategy** To find the sale price, subtract the discount ($.25) from the original price ($1.25).

**Solution** $1.25 - 0.25 = 1.00$

The sale price is $1.00 per pound.

**41. Strategy** To find the discount rate:

- Find the amount of the discount by subtracting the sale price ($12.40) from the regular price ($15.50).

© 2013 Cengage Learning. All Rights Reserved. May not be scanned, copied or duplicated, or posted to a publicly accessible website, in whole or in part.

7. (continued)

• Solve the basic percent equation for percent. The base is \$15.50 and the amount is the amount of the discount.

**Solution** $15.50 - 12.40 = 3.10$

The discount is \$4.

$$\begin{aligned} \text{Percent} \times \text{base} &= \text{amount} \\ n \times 15.50 &= 3.10 \\ n &= 3.10 \div 15.50 \\ n &= 0.2 = 20\% \end{aligned}$$

The discount rate is 20%.

## Section 6.3

### Objective A Exercises

**1a.** \$10,000

**b.** \$850

**c.** 4.25%

**d.** 2 years

**3. Strategy** To find the simple interest, multiply the principal by the annual interest rate by the time (in years).

**Solution** $8000 \times 0.06 \times 2 = 960$

The simple interest owed is \$960.

**5. Strategy** To find the simple interest, multiply the principal by the annual interest rate by the time (in years).

**Solution** $100{,}000 \times 0.045 \times \frac{9}{12} = 3375$

The simple interest due is \$3375.

**7. Strategy** To find the simple interest, multiply the principal by the annual interest rate by the time (in years).

**Solution** $20{,}000 \times 0.088 \times \frac{9}{12} = 1320$

The simple interest due is \$1320.

**9. Strategy** To find the simple interest, multiply the principal by the annual interest rate by the time (in years).

**Solution** $7500 \times 0.055 \times \frac{75}{365} \approx 84.76$

The simple interest due is \$84.76

**11. Strategy** To find the maturity value of the loan, add the principal and the simple interest.

**Solution** $4800 + 320 = 5120$

The maturity value of the loan is \$5120

**13. Strategy** To find the total amount due:

• Find the simple interest due by multiplying the principal by the annual interest rate by the time (in years).

• Find the total amount due by adding the principal and the simple interest.

**Solution** $12{,}500 \times 0.045 \times \frac{8}{12} \approx 375$

$12{,}500 + 375 = 12{,}875$

The total amount due on the loan is \$12,875.

**15. Strategy** To find the maturity value:

• Find the simple interest due by multiplying the principal by the annual interest rate by the time (in years).

© 2013 Cengage Learning. All Rights Reserved. May not be scanned, copied or duplicated, or posted to a publicly accessible website, in whole or in part.

• Find the maturity value by adding the principal and the simple interest.

**Solution** $14{,}000 \times 0.0525 \times \frac{270}{365} \approx 543.70$

$14{,}000 + 543.70 = 14{,}543.70$

The maturity value is $14,543.70.

**17.** **Strategy** To find the monthly payment, divide the sum of the loan amount ($225,000) and the interest ($72,000) by the number of payments (48).

**Solution** $\frac{225{,}000 + 72{,}000}{48} = 6187.50$

The monthly payment is $6187.50.

**19a.** **Strategy** To find the simple interest charged, multiply the principal ($12,000) by the annual interest rate by the time (in years).

**Solution** $12{,}000 \times 0.045 \times 2 = 1080$

The interest charged is $1080.

**b.** **Strategy** To find the monthly payment, divide the sum of the loan amount ($12,000) and the interest ($1080) by the number of payments (24).

**Solution** $\frac{12{,}000 + 1080}{24} = 545$

The monthly payment is $545.

**21.** **Strategy** To find the monthly payment:

• Find the simple interest due by multiplying the principal by the annual interest rate by the time (in years).

• Find the monthly payment by adding the interest due to the loan amount ($142,000) and dividing that sum by the number of payments (66).

**Solution** $142{,}000 \times 0.075 \times 5.5 = 58{,}575$

$\frac{142{,}000 + 58{,}575}{66} \approx 3039.02$

The monthly payment is $3039.02

**23a.** Student A's principal is equal to Student B's principal; the students borrowed the same amount of money.

**b.** Student A's maturity value is greater than Student B's maturity value; Student A's loan has a longer term and accumulates interest for a longer period of time.

**c.** Student A's monthly payment is less than Student B's monthly payment; the payments are spread out over a longer period of time for Student A, so Student A does not need to pay as much per month to pay off the loan.

## Objective B Exercises

**25.** **Strategy** To find the finance charge, multiply the unpaid balance by the monthly interest rate by the number of months.

**Solution** $391.64 \times 0.0175 \times 1 = 6.85$ .

The finance charge is $6.85.

**27.** **Strategy** To find the finance charge, multiply the unpaid balance by the monthly interest rate by the number of months.

**Solution** $995.04 \times 0.012 \times 1 \approx 11.94$

The finance charge is $11.94.

**29.** **Strategy** To find the difference in finance charges:

• Find the difference in monthly interest rates by subtracting the smaller rate (1.25%) from the larger rate

© 2013 Cengage Learning. All Rights Reserved. May not be scanned, copied or duplicated, or posted to a publicly accessible website, in whole or in part.

(1.75%).

• To find the difference in finance charges, multiply the unpaid balance by the difference in monthly interest rates by the number of months.

**Solution** $0.0175 - 0.0125 = 0.005$
$= 0.5\%$

$687.45 \times 0.005 \times 1 \approx 3.44$

The difference in finance charges is \$3.44.

**31.** The finance charge the first month was exactly equal to the minimum monthly payment, so no money was applied to the principal amount borrowed. The second month, the principal is the same as the first month so the finance charge will again be \$10, equal to the finance charge from the first month. No, you will not eventually pay off the balance with this payment plan.

## Objective C Exercises

**33. Strategy** To find the value of the investment after 20 years, multiply the original investment by the compound interest factor.

**Solution** $2500 \times 4.95217 \approx 12,380.43$

The value of the investment after 20 years is \$12,380.43.

**35. Strategy** To find the value of the investment after 5 years, multiply the original investment by the compound interest factor.

**Solution** $20,000 \times 1.417625 = 28,352.50$

The value of the investment after 5 years is \$28,352.50.

**37a. Strategy** To find the value of the investment in 10 years, multiply the original investment by the compound interest factor.

**Solution** $3000 \times 2.01362 = 6040.86$

The value of the investment in 10 years will be \$6040.86.

**b. Strategy** To find how much interest will be earned, subtract the original investment from the new value of the investment.

**Solution** $6040.86 - 3000 = 3040.86$

The amount of interest earned in 10 years will be \$3040.86.

**39. Strategy** To find the amount of interest earned over a 2-year period:

• Find the value of the investment after 1 year by multiplying the original investment by the compound interest factor.

• Find the value of the investment after the second year by multiplying the new investment (4245.44) by the compound interest factor.

• Subtract the original value of the investment (\$4000) from the value of the investment after 2 years.

**Solution** $4000 \times 1.06136 = 4245.44$

$4245.44 \times 1.06136 \approx 4505.94$

$4505.94 - 4000 = 505.94$

The amount of interest earned is \$505.94.

## Applying the Concepts

**41.** You received less interest during the second

© 2013 Cengage Learning. All Rights Reserved. May not be scanned, copied or duplicated, or posted to a publicly accessible website, in whole or in part.

month because there are fewer days in the month of September (30 days) than in the month of August (31 days). Using the simple interest formula:

$$500 \times 0.05 \times \frac{31}{365} \approx 2.12$$

$$502.12 \times 0.05 \times \frac{30}{365} \approx 2.06$$

Even though the principal is greater during the second month, the interest earned is less because there are fewer days in the month.

**b.** **Strategy** To find the value of the savings account after the deposit on March 1, multiply the original investment by the compound interest factor and add the deposit.

**Solution**

$$200.50 \times 0.06 \times \frac{1}{12} = 1.0025 \approx 1.00$$

$$200.50 + 1.00 + 100 = 301.50$$

The value of the account after the deposit is \$301.50.

# Section 6.4

## Objective A Exercises

**1.** **Strategy** To find the mortgage, subtract the down payment from the purchase price.

**Solution** $197{,}000 - 24{,}550 = 172{,}450$

The mortgage is \$172,450.

**3.** **Strategy** To find the down payment, solve the basic percent equation for amount. The base is \$850,000 and the percent is 25%.

**Solution** Percent × base = amount

$0.25 \times 850{,}000 = 212{,}500$

The down payment is \$212,500.

**5.** **Strategy** To find the loan origination fee, solve the basic percent equation for amount. The base is \$150,000 and the percent is $2\frac{1}{2}\%$.

**Solution** Percent × base = amount

$0.025 \times 150{,}000 = 3750$

The loan origination fee is \$3750.

**7a.** **Strategy** To find the down payment, solve the basic percent equation for amount. The base is \$350,000 and the percent is 10%.

**Solution** Percent × base = amount

$0.10 \times 350{,}000 = 35{,}000$

The down payment is \$35,000.

**b.** **Strategy** To find the mortgage, subtract the down payment from the purchase price.

**Solution** $350{,}000 - 35{,}000 = 315{,}000$

The mortgage is \$315,000.

**9.** **Strategy** To find the mortgage:

- Find the down payment by solving the basic percent equation for amount. The percent is 10% and the base is \$210,000.
- Subtract the down payment from the purchase price.

© 2013 Cengage Learning. All Rights Reserved. May not be scanned, copied or duplicated, or posted to a publicly accessible website, in whole or in part.

**Solution** Percent × base = amount

$0.10 \times 210{,}000 = 21{,}000$

$210{,}000 - 21{,}000 = 189{,}000$

The mortgage is \$189,000.

**11.** (iii); find 10% of the purchase price and subtract this amount from the purchase price.

## Objective B Exercises

**13. Strategy** To find the monthly mortgage payment, multiply the mortgage by the monthly mortgage factor.

**Solution** $90{,}000 \times 0.0071643 \approx 644.79$

The monthly mortgage payment is \$644.79.

**15. Strategy** To determine whether the podiatrist can afford the monthly mortgage payment:

• Find the monthly mortgage payment by multiplying the mortgage by the monthly mortgage factor.

• Compare the monthly mortgage payment with \$3500.

**Solution** $400{,}000 \times 0.0084386 = 3375.44$

$\$3375.44 < \$3500$

Yes, the podriatist can afford the monthly mortgage payment.

**17. Strategy** To find the monthly property tax payment, divide the annual property tax by 12.

**Solution** $1992 \div 12 = 166$

The monthly property tax is \$166.

**19a. Strategy** To find the monthly mortgage payment, multiply the mortgage by the monthly mortgage factor.

**Solution** $135{,}000 \times 0.0066530 \approx 898.16$

The monthly mortgage payment is \$898.16.

**b. Strategy** To find how much of the monthly mortgage payment is interest, subtract the amount that is principal (\$392.47) from the monthly mortgage payment.

**Solution** $898.16 - 39247 = 505.69$

The interest payment is \$505.69.

**21. Strategy** To find the total monthly payment for the mortgage and property tax:

• Find the monthly property tax payment by dividing the annual tax (\$792) by 12.

• Add the monthly property tax to the monthly mortgage payment (\$716.40).

**Solution** $1512 \div 12 = 126$

$126 + 716.40 = 842.40$

The total monthly payment for the mortgage and property tax is \$842.40.

**23. Strategy** To find the monthly mortgage payment:

• Find the mortgage amount by subtracting the down payment from the purchase price.

• Multiply the mortgage amount by the monthly mortgage factor.

**Solution** $385{,}000 - 40{,}000 = 345{,}000$

$345{,}000 \times 0.006653 \approx 2295.29$

The monthly mortgage payment is \$2295.29.

## Applying the Concepts

**25.** Choice 1: 8% for 20 years

© 2013 Cengage Learning. All Rights Reserved. May not be scanned, copied or duplicated, or posted to a publicly accessible website, in whole or in part.

100,000 × 0.0083644 = 836.44/month

Payback = 836.44 × 240 months =

$200,745.60, or 100,745.60 in interest

Choice 2: 8% for 30 years

100,000 × 0.0073376 = 733.76

Payback = 733.76 × 360 months =

$264,153.60 or 164,153.60 in interest

$164,153.60 – 100,745.60 = $63,408

By using the 20-year loan, the couple will save $63,408.

## Section 6.5

### Objective A Exercises

1. **Strategy** To determine whether Amanda has enough money for the down payment:
   - Find the down payment by solving the basic percent equation for amount. The base is $7100 and the percent is 12%.
   - Compare the required down payment with $780.

   **Solution** Percent × base = amount

   0.12 × 7100 = 852 down paymer

   $852 > $780

   No, Amanda does not have enough for the down payment.

3. **Strategy** To find how much sales tax is paid, solve the basic percent equation for amount. The base is $26,500 and the percent is 4.5%.

   **Solution** 0.045 × 26,500 = 1192.5

   The sales tax is $1192.50.

5. **Strategy** To find the state license fee, solve the basic percent equation for amount. The base is $32,500 and the percent is 2%.

   **Solution** Percent × base = amount

   0.02 × 32,500 = 650

   The license fee is $650.

7a. **Strategy** To find the sales tax, solve the basic percent equation for amount. The base is $32,000 and the percent is 3.5%.

   **Solution** Percent × base = amount

   0.035 × 32,000 = 1120

   The sales tax is $1120.

b. **Strategy** To find the total cost of the sales tax and license fee, add the sales tax ($1120) and the license fee ($275).

   **Solution** 1120 + 275 = 1395

   The total cost of the sales tax and license fee is $1395.

9a. **Strategy** To find the down payment, solve the basic percent equation for amount. The base is $16,200 and the percent is 25%.

   **Solution** Percent × base = amount

   0.25 × 16,200 = 4050

   The down payment is $4050.

b. **Strategy** To find the amount financed, subtract the down payment from the purchase price.

   **Solution** 16,200 – 4050 = 12,150

   The amount financed is $12,150.

11. **Strategy** To find the amount financed:
   - Find the amount of the down payment by solving the basic percent equation for amount. The base is $45,000 and the percent is 20%.

© 2013 Cengage Learning. All Rights Reserved. May not be scanned, copied or duplicated, or posted to a publicly accessible website, in whole or in part.

• Subtract the down payment from the purchase price ($45,000).

**Solution** Percent × base = amount
$0.20 \times 45{,}000 = 9000$
$45{,}000 - 9000 = 36{,}000$
The amount financed is $36,000.

**13.** The expression represents the total cost of buying the car.

## Objective B Exercises

**15.** To find the cost to drive 23,000 miles, multiply the number of miles by the cost per mile.

**17.** **Strategy** To find the monthly car payment, multiply the amount financed by the monthly payment factor.

**Solution** $18{,}000 \times 0.0295240 \approx 531.70$
The monthly car payment is $531.43.

**19.** **Strategy** To find the cost for the care and maintenance of tires for 14,000 miles, multiply the cost per mile by the number of miles.

**Solution** $0.018 \times 14{,}000 = 252$
The cost is $252.

**21.** **Strategy** To find the cost per mile for gasoline, divide the total cost by the number of miles.

**Solution** $2400 \div 15{,}000 = 0.16$
The cost was $0.16 per mile.

**23a.** **Strategy** To find the amount financed, subtract the down payment from the purchase price.

**Solution** $14{,}999 - 2999 = 12{,}000$
The amount financed is $12,000.

**b.** **Strategy** To find the monthly payment, multiply the amount financed by the monthly payment factor.

**Solution** $12{,}000 \times 0.0299709 \approx 359.65$.
The monthly car payment is $359.65.

**25.** **Strategy** To find the monthly car payment:
• Find the amount financed by subtracting the down payment from the purchase price.
• Multiply the amount financed by the monthly payment factor.

**Solution** $39{,}500 - 5000 = 34{,}500$
$34{,}500 \times 0.0234850 \approx 810.23$
The monthly payment is $810.23.

## Applying the Concepts

**27.** The monthly payment is $\$19{,}000 \times 0.0207584 = \$394.4096$. The total interest repaid is $\$394.4096(12 \times 5) - \$19{,}000 \approx \$4665.00$.

# Section 6.6

## Objective A Exercises

**1.** **Strategy** To find the earnings, multiply the hourly wage by the number of hours.

**Solution** $11.50 \times 40 = 460$
Lewis earns $460.

**3.** **Strategy** To find the commission, solve the basic percent equation for amount. The base is $131,000 and the percent is 3%.

**Solution** Percent × base = amount
$0.03 \times 131{,}000 = 3930$

© 2013 Cengage Learning. All Rights Reserved. May not be scanned, copied or duplicated, or posted to a publicly accessible website, in whole or in part.

The real estate agent's commission is $3930.

**5. Strategy** To find the commission, solve the basic percent equation for amount. The base is $5600 and the percent is 1.5%.

**Solution** Percent × base = amount

$0.015 \times 5600 = 84$

The stockbroker's commission is $84.

**7. Strategy** To find the monthly salary, divide the annual salary by 12.

**Solution** $38{,}928 \div 12 = 3244$

Keisha receives $3244 a month.

**9. Strategy** To find the commission, solve the basic percent equation for amount. The base is $4500 and the percent is 12%.

**Solution** Percent × base = amount

$0.12 \times 4500 = 540$

Carlos's commission was $540.

**11. Strategy** To find the earnings, multiply the earnings per hour ($15.20) by the number of hours (25).

**Solution** $15.20 \times 25 = 380$

The medical transcriptionist receives $380.

**13. Strategy** To find the chemist's hourly wage, divide the total wage by the number of hours.

**Solution** $15{,}000 \div 120 = 125$

125 The chemist's hourly wage is $125.

**15a. Strategy** To find the hourly wage for overtime, multiply the regular wage by 2 (double time).

**Solution** $10.78 \times 2 = 21.56$

Gil's overtime hourly wage is $21.56.

**b. Strategy** To find the earnings, multiply the overtime hourly wage by the number of hours.

**Solution** $21.56 \times 16 = 344.96$

Gil earns $344.96 for overtime.

**17a. Strategy** To find the increase in pay for the night shift, solve the basic percent equation for amount. The base is $8.20 and the percent is 15%.

**Solution** Percent × base = amount

$0.15 \times 8.20 = 1.23$

The increase in pay is $1.23.

**b. Strategy** To find the hourly wage for the night shift, add the increase in pay to the regular hourly wage

**Solution** $8.20 + 1.23 = 9.43$

The aide's hourly wage for the night shift is $9.43.

**19. Strategy** To find the earnings for the week:

- Find the amount of sales over $1500 by subtracting $1500 from the total sales ($3000).
- Find the commission by solving the basic percent equation for amount. The base is the sales over $1500 and the percent is 15%.
- Add the commission to the weekly salary ($250).

**Solution** $3000 - 1500 = 1500$

Percent × base = amount

$0.15 \times 1500 = 225$ commission

$250 + 225 = 475$

Nicole's earnings were $475.

© 2013 Cengage Learning. All Rights Reserved. May not be scanned, copied or duplicated, or posted to a publicly accessible website, in whole or in part.

## Applying the Concepts

**21.** Let $n$ represent the previous year's salary.

$$\text{Percent} \times \text{base} = \text{amount}$$
$$1.026 \times n = 41{,}360$$
$$n = 41{,}360 \div 1.0312$$
$$n \approx 40{,}312$$

The starting salary in the previous year for an accountant was $40,312.

**23.** Let $n$ represent the previous year's salary.

$$\text{Percent} \times \text{base} = \text{amount}$$
$$0.924 \times n = 46{,}536$$
$$n = 46{,}536 \div 0.924$$
$$n \approx 50{,}364$$

The starting salary in the previous year for a computer science major was $50,364.

# Section 6.7

## Objective A Exercises

**1.** **Strategy** To find your current checking balance, add the deposit to the old balance.

**Solution** $342.51 + 143.81 = 486.32$

Your current checking account balance is $486.32.

**3.** **Strategy** To find the current checking account balance, subtract the amount of each check from the original balance.

**Solution**

$$\begin{array}{r} 1204.63 \\ -\ 119.27 \\ \hline 1085.36 \\ -\ 260.09 \\ \hline 825.27 \end{array}$$

The nutritionist's current balance is $825.27.

**5.** **Strategy** To find the current checking account balance, add the amount of the deposit to the old balance. Then subtract the amount of each check.

**Solution**

$$\begin{array}{r} 3476.85 \\ +\ 1048.53 \\ \hline 4525.38 \\ -\ 848.37 \\ \hline 3677.01 \\ -\ 676.19 \\ \hline 3000.82 \end{array}$$

The current checking account balance is $3000.82.

**7.** **Strategy** To determine whether there is enough money in the account, compare $675 with the current balance after finding the current checking account balance.

**Solution**

$$\begin{array}{r} 404.96 \\ +\ 350.00 \\ \hline 754.96 \\ -\ 71.29 \\ \hline 683.67 \end{array}$$

$\$683.67 > \$675$

Yes, there is enough money in the nurse's account to purchase the refrigerator.

**9.** **Strategy** To determine whether there is enough money in the account to buy two wheelchairs, multiply the cost of one chair ($2215) by two and compare the total with the current checking account balance.

**Solution** $2215 \times 2 = 4430$ purchases

$\$4430 < \$5127.25$

Yes, there is enough money in the medical supply's account to buy two wheelchairs.

© 2013 Cengage Learning. All Rights Reserved. May not be scanned, copied or duplicated, or posted to a publicly accessible website, in whole or in part.

**11.** The ending balance might be less than the starting balance because the check written might be for an amount that is greater than the sum of the two deposits.

## Objective B Exercises

**13. Solution**

| | | |
|---|---|---|
| Current balance: 989.86 | | |
| Checks: 228 | | 419.32 |
| | 233 | 166.40 |
| | 235 | +288.39 |
| | | 1863.97 |
| Interest: | | +13.22 |
| | | 1877.19 |
| Service charge: | | −0.00 |
| | | 1877.19 |
| Deposits: | | −0.00 |
| Checkbook balance: 1877.19 | | |

Current bank balance from bank statement: $1877.19.

Checkbook balance: $1877.19.

The bank statement and checkbook balance.

**15. Solution**

| | | |
|---|---|---|
| Current balance: | | 1051.92 |
| Checks: 223 | | 414.83 |
| | 224 | 113.37 |
| Interest: | | +5.15 |
| | | 1585.27 |
| Service charge: | | − 0.00 |
| | | 1585.27 |
| Deposits: | | −0.00 |
| Checkbook balance: 1585.27 | | |

Current bank balance from bank statement: $1585.27.

Checkbook balance: $1585.27.

The bank statement and checkbook balance.

**17.** The ending balance on the statement is greater than the ending balance on the check register.

# Chapter 6 Concept Review

**1.** To find the unit cost, divide the total cost by the number of units. The cost is $2.96. The number of units is 4. $2.96 \div 4 = 0.74$, so the unit cost is $.74 per can.

**2.** To find the total cost, multiply the unit cost by the number of units purchased. The unit cost is $.85. The number of units purchased is 3.4. $0.85 \times 3.4 = 2.89$, so the total cost is $2.89.

**5.** To find the selling price when you know the cost and the markup, add the cost and the markup.

**4.** To find the markup when you know the markup rate, multiply the markup rate by the cost.

**5.** If you know the percent decrease, you can find the amount of decrease by multiplying the percent decrease by the original value.

**6.** If you know the regular price and the sale price, you can find the discount amount by subtracting the sale price from the regular price.

**7.** To find the discount rate, first subtract the sale price from the regular price to find the discount. Then divide the discount by the regular price.

**8.** To find simple interest, multiply the principal by the annual interest rate by the time (in years).

**9.** To find the maturity value for simple interest loans, add the principal and the interest.

**10.** Principal is the original amount deposited in an account or the original amount borrowed for a loan.

© 2013 Cengage Learning. All Rights Reserved. May not be scanned, copied or duplicated, or posted to a publicly accessible website, in whole or in part.

**11.** When you know the maturity value of an 18-month loan, you can find the monthly payment by dividing the maturity value by 18 (the length of the loan in months).

**12.** Compound interest is computed not only on the original principal but also in interest already earned.

**13.** For a fixed-rate mortgage, the monthly payment remains the same throughout the life of the loan.

**14.** The following expenses are involved in owning a car: car insurance, gas, oil, general maintenance, and the monthly car payment.

**15.** To balance a checkbook:

1. In the checkbook register, put a check mark by each check paid by the bank and by each deposit recorded by the bank.
2. Add to the current checkbook balance all checks that have been written but have not yet been paid by the bank and any interest paid on the account.
3. Subtract any service charges and any deposits not yet recorded by the bank. This is the checkbook balance.
4. Compare the balance with the bank balance listed on the bank statement. If the two numbers are equal, the bank statement and the checkbook "balance."

## Chapter 6 Review Exercises

**1.** **Strategy** To find the unit cost, divide the total cost ($3.90) by the number of units (20).

**Solution** $3.90 \div 20 = 0.195$

The unit cost is $.195 per ounce or 19.5¢ per ounce.

**2.** **Strategy** To find the cost per mile:

- Find the total cost by adding the amounts spent ($1025.58, $1805.82, $37.92, and $288.27).
- Divide the total cost by the number of miles (11,320).

**Solution** $1025.58 + 1805.82 + 37.92 + 288.27 = 3157.59$

$3157.59 \div 11{,}320 \approx 0.279$

The cost is $.279 or 27.9¢ per mile.

**3.** **Strategy** To find the percent increase:

- Find the amount of the increase by subtracting the original price ($42.375) from the increased price ($55.25).
- Solve the basic percent equation for percent. The base is $42.375 and the amount is the amount of the increase.

**Solution** $55.25 - 42.375 = 12.875$

$$n \times 42.375 = 12.875$$
$$n = 12.875 \div 42.375$$
$$\approx 0.304$$
$$= 30.4\%$$

The percent increase is 30.4%.

**4.** **Strategy** To find the markup, solve the basic percent equation for amount. The base is $21 and the percent is 40%.

**Solution** $0.40 \times 21 = n$

$8.40 = n$

The markup is $8.40.

**5.** **Strategy** To find the simple interest, multiply the principal by the annual interest rate by the time (in years).

**Solution** $100{,}000 \times 0.04 \times \dfrac{9}{12} = 3000$

© 2013 Cengage Learning. All Rights Reserved. May not be scanned, copied or duplicated, or posted to a publicly accessible website, in whole or in part.

The simple interest due is $3000.

**6. Strategy** To find the value of the investment in 10 years, multiply the original investment by the compound interest factor.

**Solution** $25{,}000 \times 1.82203 = 45{,}550.75$

The value of the investment after 10 years is $45,550.75.

**7. Strategy** To find the percent increase:

• Find the amount of the increase by subtracting the original amount ($4.12) from the increased amount ($4.73).

• Solve the basic percent equation for percent. The base is $4.12 and the amount is the increased amount.

**Solution** $4.73 - 4.12 = 0.61$

$n \times 4.12 = 0.61$

$n = 0.61 \div 4.12$

$n \approx 0.15$

$n = 15\%$

The percent increase is 15%.

**8. Strategy** To find the total monthly payment:

• Find the monthly property tax by dividing the annual tax ($2582.76) by 12.

• Add the monthly property tax payment to the monthly mortgage payment ($923.67).

**Solution** $2582.76 \div 12 = 215.23$

$215.23 + 923.67 = 1138.90$

The total monthly payment for the mortgage and property tax is $1138.90.

**9. Strategy** To find the monthly payment:

• Find the down payment by solving the basic percent equation for amount. The percent is 8% and the base is $24,450.

• Find the amount financed by subtracting the down payment from the purchase price ($24,450).

• Multiply the amount financed by the monthly payment factor.

**Solution** $0.08 \times 24{,}450 = 1956$

$24{,}450 - 1956 = 22{,}494$

$22{,}494 \times 0.0230293 \approx 518.02$

The monthly payment is $518.02.

**10. Strategy** To find the value of the investment in 1 year, multiply the original investment by the compound interest factor.

**Solution** $50{,}000 \times 1.07186 = 53{,}593$

The value of the investment will be $53,593.

**11. Strategy** To find the down payment, solve the basic percent equation for amount. The base is $195,000 and the percent is 15%.

**Solution** $0.15 \times 195{,}000 = 29{,}250$

The down payment is $29,250.

**12. Strategy** To find the total cost of the sales tax and license fee:

• Find the sales tax by solving the basic percent equation for amount. The base is $28,500 and the percent is 6.25%.

• Add the sales tax and the license fee ($315).

**Solution** $0.0625 \times 28{,}500 = 1781.25$

$1781.25 + 315 = 2096.25$

© 2013 Cengage Learning. All Rights Reserved. May not be scanned, copied or duplicated, or posted to a publicly accessible website, in whole or in part.

The total cost of the sales tax and license fee is \$2096.25.

**13. Strategy** To find the selling price:

• Find the markup by solving the basic percent equation for amount. The percent is 35% and the base is \$1540.

• Find the selling price by adding the markup to the cost.

**Solution** $0.35 \times 1540 = 539$

$539 + 1540 = 2079$

The selling price is \$2079.

**14. Strategy** To find how much of the payment is interest, subtract the principal (\$65.45) from the total payment (\$222.78).

**Solution** $222.78 - 65.45 = 157.33$

The interest paid is \$157.33.

**15. Strategy** To find the commission, solve the basic percent equation for amount. The base is \$108,000 and the percent is 3%.

**Solution** $0.03 \times 108{,}000 = n$

$3240 = n$

The commission was \$3240.

**16. Strategy** To find the sale price:

• Find the amount of the discount by solving the basic percent equation for amount. The base is \$235 and the percent is 40%.

• Subtract the discount from the original price.

**Solution** $0.40 \times 235 = n$

$94 = n$

$235 - 94 = 141$

The discount price is \$141.

**17. Strategy** To find the current checkbook balance, subtract the amount of each check and add the amount of the deposit.

**Solution**

$$\begin{array}{r} 1568.45 \\ \underline{-123.76} \\ 1444.69 \\ \underline{-756.45} \\ 688.24 \\ \underline{-88.77} \\ 599.47 \\ \underline{+344.21} \\ 943.68 \end{array}$$

The current checkbook balance is \$943.68.

**18. Strategy** To find the maturity value:

• Find the simple interest due by multiplying the principal by the annual interest rate by the time (in years).

• Find the maturity value by adding the principal and the simple interest.

**Solution** $30{,}000 \times 0.08 \times \frac{6}{12} = 1200$

$30{,}000 + 1200 = 31{,}200$

The maturity value is \$31,200.

**19. Strategy** To find the origination fee, solve the basic percent equation for amount. The base is \$75,000 and the percent is $2\frac{1}{2}\%$.

**Solution** $0.025 \times 75{,}000 = 1875$

The origination fee is \$1875.

**20. Strategy** To find the more economical purchase, compare the unit costs.

**Solution** $3.49 \div 16 \approx 0.218$

$6.99 \div 33 \approx 0.212$

The more economical purchase is 33 ounces for \$6.99.

**21. Strategy** To find the monthly mortgage

© 2013 Cengage Learning. All Rights Reserved. May not be scanned, copied or duplicated, or posted to a publicly accessible website, in whole or in part.

payment:

- Find the down payment by solving the basic percent equation for amount. The base is \$356,000 and the percent is 10%.
- Find the amount financed by subtracting the down payment from the purchase price.
- Find the monthly mortgage payment by multiplying the amount financed by the monthly mortgage factor.

**Solution** $0.10 \times 356{,}000 = 35{,}600$

$356{,}000 - 35{,}600 = 320{,}400$

$320{,}400 \times 0.006653 = 2131.62$

The monthly mortgage payment is \$2131.62.

**22. Strategy** To find the total income:

- Find the overtime wage by multiplying the regular wage by 1.5 (time and half).
- Find the number of overtime hours worked by subtracting the regular weekly schedule (40) from the total hours worked (48).
- Find the wages earned for overtime by multiplying the overtime wage by the number of overtime hours worked.
- Find the wages for the 40-hour week by multiplying the hourly rate (\$12.60) by 40.
- Add the pay from the overtime hours to the pay from the regular week.

**Solution** $1.5 \times 12.60 = 18.90$

$48 - 40 = 8;\ 8 \times 18.90 = 151.20$

$40 \times 12.60 = 504$

$504 + 151.20 = 655.20$

The total income was \$655.20.

**23. Strategy** To find the medial spa's current checkbook balance, subtract the amount of each check and add the amount of each deposit.

**Solution**

$$\begin{array}{r} 9567.44 \\ -\ 1023.55 \\ \hline 8543.89 \\ -\ 345.44 \\ \hline 8198.45 \\ -\ 23.67 \\ \hline 8174.78 \\ +\ 555.89 \\ \hline 8730.67 \\ +\ 135.91 \\ \hline 8866.58 \end{array}$$

The medical spa's checkbook balance is \$8866.58.

**24. Strategy** To find the monthly payment, divide the sum of the loan amount (\$55,000) and the interest (\$1375) by the number of payments (4).

**Solution** $\dfrac{55{,}000 + 1375}{4} = 14{,}093.75$

The monthly payment is \$14,093.75.

**25. Strategy** To find the finance charge, multiply the unpaid balance by the monthly interest rate by the number of months.

**Solution** $576 \times 0.0125 \times 1 = 7.2$

The finance charge is \$7.20.

© 2013 Cengage Learning. All Rights Reserved. May not be scanned, copied or duplicated, or posted to a publicly accessible website, in whole or in part.

## Chapter 6 Test

**1.** **Strategy** To find the cost per bottle, divide the total cost ($44.88) by the number of bottles (24).

**Solution** $44.88 \div 24 = 1.87$

The cost per bottle is $1.87.

**2.** **Strategy** To find the more economical purchase, compare the unit prices of the items.

**Solution** $7.49 \div 3$ or $12.59 \div 5$

$7.49 \div 3 \approx 2.50$

$12.59 \div 5 \approx 2.52$

The more economical purchase is 3 pounds for $7.49.

**3.** **Strategy** To find the total cost, multiply the cost per pound ($4.15) by the number of pounds (3.5).

**Solution** $4.15 \times 3.5 \approx 14.53$

The total cost is $14.53.

**4.** **Strategy** To find the percent increase:

- Find the amount of the increase by subtracting the original price ($415) from the increased price ($498).
- Solve the basic percent equation for percent. The base is $415 and the amount is the amount of the increase.

**Solution** $498 - 415 = 83$

$n \times 415 = 83$

$n = 83 \div 415$

$n = 0.20 = 20\%$

The percent increase in the cost of the exercise bicycle is 20%.

**5.** **Strategy** To find the selling price:

- Find the amount of the markup by solving the basic percent equation for amount. The percent is 40% and the base is $315.
- Add the markup to the cost ($315).

**Solution** $0.40 \times 315 = 126$

$315 + 126 = 441$

The selling price of a blu-ray disc player is $441.

**6.** **Strategy** To find the percent increase:

- Find the amount of the increase by subtracting the original value ($25.99) from the increased value ($29.99).
- Solve the basic percent equation for percent. The base is ($25.99) and the amount is the amount of the increase.

**Solution** $29.99 - 25.99 = 4$

$n \times 25.99 = 4$

$n = 4 \div 25.99$

$n \approx 0.154 = 15.4\%$

The percent decrease is 15.4%.

**7.** **Strategy** To find the percent decrease:

- Find the amount of the decrease by subtracting the decreased value ($357) from the original value ($420).
- Solve the basic percent equation for percent. The base is $420 and the amount is the amount of the decrease.

**Solution** $420 - 357 = 63$

$n \times 420 = 63$

$n = 63 \div 420$

$n = 0.15$

$n = 15\%$

The percent decrease is 15%.

**8.** **Strategy** To find the sale price:

© 2013 Cengage Learning. All Rights Reserved. May not be scanned, copied or duplicated, or posted to a publicly accessible website, in whole or in part.

• Find the amount of the discount by solving the basic percent equation for amount. The base is \$299 and the percent is 30%.

• Subtract the amount of the discount from the regular price (\$299).

**Solution**

$$0.30 \times 299 = n$$
$$897 = n$$
$$299 - 89.70 = 209.30$$

The sale price of the rolling medical cabinet is \$209.30.

**9. Strategy** To find the discount rate:

• Find the amount of the discount by subtracting the sale price (\$5.70) from the regular price (\$9.50).

• Solve the basic percent equation for percent. The base is \$9.50 and the amount is the amount of the discount.

**Solution**

$$9.50 - 5.70 = 3.80$$
$$n \times 9.50 = 3.80$$
$$n = 3.80 \div 9.50$$
$$n = 0.40$$
$$n = 40\%$$

The discount rate is 40%.

**10. Strategy** To find the simple interest due, multiply the principal by the annual interest rate by the time in years.

**Solution**

$$75{,}000 \times 0.08 \times \frac{4}{12} = 2000$$

The simple interest due is \$2000.

**11. Strategy** To find the maturity value:

• Find the simple interest due by multiplying the principal by the annual interest rate by the time (in years).

• Find the maturity value by adding the principal and the simple interest.

**Solution**

$$25{,}000 \times 0.092 \times \frac{9}{12} = 1725$$
$$25{,}000 + 1725 = 26{,}725$$

The maturity value is \$26,725.

**12. Strategy** To find the finance charge, multiply the unpaid balance by the monthly interest rate by the number of months.

**Solution**

$$374.95 \times 0.012 \times 1 = 4.50$$

The finance charge is \$4.50.

**13. Strategy** To find the interest earned:

• Find the value of the investment in 10 years by multiplying the original investment by the compound interest factor.

• Find the interest earned by subtracting the original investment from the new value of the investment.

**Solution**

$$30{,}000 \times 1.81402 = 54,\ 420.6$$
$$54{,}420.60 - 30{,}000 = 24{,}420.60$$

The amount of interest earned in 10 years will be \$24,420.60.

**14. Strategy** To find the loan origination fee, solve the basic percent equation for amount. The base is \$134,000 and the percent is $2\frac{1}{2}\%$.

**Solution**

$$0.025 \times 134{,}000 = 3350$$

The origination fee is \$3350.

**15. Strategy** To find the monthly mortgage payment, multiply the mortgage amount by the monthly mortgage factor.

© 2013 Cengage Learning. All Rights Reserved. May not be scanned, copied or duplicated, or posted to a publicly accessible website, in whole or in part.

**Solution** $222{,}000 \times 0.0077182 \approx 1713.44$

The monthly mortgage payment is $1713.44.

**16. Strategy** To find the amount financed:

- Find the amount of the down payment by solving the basic percent equation for amount. The base is $23,750 and the percent is 20%.
- Subtract the down payment from the purchase price.

**Solution**

$0.20 \times 23{,}750 = 4{,}750$

$23{,}750 - 4{,}750 = 19{,}000$

The amount financed is $19,000.

**17. Strategy** To find the monthly car payment:

- Find the amount of the down payment by solving the basic percent equation for amount. The base is $33,714 and the percent is 15%.
- Find the amount financed by subtracting the down payment from the purchase price ($33,714).
- Multiply the amount financed by the monthly mortgage factor.

**Solution**

$0.15 \times 33{,}714 = 5{,}057.10$

$33{,}714 - 5{,}057.10 = 28{,}656.90$

$28{,}656.90 \times 0.0239462 \approx 686.224$

The monthly car payment is $686.22.

**18. Strategy** To find Shaney's total weekly earnings:

- Find the hourly overtime wage for multiplying the hourly wage ($30.40) by 1.5 (time and a half).
- Find the earnings for overtime by multiplying the number of overtime hours (15) by the hourly overtime wage.
- Find the earnings for the normal hours worked by multiplying the number of hours worked (30) by the hourly rate ($30.40).
- Add the earnings from the night hours to the salary from the normal hours.

**Solution**

$30.40 \times 1.5 = 45.60$

$15 \times 45.60 = 684$

$30 \times 30.40 = 912$

$684 + 912 = 1596$

Shaney earns $1596.

**19. Strategy** Find the current checkbook balance by subtracting the checks written and adding the deposit to the original balance.

**Solution**

$$\begin{array}{r} 7349.44 \\ -1349.67 \\ \hline 5999.77 \\ -344.12 \\ \hline 5655.65 \\ +956.60 \\ \hline 6612.25 \end{array}$$

The current checkbook balance is $6612.25.

**20. Solution**

| | |
|---|---|
| Current balance: | 1106.31 |
| Checks: | 322.37 |
| | 413.45 |
| | +78.20 |
| | 1920.33 |
| Service charge: | −0.00 |
| | 1920.33 |
| Deposits: | −0.00 |
| Checkbook balance: | 1920.33 |

Current bank balance from bank statement: $1920.33.

© 2013 Cengage Learning. All Rights Reserved. May not be scanned, copied or duplicated, or posted to a publicly accessible website, in whole or in part.

Checkbook balance: \$1920.33.
The bank statement and
checkbook balance.

## Cumulative Review Exercises

**1.** $12 - (10-8)^2 \div 2 + 3$
$12 - 2^2 \div 2 + 3$
$12 - 4 \div 2 + 3$
$12 - 2 + 3$
$10 + 3 = 13$

**2.**
$$\begin{aligned} 3\frac{1}{3} &= 3\frac{8}{24} \\ 4\frac{1}{8} &= 4\frac{3}{24} \\ +1\frac{1}{12} &= 1\frac{2}{24} \\ \hline & \quad 8\frac{13}{24} \end{aligned}$$

**3.**
$$\begin{aligned} 12\frac{3}{16} &= 12\frac{9}{48} = 11\frac{57}{48} \\ -9\frac{5}{12} &= 9\frac{20}{48} = 9\frac{20}{48} \\ \hline & \qquad\qquad 2\frac{37}{48} \end{aligned}$$

**4.** $5\frac{5}{8} \times 1\frac{9}{15} = \frac{45}{8} \times \frac{24}{15}$
$$= \frac{45 \times 24}{8 \times 15}$$
$$= \frac{\cancel{3} \cdot 3 \cdot \cancel{5} \cdot \cancel{2} \cdot \cancel{2} \cdot \cancel{2} \cdot 3}{\cancel{2} \cdot \cancel{2} \cdot \cancel{2} \cdot \cancel{3} \cdot \cancel{5}} = 9$$

**5.** $3\frac{1}{2} \div 1\frac{3}{4} = \frac{7}{2} \div \frac{7}{4} = \frac{7}{2} \times \frac{4}{7} = \frac{\cancel{7} \cdot \cancel{2} \cdot 2}{\cancel{2} \cdot \cancel{7}} = 2$

**6.** $\left(\frac{3}{4}\right)^2 \div \left(\frac{3}{8} - \frac{1}{4}\right) + \frac{1}{2}$
$$= \left(\frac{3}{4} \cdot \frac{3}{4}\right) \div \left(\frac{3}{8} - \frac{2}{8}\right) + \frac{1}{2}$$
$$= \frac{9}{16} \div \frac{1}{8} + \frac{1}{2}$$
$$= \frac{9}{16} \times \frac{8}{1} + \frac{1}{2}$$
$$= \frac{9}{2} + \frac{1}{2} = \frac{10}{2} = 5$$

**7.**
$$\begin{array}{r} 52.18 \approx 52.2 \\ 0.059.\overline{)3.079.20} \\ \underline{-295} \\ 129 \\ \underline{-118} \\ 112 \\ \underline{-59} \\ 530 \\ \underline{-472} \\ 58 \end{array}$$

**8.** $\frac{17}{12} = 17 \div 12$
$$\begin{array}{r} 1.4166 \approx 1.417 \\ 12\overline{)17.0000} \\ \underline{-12} \\ 50 \\ \underline{-48} \\ 20 \\ \underline{-12} \\ 80 \\ \underline{-72} \\ 80 \\ \underline{-72} \\ 8 \end{array}$$

**9.** $\frac{\$410}{8 \text{ hours}} = \$51.25\text{/hour}$

**10.**
$$\begin{aligned} \frac{5}{n} &= \frac{16}{35} \\ 5 \times 35 &= n \times 16 \\ 175 &= n \times 16 \\ 175 \div 16 &= n \\ 10.9375 &= n \\ 10.94 &\approx n \end{aligned}$$

© 2013 Cengage Learning. All Rights Reserved. May not be scanned, copied or duplicated, or posted to a publicly accessible website, in whole or in part.

**11.** $\frac{5}{8} \times 100\% = \frac{500}{8}\% = 62.5\%$

**12.** $6.5\%$ of $420 = 0.065 \times 420 = 27.3$

**13.** $18.2 \times 0.01 = 0.182$

**14.** $n \times 20 = 8.4$
$n = 8.4 \div 20 = 0.42 = 42\%$

**15.** $0.12 \times n = 30$
$n = 30 \div 0.12 = 250$

**16.** $0.42 \times n = 65$
$n = 65 \div 0.42 \approx 154.76$

**17. Strategy** To find the total rainfall for the 3 weeks, add the 3 weekly amounts $\left(3\frac{3}{4}, 8\frac{1}{2}, \text{ and } 1\frac{2}{3} \text{ inches}\right)$.

**Solution**

$$\begin{aligned} 3\frac{3}{4} &= 3\frac{9}{12} \\ 8\frac{1}{2} &= 8\frac{6}{12} \\ +1\frac{2}{3} &= 1\frac{8}{12} \\ \hline 12\frac{23}{12} &= 13\frac{11}{12} \end{aligned}$$

The total rainfall is $13\frac{11}{12}$ inches.

**18. Strategy** Find the amount paid in taxes by multiplying the total monthly income ($4850) by the portion paid in taxes $\left(\frac{1}{5}\right)$.

**Solution** $4850 \times \frac{1}{5} = 970$

The amount paid in taxes is $970.

**19. Strategy** To find the ratio:
• Find the amount of the decrease by subtracting the decreased price ($30) from the original price ($75).
• Write in simplest form the ratio of the decrease to the original price.

**Solution** $75 - 30 = 45$

$\frac{45}{75} = \frac{3}{5}$

The ratio is $\frac{3}{5}$.

**20. Strategy** To find the number of miles driven per gallon of gasoline, divide the number of miles driven (417.5) by the number of gallons used (12.5).

**Solution** $417.5 \div 12.5 = 33.4$

The mileage was 33.4 miles per gallon.

**21. Strategy** To find the unit cost, divide the total cost ($15.40) by the number of pounds (14).

**Solution** $15.40 \div 14 \approx 1.1$

The cost is $1.10 per pound.

**22. Strategy** To find the dividend on 200 shares, write and solve a proportion.

**Solution**

$$\frac{80}{112} = \frac{200}{n}$$
$$80 \times n = 112 \times 200$$
$$80 \times n = 22{,}400$$
$$n = 22{,}400 \div 80$$
$$n = 280$$

The dividend is $280.

**23. Strategy** To find the sale price:
• Solve the basic percent equation for amount to find the amount of the discount. The base is $900 and the percent is 20%.

© 2013 Cengage Learning. All Rights Reserved. May not be scanned, copied or duplicated, or posted to a publicly accessible website, in whole or in part.

• Subtract the discount from the regular price.

**Solution** $0.20 \times 900 = 180$
$900 - 180 = 720$

The sale price is \$720.

**24. Strategy** To find the selling price:
• Find the amount of markup by solving the basic percent equation for amount. The base is \$1600 and the percent is 40%.
• Add the markup to the cost.

**Solution** $0.40 \times 1600 = 640$
$1600 + 640 = 2240$

The selling price of the EKG machine is \$2240.

**25. Strategy** To find the percent increase:
• Find the amount of the increase by subtracting the original value from the value after the increase.
• Solve the basic percent equation for the percent. The base is \$2800 and the amount is the amount of the increase.

**Solution**
$$3024 - 2800 = 224$$
$$n \times 2800 = 224$$
$$n = 224 \div 2800$$
$$n = 0.08$$
$$n = 8\%$$

The percent increase in physical therapist assistant's salary is 8%.

**26. Strategy** To find the simple interest due, multiply the principal by the annual rate by the time (in years).

**Solution**
$$120{,}000 \times 0.045 \times \frac{6}{12} = 2700$$

The simple interest due is \$2700.

**27. Strategy** To find the monthly payment:
• Find the amount financed by subtracting the down payment from the purchase price.
• Multiply the amount financed by the monthly mortgage factor.

**Solution** $26{,}900 - 2{,}000 = 24{,}900$
$24{,}900 \times 0.0317997 \approx 791.812$

The monthly car payment is \$791.81.

**28. Strategy** To find the new checking account balance, add the deposit to the original balance and subtract the check amounts.

**Solution**
$$\begin{array}{r} 1846.78 \\ +568.30 \\ \hline 2415.08 \\ -123.98 \\ \hline 2291.10 \\ -47.33 \\ \hline 2243.77 \end{array}$$

The family's new checking account balance is \$2243.77.

**29. Strategy** To find the cost per mile:
• Find the total cost by adding the expenses (\$1840, \$520, \$185, and \$432).
• Divide the total cost by the number of miles driven (10,000).

**Solution**
$$\begin{array}{r} 1840 \\ 820 \\ 185 \\ +432 \\ \hline 3277 \end{array}$$
$3277 \div 10{,}000 = 0.3277$

The cost per mile is about \$0.33.

**30. Strategy** To find the monthly mortgage

© 2013 Cengage Learning. All Rights Reserved. May not be scanned, copied or duplicated, or posted to a publicly accessible website, in whole or in part.

payment, multiply the mortgage amount by the monthly mortgage factor.

**Solution** $172{,}000 \times 0.0071643 \approx 1232.26$

The monthly mortgage payment is \$1232.26.

© 2013 Cengage Learning. All Rights Reserved. May not be scanned, copied or duplicated, or posted to a publicly accessible website, in whole or in part.

# Chapter 7: Statistics and Probability

## Prep Test

**1.** **Strategy** To find the percent of the mail that was bill-related, divide the total number of pieces of first-class mail (102 billion) by the number of pieces that were bill-related (49 billion).

**Solution** $\frac{49 \text{ billion}}{102 \text{ billion}} \approx 0.480 = 48.0\%$

48.0% was bill-related mail.

**2.** **Strategy** To determine between which two enrollment years the increase in cost is the greatest, find the difference between each pair of consecutive years.

**Solution** Between 2005 and 2006

$74{,}418 - 70{,}206 = 4212$

Between 2006 and 2007

$78{,}883 - 74{,}418 = 4465$

Between 2007 and 2008

$83{,}616 - 78{,}883 = 4733$

Between 2008 and 2009

$88{,}633 - 83{,}616 = 5017$

Between 2009 and 2010

$93{,}951 - 88{,}633 = 5318$

**a.** The greatest cost increase is between 2009 and 2010.

**b.** Between those years, there was an increase of $5318.

**3.** $\frac{45 \text{ gold}}{27 \text{ silver}} = \frac{45}{27} = \frac{5}{3}$

**4.** **Strategy** To find the fractional amount of women in the military that are in the Marine Corps:

- Find the number of women in the Marine Corps by writing and solving the basic percent equation using $n$ to represent the number of women in the Marine Corps. The percent is 6% and the base is 198,000.
- Write this amount over the total number of women in the military and reduce the fraction.

**Solution**

$$\begin{aligned} 6\% \times 198{,}000 &= n \\ 0.06 \times 198{,}000 &= n \\ 11{,}880 &= n \end{aligned}$$

11,880 women who are in the U.S. military serve in the Marine Corps.

$$\frac{11{,}880}{198{,}000} = \frac{3 \cdot 3960}{50 \cdot 3960} = \frac{3}{50}$$

The fractional amount is $\frac{3}{50}$.

## Section 7.1

### Objective A Exercises

**1.** **Strategy** To find the total:

• Read the pictograph to determine the number of patients in each age group.

• Add the three numbers.

**Solution**

$$\begin{aligned} \text{Under 5: } & 24 \times 5 = 120 \\ \text{5 - 64: } & 12 \times 5 = 60 \\ \text{65 - older: } & 6 \times 5 = \underline{30} \\ & \quad 210 \end{aligned}$$

© 2013 Cengage Learning. All Rights Reserved. May not be scanned, copied or duplicated, or posted to a publicly accessible website, in whole or in part.

210 patients visited the emergency room with asthma.

**3. Strategy** To find the percent, solve the basic percent equation for percent. The base is 210 (from Exercise 1 ) and the amount is the number under 5 (120).

**Solution** Percent × base = amount

$$n \times 210 = 120$$
$$n = 120 \div 210$$
$$n \approx 0.57$$
$$n = 57\%$$

The percent is 57%.

**5. Strategy** To find how more the rate for a certified dental assistant is than the rate for a certified nurse is, subtract the rate for certified nurse assistant ($10) from the rate for certified dental assistant ($14).

**Solution** $14 - 10 = 4$

The rate of certified dental assistant is $4 more than the rate for certified nurse assistant.

**7. Strategy** To find the number of children who said they hid vegetables under a napkin, write and solve the basic percent equation for amount. The percent is 30% and the base is 500.

**Solution** Percent × base = amount

$$0.30 \times 500 = 150$$

150 children said they hid their vegetables under a napkin.

**9.** No, the sum of the percents given in the graph is only 80%, not 100%.

**11.** Sample answers: David Koch and Charles Koch have the same net worth. Bill Gates's net worth is twice Larry Ellison's net worth. Warren Buffet's net worth is twice that of Chirsty Walton.

## Objective B Exercises

**13. Strategy** To determine whether the number of units required in anatomy/physiology is less than or greater than twice the number of units required in social/behavioral sciences:

- Multiply the number of units required in social/behavioral sciences (6) by 2.
- Compare this result to the number of units required in anatomy/physiology (8).

**Solution** $6 \times 2 = 12$

$$8 < 12$$

The number of units required in anatomy/ physiology is less than twice the number of units required in social/behavioral sciences.

**15. Strategy** To find the total:

- Read the circle graph to determine the number in each blood group.
- Add the numbers.

© 2013 Cengage Learning. All Rights Reserved. May not be scanned, copied or duplicated, or posted to a publicly accessible website, in whole or in part.

**Solution**

$$\begin{aligned} O+ &= 35 \\ O- &= 7 \\ A+ &= 30 \\ A- &= 7 \\ B+ &= 8 \\ B- &= 1 \\ AB+ &= 2 \\ AB- &= \underline{0} \\ & \phantom{=}\ 90 \end{aligned}$$

There were 90 blood donors.

**17. Strategy** To find the percent, solve the basic percent equation for percent. The base is 90 (from Exercise 15) and the amount is the number of Type A+ donors (30).

**Solution**

$$\begin{aligned} \text{Percent} \times \text{base} &= \text{amount} \\ n \times 90 &= 30 \\ n &= 30 \div 90 \\ n &\approx 33.3 \\ n &= 33.3\% \end{aligned}$$

The percent is 33.3%.

**19. Strategy** To find the amount of money allocated for housing and utilities:

- Read the circle graph to find the percent of money allocated for housing and utilities.
- Use the basic percent equation to find the amount. The base is $125,000.

**Solution** 33% is allocated of housing and utilities.

$$\begin{aligned} \text{Percent} \times \text{base} &= \text{amount} \\ 0.33 \times 125{,}000 &= n \\ 42{,}150 &= n \end{aligned}$$

$42,150 was allocated yearly for housing and utilities.

**Strategy** To find the monthly allocation for housing and utilities, divide the yearly allocation by the number of months in a year (12).

**Solution** $41{,}250 \div 12 = 3{,}437.5$

$3,437.50 is allocated monthly for housing and utilities.

**21. Strategy** To find the fractional amount allocated for food, change the percent allocated for food (15%) to a fraction in lowest terms.

**Solution** $15\% = \frac{15}{100} = \frac{3}{20}$

$\frac{3}{20}$ is allocated for food.

**23.** The age group 35 to 44 represents the largest segment.

**25. Strategy** To find the percent of the homeless population under 35, add the percent of homeless under 25 (12%) and the percent of homeless aged 25 to 34 (25%).

**Solution** 12% + 25% = 37%

The percent of the homeless population under age 35 is 37%.

**27. Strategy** To find the total number of students enrolled in health care programs:

- Read the circle graph to determine the number in each program.
- Add the five numbers.

© 2013 Cengage Learning. All Rights Reserved. May not be scanned, copied or duplicated, or posted to a publicly accessible website, in whole or in part.

**Solution**

| | |
|---|---|
| 30 | Medial Lab Technology |
| 45 | Medical Assistant |
| 125 | Nursing |
| 38 | Dental Assistant |
| 52 | Nursing Assistant |
| 290 | |

There are 290 students enrolled in Health Programs.

**29. Strategy** To find the percent:

• Read the circle graph to determine the number in the medical assistant program.

• Write and solve the basic percent equation for percent. The amount is the number in the medical assistant program and the base is the total from Exercise 27.

**Solution** The number in the medical assistant program is 45.

$$\begin{aligned} \text{Percent} \times \text{base} &= \text{amount} \\ n \times 290 &= 45 \\ n &= 45 \div 290 \\ n &\approx 0.155 \\ n &= 15.5\% \end{aligned}$$

15.5 % are enrolled in the medical assistant program.

**31. Strategy** To find the number of people living in the United States that are of Asian ethnic origin:

• Locate the percent of the population that is Asian.

• Solve the basic percent equation for amount.

**Solution** Percent that is Asian: 4.5%

$$\text{Percent} \times \text{base} = \text{amount}$$
$$0.045 \times 300{,}000{,}000 = 13{,}500{,}000$$

13,500,000 people are of Asian ethnic origin.

**33. Strategy** To find the average number of people of black ethnic origin would be in a random sample of 500,000 people living in the United States:

• Locate the percent of the population that is of black ethnic origin.

• Solve the basic percent equation.

**Solution** Percent that is of black ethnic origin: 12.9%

$$\text{Percent} \times \text{base} = \text{amount}$$
$$0.129 \times 500{,}000 = 64{,}500$$

There would be an average of 64,500 people of black ethnic origin.

## Applying the Concepts

**35.** Answers will vary. For example: The couple's largest single expense was rent.

Food represents approximately one-quarter of the month's expenditures.

Rent represents approximately one-third of the month's expenditures.

The expenditure for food is approximately the same as the expenditures for entertainment and transportation.

The couple spent more for transportation than for entertainment.

© 2013 Cengage Learning. All Rights Reserved. May not be scanned, copied or duplicated, or posted to a publicly accessible website, in whole or in part.

## Section 7.2

### Objective A Exercises

**1. Strategy** To find the number of Americans over 65 with diabetes, read the bar graph to determine the height.

**Solution** Approximately 27% of Americans over 65 have diabetes.

**3. Strategy** To find the ratio of the age 45 – 64 to ages 20 - 44:

- Read the bar graph to determine the percents for these groups.
- Write the ratio and simplify.

**Solution** 45 – 64: 14%

20 – 44: 4%

$$\frac{14\%}{4\%} = \frac{7}{2}$$

The ratio is 7 to 2.

**5. Strategy** To find the difference:

- Read the bar graph to find the life expectancy in 2010 and the life expectancy in 1930.
- Subtract the two numbers.

**Solution**

$$\begin{array}{rl} 76 & \quad 2010 \\ \underline{-58} & \quad 1930 \\ 18 & \end{array}$$

The difference is 18 years.

**7. Strategy** To estimate the difference between the maximum and minimum salaries for a physical therapist?

- Read the double-bar graph for the maximum salary for a physical therapist and the minimum salary.
- Subtract to find the difference between the two salaries.

**Solution**

$$\begin{array}{lr} \text{Maximum salary:} & 70 \\ \text{Minimum salary:} & \underline{-55} \\ & 15 \end{array}$$

The maximum salary for a physical therapist is $15,000 more than the minimum salary.

**9. Strategy** To find which occupation has the greatest difference between the maximum salary and the minimum salary.

- Read the double-bar graph to find maximum salaries and minimum salaries for each group.
- Subtract the minimum salary from the maximum.

**Solution** Physical Therapist.:

70 – 55 = 15

Medical Lab Technologist:

56 – 41 = 14

Occupational Therapist:

65 – 50 = 15

Dental Hygienist:

78 – 56 = 22

Physician Assistant:

88 – 70 = 18

The greatest difference in salaries is for Dental Hygienist.

**11.** (iii)

### Objective B Exercises

**13. Strategy** To find the blood glucose level, read the broken-line graph for 10 P.M. Tuesday.

© 2013 Cengage Learning. All Rights Reserved. May not be scanned, copied or duplicated, or posted to a publicly accessible website, in whole or in part.

| | | |
|---|---|---|
| | **Solution** | The blood glucose level at 10 P.M. Tuesday was 200 milligrams/deciliter. |
| **15.** | **Strategy** | To find number of readings that are outside the normal range, count the number of readings that are above 125 or below 50. |
| | **Solution** | 6 readings are outside the normal range. |
| **17.** | **Strategy** | To find the percent of adults in 2007, read the broken-line graph for 2007. |
| | **Solution** | In 2007, 30% of adults over 18 years old took the influenza vaccine. |
| **19.** | **Strategy** | To find the percent increase between 2008 and 2009:<br>• Find the percents for 2008 and 2009.<br>• Find the difference. |
| | **Solution** | 2008: 32%<br>2009: 34%<br>34% − 32% = 2%<br>There was a 2% increase in the number vaccines between 2008 and 2009. |
| **21.** | **Strategy** | To find what age and gender has the lowest number of recommended Calories, read the double broken-line graph and select the age and gender beneath the lowest point. |
| | **Solution** | The age and gender that has the lowest number of recommended Calories is for women age 75+. |

**23.** True

**24.** True

## Applying the Concepts

**25.**

| Year | Wind Power Capacity in Texas (megawatts) | Wind Power Capacity in California (megawatts) |
|---|---|---|
| 2000 | 200 | 1600 |
| 2001 | 1100 | 1700 |
| 2002 | 1100 | 1800 |
| 2003 | 1300 | 2000 |
| 2004 | 1300 | 2100 |
| 2005 | 2000 | 2200 |
| 2006 | 2700 | 2400 |
| 2007 | 4300 | 2400 |

# Section 7.3

## Objective A Exercises

| | | |
|---|---|---|
| **1.** | **Strategy** | Read the histogram to find the number of account balances between $1500 and $2000. |
| | **Solution** | 13 account balances were between $1500 and $2000. |
| **3.** | **Strategy** | To find the percent:<br>• Read the histogram to find the number of account balances between $2000 and $2500.<br>• Solve the basic percent equation for percent. The base is 50 and the amount is the number of account balances between $2000 and $2500. |
| | **Solution** | Number of account balances between $2000 and $2500: 11 |

© 2013 Cengage Learning. All Rights Reserved. May not be scanned, copied or duplicated, or posted to a publicly accessible website, in whole or in part.

Percent × base = amount

$n \times 50 = 11$

$n = 11 \div 50$

$n = 0.22$

The percent is 22%.

**5. Strategy** To find the number of temperatures below 98.6°,

• Read the histogram to find the number of temperatures between 95.5° and 96.5°, between 96.5° and 97.5° and between 97.5° and 98.5°.

• Add the three numbers.

**Solution**

95.5° to 96.5°: 1 patient

96.5° to 97.5°: 7 patients

97.5° to 98.5°: + 13 patients

21 patients

There were 21 adults with temperatures below normal.

**7. Strategy** To find the ratio:

• Read the histogram to find the number adults with temperatures between 96.5° and 97.5°.

• Add all of the numbers to find the total number of adults.

• Write the ratio of the number between 96.5° and 97.5° to the total in simplest terms.

**Solution** Between 96.5° and 97.5°: 7

Total: 1 + 7 + 13 + 9 = 30

$\frac{7}{30}$

The ratio is 7 to 30.

**9.** The largest number of adults had a temperature between 97.5° and 98.5°, so it would seem that a "normal" temperature would be within that range.

**11. Strategy** To find the total under 200:

• Read the histogram to find the number of patients with readings between 0 and 100 and the number between 100 and 200.

• Add the two numbers.

**Solution** Between 0 and 100: 8

Between 100 and 200: 13

8 + 13 = 21

21 patients had readings lower than 200.

## Objective B Exercises

**13. Strategy** To find the number of runners, find the sum of all the runners who had finishing times between 2 ½ hours and 6 hours.

**Solution**

1000

5500

8000

4000

2000

1000

+500

22,000

There were 22,000 finishers.

**15.** Yes

**17. Strategy** To find the percent:

• Read the frequency polygon to find how many people were taller than 68 inches.

• Add all of the frequencies to get the total number of women.

• Solve the basic percent equation for percent. The base is total number of women and the amount is the number of women over 68 inches.

**Solution** Total: 8 + 9 + 6 + 1 + 1 = 25

Over 68 inches: 1 + 1 = 2

© 2013 Cengage Learning. All Rights Reserved. May not be scanned, copied or duplicated, or posted to a publicly accessible website, in whole or in part.

Percent × base = amount

$n \times 25 = 2$

$n = 2 \div 25$

$n = 0.08$

$n = 8\%$

8% of the women are over 68 inches tall.

**19.** **Strategy** To find the number of students who scored between 700 and 800, read the frequency polygon.

**Solution** 100,000 students scored between 700 and 800.

**21.** **Strategy** To find the number of students:

- Read the frequency polygon to find the number of students who scored between 200 and 300, between 300 and 400, and between 400 and 500.
- Add the three numbers.

**Solution**

| | |
|---|---|
| Between 200 and 300: | 40,000 |
| Between 300 and 400: | 190,000 |
| Between 400 and 500: | + 460,000 |
| | 690,000 |

690,000 students scored below 500.

# Section 7.4

## Objective A Exercises

**1a.** Median

**b.** Mean

**c.** Mode

**d.** Median

**e.** Mode

**f.** Mean

**3.** **Strategy** To find the mean value of the amount of sugar:

- Find the sum of amounts of sugar.
- Divide the sum by the number of soft drinks (6).

**Solution**

$$\begin{array}{r} 40.5 \\ 40 \\ 47 \\ 40 \\ 39 \\ +41 \\ \hline 217.5 \end{array} \qquad \begin{array}{r} 41.25 \\ 6\overline{)217.50} \end{array}$$

The mean of the number of calories s 41.25 calories.

**Strategy** To find the median value of the number of calories, arrange the numbers in order from smallest to largest. The median is the mean of the two middle numbers.

**Solution**

$$\left.\begin{array}{l} 39 \\ 40 \end{array}\right\} \text{2 numbers}$$

$$\left.\begin{array}{l} 40 \\ 40.5 \end{array}\right\} \text{Middle numbers}$$

$$\left.\begin{array}{l} 41 \\ 39 \end{array}\right\} \text{2 numbers}$$

$$\frac{40 + 40.5}{2} = 40.25$$

The median of the number of calories is 40.25 calories.

**Strategy** To find the mode, look at the number of calories and locate the number that occurs most frequently.

**Solution** Since 40 appears the most often, the mode is 40 calories.

**5.** **Strategy** To find the mean cost:

- Find the sum of the costs.
- Divide the total costs by the number of purchases (8).

**Solution**

$$\begin{array}{r} 85.89 \\ 92.12 \\ 81.43 \\ 80.67 \\ 88.73 \\ 82.45 \\ 87.81 \\ +\,85.82 \\ \hline 684.92 \end{array} \qquad \begin{array}{r} 85.615 \\ 8\overline{)684.920} \end{array}$$

The mean cost is \$85.615.

© 2013 Cengage Learning. All Rights Reserved. May not be scanned, copied or duplicated, or posted to a publicly accessible website, in whole or in part.

**Strategy** To find the median cost, arrange the costs in order from smallest to largest. The median is the mean of the two middle numbers.

**Solution**

$$\left.\begin{matrix}80.67\\81.43\\82.45\end{matrix}\right\}\text{3 numbers}$$
$$\left.\begin{matrix}85.82\\85.89\end{matrix}\right\}\text{middle numbers}$$
$$\left.\begin{matrix}87.81\\88.73\\92.12\end{matrix}\right\}\text{3 numbers}$$

$$\frac{85.82+85.88}{2}=85.85$$

The median cost is $85.85

The median is 28 years.

**7.** **Strategy** To find the mean monthly rate:

- Find the sum of the monthly rates.
- Divide the sum by the number of plans (8).

**Solution**

$$\begin{array}{r}423\\390\\405\\396\\426\\355\\404\\+\,430\\\hline 3{,}229\end{array}\qquad 8\overline{)3{,}229.000}\ \ 403.625$$

The mean monthly rate is $403.625.

**Strategy** To find the median monthly rate, write the rates in order from smallest to largest. The median is the mean of the two middle terms.

**Solution**

$$\left.\begin{matrix}355\\390\\396\end{matrix}\right\}\text{3 numbers}$$
$$\left.\begin{matrix}404\\405\end{matrix}\right\}\text{middle numbers}$$
$$\left.\begin{matrix}423\\426\\430\end{matrix}\right\}\text{3 numbers}$$

$$\frac{404+405}{2}=404.50$$

The median monthly rate is $404.50.

**9a.** **Strategy** To find the mean life expectancy:

- Find the sum of the years.
- Divide the sum by the number of countries (10).

**Solution**

$$\begin{array}{r}72\\77\\77\\77\\70\\75\\70\\67\\76\\+73\\\hline 734\end{array}\qquad 10\overline{)734.0}\ \ 73.4$$

The mean life expectancy is 73.4 years.

**b.** **Strategy** To find the median life expectancy, write the years in order from lowest to highest. The median is the mean of the two middle numbers.

**Solution**

$$\left.\begin{matrix}67\\70\\70\\72\end{matrix}\right\}\text{4 numbers}$$
$$\left.\begin{matrix}73\\75\end{matrix}\right\}\text{middle numbers}$$
$$\left.\begin{matrix}76\\77\\77\\77\end{matrix}\right\}\text{4 numbers}$$

$$\frac{73+75}{2}=74$$

The median life expectancy is 74 years.

**11.** No, the mean scores of the two students are not the same. The mean score of the second student is 5 points higher than the mean score of the first student.

© 2013 Cengage Learning. All Rights Reserved. May not be scanned, copied or duplicated, or posted to a publicly accessible website, in whole or in part.

## Objective B Exercises

**13a.** 25%

**b.** 75%

**c.** 75%

**d.** 25%

**f.** **Strategy** Find the range by subtracting the youngest from the oldest.

**Solution** Range: 69–42 = 27 years

**g.** **Strategy** Interquartile range = $Q_3 - Q_1$.

**Solution** Interquartile range = 58 – 51 = 7 years

**15.** **Strategy**
- Read the lowest value, the highest value, the first quartile, the third quartile, the median directly from the box-and-whiskers plot.
- Find the range by subtracting the lowest from the highest.
- Interquartile range = $Q_3 - Q_1$.

**Solution** Lowest is \$46,596.
Highest is \$82,879.
$Q_1$ = \$56,067
$Q_3$ = \$66,507
Median = \$61,036
Range: 82,879 – 46,596 = \$36,283
Interquartile range:
66,507 – 56,067 = \$10,440

**17a.** **Strategy** To find the number of adults who had a cholesterol level above 217, the median, solve the basic percent equation for the amount, where the base is 80 and the percent is 50%.

**Solution** Percent × base = amount
$0.50 \times 80 = 40$
There were 40 adults who had cholesterol levels above 217.

**b.** **Strategy** To find the number of adults who had a cholesterol level below 254, the third quartile, solve the basic percent equation for the amount, where the base is 80 and the percent is 75%.

**Solution** Percent × base = amount
$0.75 \times 80 = 60$
There were 60 adults who had cholesterol levels below 254.

**c.** **Strategy** To find the number of cholesterol levels represented in each quartile, solve the basic percent equation for the amount, where the base is 80 and the percent is 25%.

**Solution** Percent × base = amount
$0.25 \times 80 = 20$
There are 20 cholesterol levels in each quartile.

**d.** The first quartile is at 198. So 25% of the adults had cholesterol levels not more than 198.

© 2013 Cengage Learning. All Rights Reserved. May not be scanned, copied or duplicated, or posted to a publicly accessible website, in whole or in part.

**19a. Strategy**
- Arrange the data from smallest to largest.
- Find the range.
- Find $Q_1$, the median of the lower half of the data.
- Find $Q_3$, the median of the upper half of the data.
- Interquartile range = $Q_3 - Q_1$.

**Solution**

| | | | | |
|---|---|---|---|---|
| 0.45 | 0.47 | 0.59 | 0.64 | 0.81 |
| 1.26 | 1.34 | 1.52 | 5.01 | 6.05 |

Range: 6.05 – 0.45 = 5.6 million metric tons

$Q_1$ = 0.59 million metric tons

$Q_3$ = 1.52 million metric tons

$$\begin{aligned}\text{Interquartile range} &= Q_3 - Q_1 \\ &= 1.52 - 0.59 \\ &= 0.93 \text{ million metric tons}\end{aligned}$$

**b.** Median $= \dfrac{0.81 + 1.26}{2} \approx 0.643$

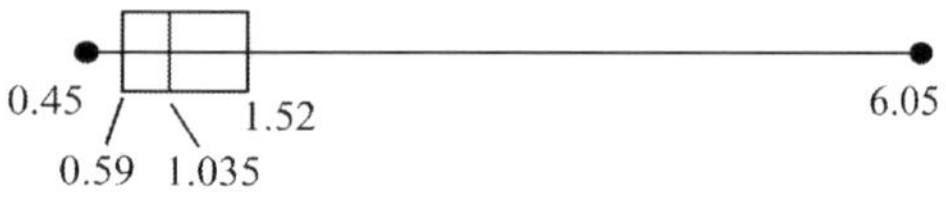


**c.** 6.05

**21a. Strategy** To determine whether the difference in means is greater than 1 inch:
- Find the sum of the rainfall in Orlando.
- Divide the sum by the number of months (12) to find the mean.
- Find the sum of the rainfall in Portland.
- Divide the sum by the number of months (12) to find the mean.
- Find the difference in the means.

**Solution**

| Orlando | | Portland | |
|---|---|---|---|
| 2.1 | | 6.2 | |
| 2.8 | | 3.9 | |
| 3.2 | | 3.6 | |
| 2.2 | | 2.3 | |
| 4.0 | | 2.1 | |
| 7.4 | | 1.5 | |
| 7.8 | | 0.5 | |
| 6.3 | $\begin{array}{r} 4.0 \\ 12\overline{)47.8} \end{array}$ | 1.1 | $\begin{array}{r} 3.1 \\ 12\overline{)37.5} \end{array}$ |
| 5.6 | | 1.6 | |
| 2.8 | | 3.1 | |
| 1.8 | | 5.2 | |
| + 1.8 | | + 6.4 | |
| 47.8 | | 37.5 | |

© 2013 Cengage Learning. All Rights Reserved. May not be scanned, copied or duplicated, or posted to a publicly accessible website, in whole or in part.

4.0 – 3.1 = 0.9

No, the difference in the means is not greater than 1 inch.

**b.** **Strategy** To find the difference between the medians, write the rainfall in order from lowest to highest. The median is the mean of the two middle numbers. Find the difference between the Orlando median and Portland median.

**Solution**

| Orlando | | Portland | |
|---|---|---|---|
| 1.8, 1.8, 2.1, 2.2, 2.8 | 5 numbers | 0.5, 1.1, 1.5, 1.6, 2.1 | 5 numbers |
| 2.8, 3.2 | middle | 2.3, 3.1 | middle |
| 4.0, 5.6, 6.3, 7.4, 7.8 | 5 numbers | 3.6, 3.9, 5.2, 6.2, 6.4 | 5 numbers |

For Orlando, $\dfrac{2.8 + 3.2}{2} = 3.0$

For Portland, $\dfrac{2.3 + 3.1}{2} = 2.7$

$3.0 - 2.7 = 0.3$

The difference in medians is 0.3 inch.

**c.** **Strategy** To draw box-and-whiskers:

- Find $Q_1$ and $Q_3$ in Orlando.
- Find $Q_1$ and $Q_3$ in Portland.

**Solution**

For Orlando, $Q_1 = \dfrac{2.1 + 2.2}{2} = 2.15$,

$Q_3 = \dfrac{5.6 + 6.3}{2} = 5.95$

For Portland, $Q_1 = \dfrac{1.5 + 1.6}{2} = 1.55$,

$Q_3 = \dfrac{3.9 + 5.2}{2} = 4.55$

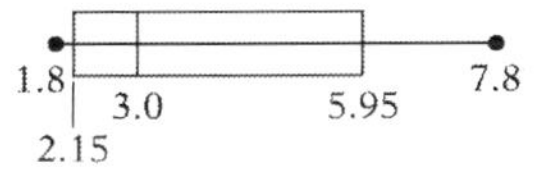


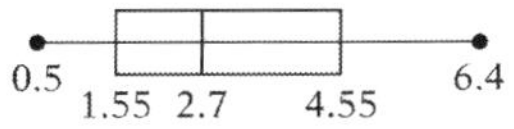


**d.** Answers will vary. For example, the distribution of the data is relatively similar for the two cities. However, the value of each of the 5 points on the boxplot for the Portland data is less than the corresponding value on the boxplot for the Orlando data. The average monthly rainfall in Portland is less than the average monthly rainfall in Orlando.

© 2013 Cengage Learning. All Rights Reserved. May not be scanned, copied or duplicated, or posted to a publicly accessible website, in whole or in part.

**23.** Answers will vary. For example, 55, 55, 55, 55, 55, or 50, 55, 55, 55, 60

## Applying the Concepts

**25a.** $Q_1$ is the number that one-quarter of the data lie below.

**b.** $Q_3$ is the number that one-quarter of the data lie above.

**c.** $\bar{x}$ is the symbol for the mean of a set of data.

**27.** Answers will vary. For example, 20, 21, 22, 24, 26, 27, 29, 31, 31, 32, 32, 33, 33, 36, 37, 37, 39, 40, 41, 43, 45, 46, 50, 54, 57

# Section 7.5

## Objective A Exercises

**1.** The possible outcomes of tossing a coin four times: {(HHHH), (HHHT), (HHTT), (HHTH), (HTTT), (HTHH), (HTTH), (HTHT), (TTTT), (TTTH), (TTHH), (THHH), (TTHT), (THHT), (THTT), (THTH)}

**3.** The possible outcomes of tossing two tetrahedral dice: {(1, 1), (1, 2), (1, 3), (1, 4), (2, 1), (2, 2), (2, 3), (2, 4), (3, 1), (3, 2), (3, 3), (3, 4), (4, 1), (4, 2), (4, 3), (4, 4)}

**5a.** The sample space is {1, 2, 3, 4, 5, 6, 7, 8}.

**b.** The outcomes in the event the number is less than 4 is {1, 2, 3}.

**7a.** **Strategy** To calculate the probability:
- Count the number of possible outcomes. See the table on p. 323.
- Count the number of favorable outcomes.
- Use the probability formula.

**Solution** There are 36 possible outcomes.
There are 4 favorable outcomes: (1, 4), (4, 1), (2, 3), (3, 2).

$$\text{Probability} = \frac{4}{36} = \frac{1}{9}$$

The probability that the sum is 5 is $\frac{1}{9}$.

**b.** **Strategy** To calculate the probability:
- Count the number of possible outcomes. See the table on p. 323.
- Count the number of favorable outcomes.
- Use the probability formula.

**Solution** There are 36 possible outcomes.
There are 0 favorable outcomes.

$$\text{Probability} = \frac{0}{36} = 0$$

The probability that the sum is 15 is 0.

**c.** **Strategy** To calculate the probability:
- Count the number of possible outcomes. See the table on p. 323.
- Count the number of favorable outcomes.
- Use the probability formula.

**Solution** There are 36 possible outcomes.
There are 36 favorable outcomes.

$$\text{Probability} = \frac{36}{36} = 1$$

The probability that the sum is less than 15 is 1.

© 2013 Cengage Learning. All Rights Reserved. May not be scanned, copied or duplicated, or posted to a publicly accessible website, in whole or in part.

**d. Strategy** To calculate the probability:

• Count the number of possible outcomes. See the table on p. 323.

• Count the number of favorable outcomes.

• Use the probability formula.

**Solution** There are 36 possible outcomes. There is 1 favorable outcome: (1, 1).

$$\text{Probability} = \frac{1}{36}$$

The probability that the sum is 2 is $\frac{1}{36}$.

**9a. Strategy** To calculate the probability:

• Count the number of possible outcomes.

• Count the number of favorable outcomes.

• Use the probability formula.

**Solution** A dodecahedral die has 12 sides. There are 3 favorable outcomes: 4, 8, 12.

$$\text{Probability} = \frac{3}{12} = \frac{1}{4}$$

The probability that the number is divisible by 4 is $\frac{1}{4}$.

**b. Strategy** To calculate the probability:

• Count the number of possible outcomes.

• Count the number of favorable outcomes.

• Use the probability formula.

**Solution** A dodecahedral die has 12 sides. There are 4 favorable outcomes: 3, 6, 9, 12.

$$\text{Probability} = \frac{4}{12} = \frac{1}{3}$$

The probability that the number is a multiple of 3 is $\frac{1}{3}$.

**11. Strategy** To calculate the probability:

• Count the number of possible outcomes. See the table on p. 323.

• Count the number of favorable outcomes.

• Use the probability formula.

• Compare the probabilities.

**Solution** There are 36 possible outcomes. For a sum of 10, there are 3 favorable outcomes: (5, 5), (4, 6), (6, 4).

$$\text{Probability} = \frac{3}{36}$$

For a sum of 5, there are 4 favorable outcomes: (1, 4), (4, 1), (2, 3), (3, 2).

$$\text{Probability} = \frac{4}{36}$$

$$\frac{4}{36} > \frac{3}{36}$$

The probability of throwing a sum of 5 is greater.

**13a. Strategy** To calculate the probability:

• Count the number of possible outcomes.

• Count the number of favorable outcomes.

• Use the probability formula.

**Solution** There are 11 possible outcomes. There are 4 favorable outcomes.

$$\text{Probability} = \frac{4}{11}$$

The probability is $\frac{4}{11}$ that the

© 2013 Cengage Learning. All Rights Reserved. May not be scanned, copied or duplicated, or posted to a publicly accessible website, in whole or in part.

letter $I$ is drawn.

**Strategy** To calculate the probability:

- Count the number of possible outcomes.
- Count the number of favorable outcomes.
- Use the probability formula.
- Compare the probabilities.

**Solution** There are 11 possible outcomes. There are 4 favorable outcomes of choosing an $S$.

$$\text{Probability} = \frac{4}{11}$$

There are 2 favorable outcomes of choosing a $P$.

$$\text{Probability} = \frac{2}{11}$$

$$\frac{4}{11} > \frac{2}{11}$$

The probability of choosing an $S$ is greater.

**15.** The letter $M$ appears one time in the word *MISSISSIPPI,* so $\frac{1}{11}$ represents the probability that the card has the letter $M$ on it.

**17.** **Strategy** To calculate the probability:

- Count the number of possible outcomes.
- Count the number of favorable outcomes.
- Use the probability formula.
- Compare the probabilities.

**Solution** There are 52 possible outcomes. There are 12 favorable outcomes of drawing a jack, queen, or king.

$$\text{Probability} = \frac{12}{52} = \frac{3}{13}$$

There are 13 favorable outcomes of drawing a spade.

$$\text{Probability} = \frac{13}{52} = \frac{1}{4}$$

$$\frac{13}{52} > \frac{12}{52}$$

The probability of drawing a spade is greater.

**19.** **Strategy** To calculate the empirical probability, use the probability formula and divide the number of observations (63) by the total number of observations (3328). Write the answer as a percent.

**Solution**

$$\text{Probability} = \frac{63}{3328} \approx 0.019$$
$$= 1.9\%$$

The probability of death after bariatric surgery is 1.9%.

**21a.** **Strategy** To calculate the number who experience headaches, solve the expected value equation. The probability is 14% and $n$ is 35.

**Solution** $14\% \times 35 =$

$0.14 \times 35 = 4.9 \approx 5$

About 5 patients will experience headaches.

**b.** **Strategy** To calculate the expected number who should experience dizziness, solve the expected value equation. The probability is 10% and $n = 65$. Compare this to 5.

$10\% \times 65 = 0.10 \times 65 = 6.5$

$5 < 6.5$

5 is less than the expected value.

© 2013 Cengage Learning. All Rights Reserved. May not be scanned, copied or duplicated, or posted to a publicly accessible website, in whole or in part.

### Applying the Concepts

**23.** The mathematical probability of an event is a number from 0 to 1. Because $\frac{5}{3} = 1\frac{2}{3}, \frac{5}{3} > 1.$

The probability of an even cannot be $\frac{5}{3}$ because the probability cannot be greater than 1.

## Chapter 7 Concept Review

**1.** A sector of a circle is one of the "pieces of the pie" into which a circle graph is divided.

**2.** A pictograph uses symbols to represent numerical information.

**3.** A jagged portion of the vertical axis on a bar graph is used to indicate that the vertical scale is missing numbers from 0 to the lowest number shown on the vertical axis.

**4.** In a broken-line graph, points are connected by line segments to show data trends. If a line segment goes up from left to right, it indicates an increase in the quantity represented on the vertical axis during that time period. If a line segment goes down from left to right, it indicates a decrease in the quantity represented on the vertical axis during that time period.

**5.** Class frequency in a histogram is the number of occurrences of data in each class interval.

**6.** A class interval in a histogram is a range of numbers that corresponds to the width of each bar.

**7.** A class midpoint is the center of a class interval in a frequency polygon.

**8.** The formula for the mean is

$$\bar{x} = \frac{\text{sum of the data values}}{\text{number of data values}}.$$

**9.** To find the median, the data must be arranged in order from least to greatest in order to determine the "middle" number, or the number which separates the data so that half of the numbers are less than the median and half of the numbers are greater than the median.

**10.** If a set of numbers has no number occurring more than once, then the data have no mode.

**11.** A box-and-whisker plot shows the least number in the data; the first quartile, $Q_1$; the median; the third quartile, $Q_3$; and the greatest number in the data.

**12.** To find the first quartile, find the median of the data values that lie below the median.

**13.** The empirical probability formula states that the empirical probability of an event is the ratio of the number of observations of the event to the total number of observations.

**14.** The theoretical probability formula states that the theoretical probability of an event is a fraction with the number of favorable outcomes of the experiment in the numerator and the total number of possible outcomes in the denominator.

© 2013 Cengage Learning. All Rights Reserved. May not be scanned, copied or duplicated, or posted to a publicly accessible website, in whole or in part.

## Chapter 7 Review Exercises

1. Strategy To find the amount of money:
   - Read the circle graph to determine the amounts of money spent.
   - Add the amounts.

   Solution

| | |
|---|---|
| Hospital Inpatient | 139.3 |
| Skilled Nursing | 26.2 |
| Physician Fee | 67.3 |
| Hospital Outpatient | 31.1 |
| Group Plans | 116.2 |
| Prescription Drugs | 58.2 |
| Home Health Agencies | 19.6 |
| Other | +63.0 |
| | 520.9 |

   Medicare Benefits totaled $520.9 billion in 2010.

2. **Strategy** To find the ratio:
   - Read the circle graph to find the amount spent on the skilled nursing facilities and on prescription drugs.
   - Write, in simplest form, the ratio of the amount spent on skilled nursing facilities to the amount spent on prescription drugs.

   **Solution** Skilled Nursing: $26.2 billion
   Prescription Drugs: $58.2 billion

   $$\frac{26.2 \text{ billion}}{58.2 \text{ billion}} = \frac{131}{291}$$

   The ratio is $\frac{131}{291}$.

3. **Strategy** To find the percent, solve the basic percent equation for percent. The base is the total amount spent ($520.9 billion) and the amount is the amount spent for hospital inpatient services ($139.3 billion)

   **Solution** Percent × base = amount

   $$n \times 520.9 \text{ billion} = 58.2 \text{ billion}$$
   $$n = 58.2 \div 520.9$$
   $$n \approx 0.2675$$
   $$n \approx 26.7\%$$

   26.7%of the total amount of money was spent on hospital inpatient services.

4. Texas had the larger population.

5. **Strategy** To find the difference in populations:
   - Read the double broken-line graph to find the Texas population and the California population in 2000.
   - Subtract the population of Texas from the population of California.

   **Solution**

| | |
|---|---|
| California : | 32.5 |
| Texas : | −20.0 |
| | 12.5 |

   The population of California is 12.5 million people more than the population of Texas.

6. **Strategy** To find which 25-year period Texas had the smallest increase in population.
   - Read the double-line graph to find the population for each 25-year period.
   - Subtract the two numbers.

   **Solution** 1900 to 1925:
   6 – 2.5 = 3.5 million
   1925 to 1950:
   8 – 6 = 2 million
   1950 to 1975:

© 2013 Cengage Learning. All Rights Reserved. May not be scanned, copied or duplicated, or posted to a publicly accessible website, in whole or in part.

12 – 8 = 4 million

1975 to 2000:

21 – 12 = 9 million

The Texas population increased the least from 1925 to 1950.

**7. Strategy** To find the number of women that are shorter than 65 inches:

- Read the frequency polygon to find the number of women between 60 – 65 inches and between 55 – 60 inches.
- Add the two numbers.

**Solution**

| | |
|---|---|
| 60 – 65 inches: | 19 women |
| 55 – 60 inches: | + 3 women |
| | 22 women |

There were 22 women under 65 inches.

**8. Strategy** To find the ratio:

- Read the frequency polygon to find the number of women between 55 and 60 inches and between 70 and 75 inches.
- Write in simplest form the ratio of the number of women between 55 and 60 inches and between 70 and 75 inches.

**Solution** 55 to 60 inches : 3 women

70 to 75 inches: 1 woman

$$\frac{3 \text{ woman}}{1 \text{ woman}} = \frac{3}{1}$$

The ratio is $\frac{3}{1}$.

**9. Strategy** To find the percent:

- Read the frequency polygon to find the number of women between 65 to 70 inches and between 70 and 75 inches.
- Add the two numbers.
- Solve the basic percent equation for percent. The base is total number of women and the amount is the number of women over 65 inches tall.

**Solution**

| | |
|---|---|
| 55 to 60 inches: | 3 |
| 60 to 65 inches: | 19 |
| 65 to 70 inches: | 13 |
| 70 to 75 inches: | + 1 |
| Total number: | 36 |

| | |
|---|---|
| 65 to 70 inches: | 13 |
| 70 to 75 inches: | + 1 |
| Total Under 65: | 14 |

Percent × base = amount

$$n \times 36 = 14$$
$$n = 14 \div 36$$
$$n \approx 0.3888$$
$$n = 38.9\%$$

The percent is 38.9%.

**10.** From the pictograph, O'Hare airport has 10 million more passengers than Los Angeles airport.

**11. Strategy** To find the ratio:

- Read the pictograph to find the number of passengers going through Hartsfield airport and the number of passengers going through Dallas/ Ft. Worth airport.
- Write in simplest form the ratio of the number of passengers going through Hartsfield airport to the number of passengers going through Dallas/Ft. Worth airport.

**Solution** Hartsfield: 40

Dallas = Ft. Worth: 30

$$\frac{40}{30} = \frac{4}{3} = 4:3$$

The ratio is 4 : 3.

© 2013 Cengage Learning. All Rights Reserved. May not be scanned, copied or duplicated, or posted to a publicly accessible website, in whole or in part.

**12.** **Strategy** To find the difference between the Non-Hispanic white boys who were classified as obese in 1988 to 1994 and in 2007 to 2008:

• Read the double-bar graph for the percent in 1988 to 1994 and the percent in 2007 to 2008.

• Subtract the two numbers.

**Solution**

$$\begin{array}{lr} \text{2007 to 2008:} & 17\% \\ \text{1988 to 1994:} & \underline{-\ 12\%} \\ & 5\% \end{array}$$

The difference was 5%.

**13.** **Strategy** To find the number:

• Read the double-bar graph to find the percent of Non-Hispanic black boys that were classified as obese in 1988 to 1994.

• Solve the basic percent equation for percent. The base is the number of boys studied (150) and percent is the percent of Non-Hispanic black boys that were classified as obese in 1988 to 1994.

**Solution** Number studied: 150

Percent: 10%

$$\begin{aligned} \text{Percent} \times \text{base} &= \text{amount} \\ 10\% \times 150 &= n \\ 0.10 \times 150 &= n \\ 15 &= n \end{aligned}$$

There will be 15 obese boys.

**14.** **Strategy** To determine which group has the largest increase, read the graph and select the group with the largest difference between the two bars.

**Solution** Mexican Americans had the largest increase.

**Strategy** To determine the increase:

• Read the double-bar graph to determine the percent in 1988 to 1994 and the percent in 2007 – 2008.

• Subtract the two numbers.

**Solution**

$$\begin{array}{lr} \text{2007 to 2008:} & 26\% \\ \text{1988 to 1994:} & \underline{-13\%} \\ & 13\% \end{array}$$

There was a 13% increase.

**15.** **Strategy** To calculate the probability:

• Count the number of possible outcomes.

• Count the number of favorable outcomes.

• Use the probability formula.

**Solution** There are 16 possible outcomes.

There are 4 favorable outcomes: THHH, HHHT, HHTH, HTHH.

$$\text{Probability} = \frac{4}{16} = \frac{1}{4}$$

The probability of one tail and three heads is $\frac{1}{4}$.

**16.** **Strategy** To find the number of people who slept 8 hours or more:

• Read the histogram to find the number of people who slept 8 hours, 9 hours, or more than 9 hours.

• Add the three numbers.

**Solution**

$$\begin{array}{lr} \text{Slept 8 hours:} & 12 \\ \text{Slept 9 hours:} & 2 \\ \text{Slept more than 9 hours:} & \underline{+\ 1} \\ & 15 \end{array}$$

© 2013 Cengage Learning. All Rights Reserved. May not be scanned, copied or duplicated, or posted to a publicly accessible website, in whole or in part.

There were 15 people who slept 8 or more hours.

**17. Strategy** To find the percent:

- Read the histogram to find the number of people who slept 7 hours.
- Solve the basic percent equation for percent. The base is 46 and the amount is the number of people who slept 7 hours.

**Solution** Slept 7 hours: 13

Percent × base = amount

$$n \times 46 = 13$$
$$n = 13 \div 46$$
$$n \approx 0.2826$$

The percent is 28.3%.

**18a. Strategy** To find the mean heart rates:

- Find the sum of the heart rates.
- Divide the sum by the number of women (24).

**Solution**

$$\begin{array}{r} 80 \\ 82 \\ 99 \\ 91 \\ 93 \\ 87 \\ 103 \\ 94 \\ 73 \\ 96 \\ 86 \\ 80 \\ 97 \\ 94 \\ 108 \\ 81 \\ 100 \\ 109 \\ 91 \\ 84 \\ 78 \\ 96 \\ 96 \\ +\ 100 \\ \hline 2198 \end{array}$$

$$\begin{array}{r} 91.58 \approx 91.6 \\ 24\overline{)2198.00} \\ \underline{-216} \\ 38 \\ \underline{-24} \\ 140 \\ \underline{-120} \\ 200 \\ \underline{-192} \\ 8 \end{array}$$

The mean heart rate is 91.6 heartbeats per minute.

© 2013 Cengage Learning. All Rights Reserved. May not be scanned, copied or duplicated, or posted to a publicly accessible website, in whole or in part.

**Strategy** To find the median heart rate: write the heart rates in order from smallest to largest. The median is the mean of the two middle numbers.

**Solution**

73, 78, 80, 80, 81, 82, 84, 86, 87, 91, 91 } 11 numbers

93, 94 } middle numbers

94, 96, 96, 96, 97, 99, 100, 100, 103, 108, 109 } 11 numbers

$$\frac{93+94}{2} = 93.5$$

The median heart rate is 93.5 heartbeats per minute.

**Strategy** To find the mode, look at the heart rates and identify the number that occurs most frequently.

**Solution** The mode is 96 heartbeats per minute, the number that occurs most frequently.

**b.** **Strategy**
- Arrange the data from smallest to largest. Then find the range.
- Find $Q_1$, the median of the lower half of the data.
- Find $Q_3$, the median of the upper half of the data.
- Interquartile range = $Q_3 - Q_1$.

**Solution** Use the list in part a.

Range = 109 – 73 = 36

The range is 36 heartbeats per minute.

$$Q_1 = \frac{82+84}{2} = 83$$

$$Q_3 = \frac{97+99}{2} = 98$$

$$Q_3 - Q_1 = 98 - 83 = 15$$

The interquartile range is 15 heartbeats per minute.

# Chapter 7 Test

**1.** **Strategy** To find the number of students who spent between \$45 and \$75 each week:
- Read the frequency polygon to find the number of students who spent between \$45 and \$60 and the number who spent between \$60 and \$75.
- Add the two numbers.

**Solution**

| | |
|---|---|
| Number between \$45 – \$60: | 12 |
| Number between \$60 – \$75: | + 7 |
| | 19 |

19 students spent between \$45 and \$75 each week.

© 2013 Cengage Learning. All Rights Reserved. May not be scanned, copied or duplicated, or posted to a publicly accessible website, in whole or in part.

**2.** **Strategy** To find the ratio:

• Read the frequency polygon to find the number of students who spent between \$30 and \$45 and the number who spent between \$45 and \$60.

• Write in simplest form the ratio of the number of students who spent between \$30 and \$45 to the number of students who spent between \$45 and \$60.

**Solution** Between \$30 and \$45: 8 students

Between \$45 and \$60: 12 students

$$\frac{8 \text{ students}}{12 \text{ students}} = \frac{2}{3}$$

The ratio is $\frac{2}{3}$.

**3.** **Strategy** To find the percent:

• Read the frequency polygon to find the number of students who spent between \$0 to \$15, between \$15 and \$30, and between \$30 and \$45 each week.

• Add the three numbers.

• Solve the basic percent equation for percent. The base is 40 and the amount is the number of students who spent less than \$45 per week.

**Solution**

| | |
|---|---|
| Between \$0 and \$15: | 4 students |
| Between \$15 and \$30: | 6 students |
| Between \$30 and \$45: | + 8 students |
| | 18 students |

$$\begin{aligned} \text{Percent} \times \text{base} &= \text{amount} \\ n \times 40 &= 18 \\ n &= 18 \div 40 \\ n &= 0.45 \end{aligned}$$

The percent is 45%.

**4.** **Strategy** To find the number of people surveyed:

• Read the pictograph to determine the number of people for each letter grade.

• Add the four numbers.

**Solution**

| | |
|---|---|
| Number of A grades: | 21 |
| Number of B grades: | 10 |
| Number of C grades: | 4 |
| Number of D grades: | + 1 |
| | 36 |

There were 36 people that were surveyed for the Gallup poll.

**5.** **Strategy** To find the ratio:

• Read the pictograph to find the number of people who gave their marriage a B grade and the number who gave their marriage a C grade.

• Write in simplest form the ratio of the number of people who gave their marriage a B grade to the number of people who gave their marriage a C grade.

**Solution** Number of B grades: 10 people

Number of C grades: 4 people

$$\frac{10 \text{ people}}{4 \text{ people}} = \frac{5}{2}$$

The ratio is $\frac{5}{2}$.

**6.** **Strategy** To find the percent:

• Read the pictograph to find the number of people who gave their marriage an A grade.

• Solve the basic percent equation for percent. The base is 36 (from Exercise 4 ) and the amount is the number of people who gave their marriage an A grade.

© 2013 Cengage Learning. All Rights Reserved. May not be scanned, copied or duplicated, or posted to a publicly accessible website, in whole or in part.

**Solution** Number of A grades: 21 people

Percent × base = amount

$n \times 36 = 21$

$n = 21 \div 36$

$n \approx 0.583$

The percent is 58.3%.

**7. Strategy** Read the bar graph to job growth rate for Medical Assistants.

**Solution** The job rate growth for Medical Assistants was 34%.

**8. Strategy** To find the two occupations that have job rate growths slightly higher than 205, read the bar graph to determine the two groups.

**Solution** Licensed practical nurses and registered nurses have job growth rates slightly above 20%.

**9. Strategy** To find difference

- Read the bar graph to determine the job rate growth for home health aides and for nursing aides.
- Subtract the two numbers.

**Solution**

| | |
|---|---|
| Home Health Aides: | 50% |
| Nursing Aides: | −19% |
| | 31% |

The difference is 31%.

**10. Strategy** To find how many more made C's than A's:

- Read the circle graph to find the number of who made C's and the number who made A's.
- Subtract the two numbers.

**Solution**

| | |
|---|---|
| C: | 47 |
| A: | − 15 |
| | 32 |

There were 32 more students who made C's.

**11. Strategy** To find the percent who earned B's:

- Read the circle graph to find the number of students that made each grade and add the numbers to get the total number of students.
- Read the circle graph to find the number of students that made B's.
- Write and solve the basic percent equation for the percent. The base is the total number of students and the amount is the number of B's.

**Solution**

| | |
|---|---|
| A: | 15 |
| B: | 27 |
| C: | 47 |
| D: | 21 |
| F: | 10 |
| | 120 |

B: 27

Percent × base = amount

$n \times 120 = 27$

$n = 27 \div 120$

$n = 0.225$

$n = 22.5\%$

22.5% made B's.

**12. Strategy** To find the percent of who made below C:

- Read the circle graph to find the number of students that made each grade and add the numbers to get the total number of students.
- Read the circle graph to find the number of students that made D's and F's and add those numbers.
- Write and solve the basic percent equation for the percent.

© 2013 Cengage Learning. All Rights Reserved. May not be scanned, copied or duplicated, or posted to a publicly accessible website, in whole or in part.

The base is the total number of students and the amount is the number below a C.

**Solution**

A: 15
B: 27
C: 47
D: 21
F: 10
120

D: 21
F: 10
31

Percent × base = amount

$n \times 120 = 31$

$n = 31 \div 120$

$n \approx 0.258$

25.8% made below C.

**13. Strategy** To find the number of states with median income between \$40,000 and \$60,000.

• Read the histogram to find the number of states with per capita income between \$40,000 and \$50,000 and between \$50,000 and \$60,000.

• Add the two numbers.

**Solution**

| | |
|---|---|
| \$40,000 to \$50,000: | 5 states |
| \$50,000 to \$60,000: | + 19 states |
| | 24 states |

There are 24 states that have a median income between \$40,000 and \$60,000.

**14. Strategy** To find the percent of the states with a median income between \$50,000 and \$70,000:

• Read the histogram to find the number of states with median incomes between \$50,000 and \$60,000 and between \$60,000 and \$70,000.

• Add the two numbers.

• Solve the basic percent equation for percent. The base is 50 and the amount is the number of states with a median income between \$50,000 and \$70,000.

**Solution**

| | |
|---|---|
| \$50,000 to \$60,000: | 19 states |
| \$60,000 to \$70,000: | + 17 states |
| | 36 states |

Percent × base = amount

$n \times 50 = 36$

$n = 36 \div 50$

$n = 0.72$

The percent is 72%.

**15. Strategy** To find the percent:

• Read the histogram to find the number of states that have a median income between \$70,000 and \$80,000 and between \$80,000 and \$90,000.

• Add the two numbers.

• Solve the basic percent equation for percent. The base is 50 and the amount is the number of states with a median income above \$70,000.

**Solution**

| | |
|---|---|
| \$70,000 – \$80,000: | 5 states |
| \$80,000 – \$90,000: | + 4 states |
| | 9 states |

Percent × base = amount

$n \times 50 = 9$

$n = 9 \div 50$

$n = 0.18$

The percent is 18%.

**16. Strategy** To calculate the probability:

• Count the number of possible outcomes.

• Count the number of favorable outcomes.

• Use the probability formula.

**Solution** There are 50 possible outcomes.

© 2013 Cengage Learning. All Rights Reserved. May not be scanned, copied or duplicated, or posted to a publicly accessible website, in whole or in part.

There are 15 favorable outcomes.

$$\text{Probability} = \frac{15}{50} = \frac{3}{10}$$

The probability is $\frac{3}{10}$ that the ball chosen is red.

**17. Strategy** To find which decade had the smallest increase in enrollment.

- Read the line graph to find the enrollment for each decade.
- Subtract the two numbers.

**Solution** 1960 to 1970:

8 – 4 = 4 million

1970 to 1980:

12 – 8 = 4 million

1980 to 1990:

14 – 12 = 2 million

1990 to 2000:

15 – 14 = 1 million

The student enrollment increased the least during the 1990s.

**18. Strategy** To approximate the increase in enrollment:

- Read the enrollment for 1960 and 2000.
- Subtract the two numbers.

**Solution**

$$\begin{array}{lr} 2000: & 15 \text{ million} \\ 1960: & \underline{-\ 4 \text{ million}} \\ & 11 \text{ million} \end{array}$$

The increase in enrollment was 11 million students.

**19a. Strategy** To find the mean lifetime of the batteries:

- Find the sum of the times.
- Divide the sum by the number of batteries tested (20).

**Solution**

$$\begin{array}{r} 2.9 \\ 2.4 \\ 3.1 \\ 2.5 \\ 2.6 \\ 2.0 \\ 3.0 \\ 2.3 \\ 2.4 \\ 2.7 \\ 2.0 \\ 2.4 \\ 2.6 \\ 2.7 \\ 2.1 \\ 2.9 \\ 2.8 \\ 2.4 \\ 2.0 \\ \underline{+\ 2.8} \\ 50.6 \end{array}$$

$$20\overline{)50.60} = 2.53$$

The mean time is 2.53 days.

**b. Strategy** To find the median lifetime of the batteries, write times in order from lowest to highest. The median is the mean of the two middle numbers.

© 2013 Cengage Learning. All Rights Reserved. May not be scanned, copied or duplicated, or posted to a publicly accessible website, in whole or in part.

**Solution**

2.0
2.0
2.0
2.1
2.3 } 9 numbers
2.4
2.4
2.4
2.4

2.5
2.6 } middle numbers

2.6
2.7
2.7
2.8
2.8 } 9 numbers
2.9
2.9
3.0
3.1

$$\frac{2.5 + 2.6}{2} = 2.55$$

The median time is 2.55 days.

**c. Strategy** The data is arranged from smallest to largest in part b.

- Find $Q_1$, the median of the lower half of the data.
- Find $Q_3$, the median of the upper half of the data.
- Draw the box-and-whiskers plot.

**Solution**

$$Q_1 = \frac{2.3 + 2.4}{2} = 2.35$$

$$Q_3 = \frac{2.8 + 2.8}{2} = 2.8$$

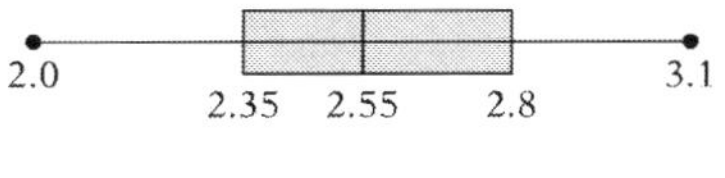


# Cumulative Review Exercises

**1.** $2^2 \cdot 3^3 \cdot 5 = (2 \cdot 2) \cdot (3 \cdot 3 \cdot 3) \cdot (5)$
$= 4 \cdot 27 \cdot 5 = 540$

**2.** $3^2 \cdot (5 - 2) \div 3 + 5$
$= 9 \cdot (3) \div 3 + 5$
$= 27 \div 3 + 5$
$= 9 + 5$
$= 14$

**3.**

| | 2 | 3 | 5 |
|---|---|---|---|
| 24 = | (2 · 2 · 2) | (3) | |
| 40 = | 2 · 2 · 2 | | (5) |

LCM $= 2 \cdot 2 \cdot 2 \cdot 3 \cdot 5 = 120$

**4.** $\dfrac{60}{144} = \dfrac{\cancel{2} \cdot \cancel{2} \cdot \cancel{3} \cdot 5}{\cancel{2} \cdot \cancel{2} \cdot 2 \cdot 2 \cdot \cancel{3} \cdot 3} = \dfrac{5}{12}$

**5.**
$$\begin{aligned} 4\tfrac{1}{2} &= 4\tfrac{20}{40} \\ 2\tfrac{3}{8} &= 2\tfrac{15}{40} \\ +5\tfrac{1}{5} &= 5\tfrac{5}{40} \\ \hline &\quad 11\tfrac{43}{40} = 12\tfrac{3}{40} \end{aligned}$$

**6.**
$$\begin{aligned} 12\tfrac{5}{8} &= 12\tfrac{15}{24} = 11\tfrac{39}{24} \\ -7\tfrac{11}{12} &= 7\tfrac{22}{24} = 7\tfrac{22}{24} \\ \hline &\quad 4\tfrac{17}{24} \end{aligned}$$

**7.** $\dfrac{5}{8} \times 3\dfrac{1}{5} = \dfrac{5}{8} \times \dfrac{16}{5}$
$= \dfrac{5 \cdot 16}{8 \cdot 5}$
$= \dfrac{\cancel{5} \cdot \cancel{2} \cdot \cancel{2} \cdot \cancel{2} \cdot 2}{\cancel{2} \cdot \cancel{2} \cdot \cancel{2} \cdot \cancel{5}} = 2$

**8.** $3\dfrac{1}{5} \div 4\dfrac{1}{4} = \dfrac{16}{5} \div \dfrac{17}{4} = \dfrac{16}{5} \times \dfrac{4}{17} = \dfrac{16 \cdot 4}{5 \cdot 17} = \dfrac{64}{85}$

© 2013 Cengage Learning. All Rights Reserved. May not be scanned, copied or duplicated, or posted to a publicly accessible website, in whole or in part.

**9.** $\frac{5}{8} \div \left(\frac{3}{4} - \frac{2}{3}\right) + \frac{3}{4} = \frac{5}{8} \div \left(\frac{9}{12} - \frac{8}{12}\right) + \frac{3}{4}$

$$= \frac{5}{8} \div \frac{1}{12} + \frac{3}{4}$$

$$= \frac{5}{8} \times \frac{12}{1} + \frac{3}{4}$$

$$= \frac{5 \cdot \overset{1}{\cancel{2}} \cdot \overset{1}{\cancel{2}} \cdot 3}{\underset{1}{\cancel{2}} \cdot \underset{1}{\cancel{2}} \cdot 2} + \frac{3}{4}$$

$$= \frac{15}{2} + \frac{3}{4} = \frac{30}{4} + \frac{3}{4} = \frac{33}{4} = 8\frac{1}{4}$$

**10.** 209.305

**11.**
$$\begin{array}{r} 4.092 \\ \times\ 0.69 \\ \hline 36828 \\ 24552\phantom{0} \\ \hline 2.82348 \end{array}$$

**12.** $16\frac{2}{3} = \frac{50}{3}$

$$\begin{array}{r} 16.666 \approx 16.67 \\ 3\overline{)50.000} \\ \underline{-3}\phantom{0.000} \\ 20\phantom{.000} \\ \underline{-18}\phantom{.000} \\ 20\phantom{00} \\ \underline{-18}\phantom{00} \\ 20\phantom{0} \\ \underline{-18}\phantom{0} \\ 20 \\ \underline{-18} \\ 20 \end{array}$$

**13.** $\frac{330 \text{ miles}}{12.5 \text{ gal}} = 24.6$ miles/gallon

**14.**
$$\frac{n}{5} = \frac{16}{55}$$
$$n \times 25 = 5 \times 16$$
$$n \times 25 = 80$$
$$n = 80 \div 25 = 3.2$$

**15.** $\frac{4}{5} \times 100\% = 80\%$

**16.**
$$10\% \times n = 8$$
$$0.10 \times n = 8$$
$$n = 8 \div 0.10 = 80$$

**17.**
$$38\% \times 43 = n$$
$$0.38 \times 43 = n$$
$$16.34 = n$$

**18.**
$$n \times 75 = 30$$
$$n = 30 \div 75 = 0.40 = 40\%$$

**19. Strategy** To find the income for the week:

- Find the commission earned on sales by solving the basic percent equation for amount. The base is \$27,500 and the percent is 2%.
- Find the total income by adding the base salary (\$100) to the commission.

**Solution**
$$2\% \times 27{,}500 = n$$
$$0.02 \times 27{,}500 = n$$
$$550 = n$$

$100 + 550 = 650$

The salesperson's income for the week was \$650.

**20. Strategy** To find the cost, write and solve a proportion.

**Solution**
$$\frac{8.15}{1000} = \frac{n}{50{,}000}$$
$$8.15 \times 50{,}000 = n \times 1000$$
$$407{,}500 = n \times 1000$$
$$407{,}500 \div 1000 = n$$
$$407.50 = n$$

The cost is \$407.50.

**21. Strategy** To find the interest due, multiply the principal by the annual interest rate and the time (in years).

**Solution** $125{,}000 \times 0.06 \times \frac{6}{12} = 3750$

The interest due is \$3750.

© 2013 Cengage Learning. All Rights Reserved. May not be scanned, copied or duplicated, or posted to a publicly accessible website, in whole or in part.

**22. Strategy** To find the markup rate of the wheelchair:
• Find the markup amount by subtracting the cost ($180) from the selling price ($279).
• Solve the basic percent equation for percent. The base is $180 and the amount is the amount of the markup.

**Solution** $279 - 180 = 99$

$$\begin{aligned} \text{Percent} \times \text{base} &= \text{amount} \\ n \times 180 &= 99 \\ n &= 99 \div 180 \\ &= 0.55 = 55\% \end{aligned}$$

The markup rate is 55%.

**23. Strategy** To find how much is budgeted for food:
• Read the circle graph to find what percent of the budget is spent on food.
• Solve the basic percent equation for amount. The base is $4500 and the rate is the percent of the budget that is spent on food.

**Solution** Amount spent on food: 19%

$$\begin{aligned} \text{Percent} \times \text{base} &= \text{amount} \\ 19\% \times 4500 &= \text{amount} \\ 0.19 \times 4500 &= 855 \end{aligned}$$

The amount budgeted for food is $855.

© 2013 Cengage Learning. All Rights Reserved. May not be scanned, copied or duplicated, or posted to a publicly accessible website, in whole or in part.

**24. Strategy** To find the difference:

• Read the double-broken-line graph to find the number of problems student 1 answered correctly on test 1 and the number of problems student 2 answered correctly on test 1.

• Subtract the student 1 total from the student 2 total to find the difference.

**Solution**

$$\begin{array}{ll} \text{student 2:} & 27 \text{ answered correctly} \\ \text{student 1:} & \underline{-15 \text{ answered correctly}} \\ & 12 \text{ answered correctly} \end{array}$$

The difference in the number answered correctly is 12 problems.

**25. Strategy** To find the mean length of stay:

• Find the sum of the lengths.

• Divide the sum of the lengths by the number of patients (10).

• Compare the average to the national average (4.8)

**Solution**

$$\begin{array}{r} 6 \\ 2 \\ 1 \\ 3 \\ 4 \\ 5 \\ 6 \\ 7 \\ 5 \\ \underline{+2} \\ 41 \end{array} \qquad \begin{array}{r} 4.1 \\ 10\overline{)41.0} \end{array}$$

$4.1 < 4.8$

The average length of stay is 4.1 days. This is less than the national average.

**26. Strategy** To calculate the probability:

• Count the number of possible outcomes.

• Count the number of favorable outcomes.

• Use the probability formula.

**Solution** There are 36 possible outcomes. There are 5 favorable outcomes: (2, 6), (6, 2), (3, 5), (5, 3), (4, 4).

$$\text{Probability} = \frac{5}{36}$$

The probability is $\frac{5}{36}$ that the sum of the dots on the two dice is 8.

© 2013 Cengage Learning. All Rights Reserved. May not be scanned, copied or duplicated, or posted to a publicly accessible website, in whole or in part.

# Chapter 8: U.S. Customary Units of Measurement

## Prep Test

**1.**
$$\begin{array}{r} 485 \\ +217 \\ \hline 702 \end{array}$$

**2.**
$$\begin{array}{r} 145 \\ -87 \\ \hline 58 \end{array}$$

**3.** $36 \times \frac{1}{9} = 4$

**4.** $\frac{5}{3} \times 6 = \frac{5}{3} \times \frac{6}{1} = \frac{5 \cdot 2 \cdot \overset{1}{\cancel{3}}}{\underset{1}{\cancel{3}}} = 10$

**5.** $400 \times \frac{1}{8} \times \frac{1}{2} = \frac{400}{1} \times \frac{1}{8} \times \frac{1}{2}$

$= \frac{\overset{1}{\cancel{2}} \cdot \overset{1}{\cancel{2}} \cdot \overset{1}{\cancel{2}} \cdot \overset{1}{\cancel{2}} \cdot 5 \cdot 5}{\underset{1}{\cancel{2}} \cdot \underset{1}{\cancel{2}} \cdot \underset{1}{\cancel{2}} \cdot \underset{1}{\cancel{2}}} = 25$

**6.** $5\frac{3}{4} \times 8 = \frac{23}{4} \times \frac{8}{1} = \frac{23 \cdot \overset{1}{\cancel{2}} \cdot \overset{1}{\cancel{2}} \cdot 2}{\underset{1}{\cancel{2}} \cdot \underset{1}{\cancel{2}}} = 46$

**7.** $3\overline{)714}$ = 238

**8.** $12\overline{)18.0}$ = 1.5

## Section 8.1

### Objective A Exercises

**1.** Greater than

**3.** Greater than

**5.** $9 \text{ ft} = 9 \cancel{\text{ ft}} \times \frac{12 \text{ in.}}{1 \cancel{\text{ ft}}} = 108 \text{ in.}$

**7.** $64 \text{ in.} = 64 \cancel{\text{ in.}} \times \frac{1 \text{ ft}}{12 \cancel{\text{ in.}}} = 5\frac{1}{3} \text{ ft}$

**9.** $4\frac{1}{2} \text{ yd} = 4\frac{1}{2} \cancel{\text{ yd}} \times \frac{3 \text{ ft}}{1 \cancel{\text{ yd}}} = 13\frac{1}{2} \text{ ft}$

**11.** $4\frac{1}{2} \text{ ft} = 4\frac{1}{2} \cancel{\text{ ft}} \times \frac{1 \text{ yd}}{3 \cancel{\text{ ft}}} = 1\frac{1}{2} \text{ yd}$

**13.** $5 \text{ yd} = 5 \cancel{\text{ yd}} \times \frac{36 \text{ in.}}{1 \cancel{\text{ yd}}} = 180 \text{ in.}$

**15.** $1\frac{1}{2} \text{ mi} = 1\frac{1}{2} \cancel{\text{ mi}} \times \frac{5280 \text{ ft}}{1 \cancel{\text{ mi}}} = 7920 \text{ ft}$

### Objective B Exercises

**17.** 5280

**19.**
$$\begin{array}{r} \text{1 mi 1120 ft} \\ 5280\overline{)6400} \\ -5280 \\ \hline 1120 \end{array}$$

6400 ft = 1 mi 1120 ft

**21.**
$$\begin{array}{r} 9 \text{ ft } 11 \text{ in.} \\ +\ 3 \text{ ft } 6 \text{ in.} \\ \hline 12 \text{ ft } 17 \text{ in.} = 13 \text{ ft } 5 \text{ in.} \end{array}$$

**23.** $4\frac{2}{3} \text{ ft} + 6\frac{1}{2} \text{ ft} = 4\frac{4}{6} \text{ ft} + 6\frac{3}{6} \text{ ft}$

$= 10\frac{7}{6} \text{ ft}$

$= 11\frac{1}{6} \text{ ft}$

**25.**
$$\begin{array}{r} 8 \text{ yd } 4 \text{ ft} \\ 9 \cancel{\text{ yd}}\ 1 \cancel{\text{ ft}} \\ -3 \text{ yd } 2 \text{ ft} \\ \hline 5 \text{ yd } 2 \text{ ft} \end{array}$$

**27.** $3\frac{2}{3} \text{ ft} \times 4 = \frac{11}{3} \text{ ft} \times 4$

$= \frac{44}{3} \text{ ft}$

$= 14\frac{2}{3} \text{ ft}$

© 2013 Cengage Learning. All Rights Reserved. May not be scanned, copied or duplicated, or posted to a publicly accessible website, in whole or in part.

**29.** $12\frac{1}{2}\text{ in.} \div 3 = 12\frac{1}{2}\text{ in.} \times \frac{1}{3}$

$= \frac{25}{2}\text{ in.} \times \frac{1}{3}$

$= \frac{25}{6}\text{ in.}$

$= 4\frac{1}{6}\text{ in.}$

## Objective C Exercises

**31. Strategy** To convert the height to feet and inches, divide the length (71 inches) by the number of inches in a foot (12). Leave the remainder as inches.

**Solution**

$$\begin{array}{r} 5\text{ ft }11\text{ in} \\ 12\overline{)71} \\ \underline{60} \\ 11 \end{array}$$

The patient is 5 ft 11 in.

**33. Strategy** To determine if the recruit meets the requirements,

- Convert the height to feet and inches, divide the height (78 in) by the number of inches in a foot (12) and leave the remainder in inches.
- Compare the recruit's height in inches to the requirements (between 5 ft 4 in and 6 ft 5 in).

**Solution**

$$\begin{array}{r} 6\text{ ft }6\text{ in} \\ 12\overline{)78} \\ \underline{72} \\ 6 \end{array}$$

6 ft 6 in > 6 ft 5 in

The applicant does not qualify.

**35. Strategy** To find the difference, subtract the Mary' height (3 ft 8 in) from Evan's height (4 ft 3 in).

**Solution**

$$\begin{array}{r} 3\text{ ft }15\text{ in} \\ 4\text{ ~~ft~~ }3\text{ in} \\ \underline{-3\text{ft }8\text{ in}} \\ 7\text{ in} \end{array}$$

Evan is 7 in taller than Mary.

**37. Strategy** To find the height, subtract 3 in from the minimum height (3 ft 1 in).

**Solution**

$$\begin{array}{r} 2\text{ ft }13\text{ in} \\ 3\text{ ~~ft~~ }1\text{ in} \\ \underline{-\quad 3\text{ in}} \\ 2\text{ ft }10\text{ in} \end{array}$$

The height is 2 ft 10 in.

**39. Strategy** To find the number of 12 in pieces that can be cut,

- Convert the length of the tape (12 yd) to in.
- Divide the length of the tape in inches by 12 in.

**Solution** $12\text{ yd} = 12\ \cancel{\text{yd}} \times \frac{36\text{ in.}}{1\ \cancel{\text{yd}}} = 432\text{ in}$

$$\begin{array}{r} 36 \\ 12\overline{)432} \\ \underline{36} \\ 72 \\ \underline{72} \\ 0 \end{array}$$

One package will serve 36 patients.

**41. Strategy** To the difference, subtract his height $\left(8\text{ ft }11\frac{1}{10}\text{ in}\right)$ from his arm span $\left(9\text{ ft }5\frac{3}{4}\text{ in}\right)$.

© 2013 Cengage Learning. All Rights Reserved. May not be scanned, copied or duplicated, or posted to a publicly accessible website, in whole or in part.

**Solution**

$$\begin{array}{r} 8 \text{ ft } 17\frac{15}{20} \text{ in} \\ 9\text{ft} \quad 5\frac{3}{4} \text{ in} = 9 \not{\text{ft}} \quad 5\frac{15}{20} \text{ in} \\ -8 \text{ ft } 11\frac{1}{10} \text{ in} = 8 \text{ ft } 11\frac{2}{20} \text{ in} \\ \hline 6\frac{13}{20} \text{ in} \end{array}$$

The difference is $6\frac{13}{20}$ in.

**43.** True; if the gauze is 15 ft long and cut into five equal pieces, then each piece is 3 ft, or 2 ft 12 in., which is not the case.

# Section 8.2

## Objective A Exercises

**1.** Less than

**3.** Greater than

**5.** $36 \text{ oz} = 36 \not{\text{oz}} \times \frac{1 \text{ lb}}{16 \not{\text{oz}}} = 2\frac{1}{4} \text{ lb}$

**7.** $7 \text{ lb} = 7 \not{\text{lb}} \times \frac{16 \text{ oz}}{1 \not{\text{lb}}} = 112 \text{ oz}$

**9.** $9000 \text{ lb} = 9000 \not{\text{lb}} \times \frac{1 \text{ ton}}{2000 \not{\text{lb}}} = 4\frac{1}{2} \text{ tons}$

**11.** $1\frac{1}{4} \text{ tons} = 1\frac{1}{4} \not{\text{tons}} \times \frac{2000 \text{ lb}}{1 \not{\text{ton}}} = 2500 \text{ lb}$

**13.** $90 \text{ oz} = 90 \not{\text{oz}} \times \frac{1 \text{ lb}}{16 \not{\text{oz}}} = 5\frac{5}{8} \text{ lb}$

**15.** $2\frac{5}{8} \text{ lb} = 2\frac{5}{8} \not{\text{lb}} \times \frac{16 \text{ oz}}{1 \not{\text{lb}}} = 42 \text{ oz}$

**17.** $5000 \text{ lb} = 5000 \not{\text{lb}} \times \frac{1 \text{ ton}}{2000 \not{\text{lb}}} = 2\frac{1}{2} \text{ tons}$

## Objective B Exercises

**19.** 2000

**21.**

$$\begin{array}{r} 4 \text{ tons } 1000 \text{ lb} \\ 2000\overline{)9000} \\ -8000 \\ \hline 1000 \end{array}$$

9000 lb = 4 tons 1000 lb

**23.**

$$\begin{array}{r} 4 \text{ lb } 7 \text{ oz} \\ +3 \text{ lb } 12 \text{ oz} \\ \hline 7 \text{ lb } 19 \text{ oz} = 8 \text{ lb } 3 \text{ oz} \end{array}$$

**25.**

$$\begin{array}{r} \overset{6}{\not{7}} \text{ lb } \overset{21}{\not{5}} \text{ oz} \\ -3 \text{ lb } 8 \text{ oz} \\ \hline 3 \text{ lb } 13 \text{ oz} \end{array}$$

**27.**

$$\begin{array}{r} 6\frac{3}{8} \text{ lb} = 6\frac{9}{24} \text{ lb} = 5\frac{33}{24} \text{ lb} \\ -2\frac{5}{6} \text{ lb} = 2\frac{20}{24} \text{ lb} = 2\frac{20}{24} \text{ lb} \\ \hline 3\frac{13}{24} \text{ lb} \end{array}$$

**29.**

$$\begin{aligned} 5\frac{1}{2} \text{ lb} \times 6 &= \frac{11}{2} \text{ lb} \times 6 \\ &= \frac{66}{2} \text{ lb} \\ &= 33 \text{ lb} \end{aligned}$$

**31.**

$$\begin{array}{r} 1 \text{ lb } 12 \text{ oz} \\ 2\overline{)3 \text{ lb } \; 8 \text{ oz}} \\ -2 \text{ lb} \\ \hline 1 \text{ lb} = 16 \text{ oz} \\ 24 \text{ oz} \\ -24 \text{ oz} \\ \hline 0 \end{array}$$

## Objective C Exercises

**33.** Greater than

**35.** **Strategy** To find the total weight of the triplets, add the three weights (4 lb 3 oz, 3 lb 14 oz, and 4 lb 1 oz).

© 2013 Cengage Learning. All Rights Reserved. May not be scanned, copied or duplicated, or posted to a publicly accessible website, in whole or in part.

**Solution**

$$\begin{array}{r} 4\text{ lb } \ \ 3\text{ oz} \\ 3\text{ lb } 14\text{ oz} \\ +4\text{ lb } \ \ 1\text{ oz} \\ \hline 11\text{ lb } 18\text{ oz} = 12\text{ lb } 2\text{ oz} \end{array}$$

The total weight is 12 lb 2 oz.

**37. Strategy** To find the total weight of the textbooks:

• Multiply the number of textbooks (1200) by the weight of one textbook (9 oz).

• Convert the number of ounces to pounds.

**Solution**

$$\begin{array}{r} 1200 \\ \times \quad 9\text{ oz} \\ \hline 10{,}800\text{ oz} \end{array}$$

$$10{,}800\ \cancel{\text{oz}} \times \frac{1\text{ lb}}{16\ \cancel{\text{oz}}} = 675\text{ lb}$$

The total weight of the textbooks is 675 lb.

**39. Strategy** To find the weight of the case in pounds:

• Find the weight in ounces by multiplying the weight of each can (6 oz) by the number of cans (24).

• Convert the weight in ounces to pounds.

**Solution**

$$\begin{array}{r} 6\text{ oz} \\ \times \quad 24 \\ \hline 144\text{ oz} \end{array}$$

$$144\ \cancel{\text{oz}} \times \frac{1\text{ lb}}{16\ \cancel{\text{oz}}} = 9\text{ lb}$$

The weight of the case of soft drinks is 9 lb.

**41. Strategy** To find the baby's weight, multiply the birth rate (6 lb 11 oz) by 3.

**Solution**

$$\begin{array}{r} 6\text{ lb } 11\text{ oz} \\ \times \qquad 3 \\ \hline 18\text{ lb } 33\text{ oz} = 20\text{ lb } 1\text{ oz} \end{array}$$

The baby's weight at 12 months is 20 lb 1 oz.

**43. Strategy** To find the number of tons of plastic bottles that are not recycled each year, convert the number of pounds of plastic bottles (2 billion lb) to tons.

**Solution**

$$2\text{ billion lb} \times \frac{1\text{ ton}}{2000\text{ lb}}$$

$$= \frac{\cancel{2000}\text{ million }\cancel{\text{lb}}}{1} \times \frac{1\text{ ton}}{\cancel{2000}\ \cancel{\text{lb}}}$$

$$= 1\text{ million tons}$$

1 million tons of plastic bottles are not recycled each year.

**45. Strategy** To find the cost of mailing the knee brace:

• Convert 2 lb 3 oz to ounces.

• Multiply the number of ounces by the postage rate per ounce ($.34)

**Solution**

$$2\text{ lb } 3\text{ oz} = 35\text{ oz}$$

$$\begin{array}{r} 0.34 \\ \times \quad 35 \\ \hline 11.90 \end{array}$$

The cost of mailing the knee brace is $11.90.

## Section 8.3

### Objective A Exercises

**1.** Greater than

**3.** Less than

**5.** $48\text{ fl oz} = 48\ \cancel{\text{fl oz}} \times \frac{1\text{ c}}{8\ \cancel{\text{fl oz}}} = 6\text{ c}$

**7.** $2\frac{1}{2}\text{c} = 2\frac{1}{2}\ \cancel{\text{c}} \times \frac{8\text{ fl oz}}{1\ \cancel{\text{c}}} = 20\text{ fl oz}$

© 2013 Cengage Learning. All Rights Reserved. May not be scanned, copied or duplicated, or posted to a publicly accessible website, in whole or in part.

**9.** $5\text{ c} = 5\,\cancel{\text{c}} \times \dfrac{1\text{ pt}}{2\,\cancel{\text{c}}} = 2\dfrac{1}{2}\text{ pt}$

**11.** $12\text{ pt} = 12\,\cancel{\text{pt}} \times \dfrac{1\text{ qt}}{2\,\cancel{\text{pt}}} = 6\text{ qt}$

**13.** $10\text{ qt} = 10\,\cancel{\text{qt}} \times \dfrac{1\text{ gal}}{4\,\cancel{\text{qt}}} = 2\dfrac{1}{2}\text{ gal}$

**15.** $7\text{ gal} = 7\,\cancel{\text{gal}} \times \dfrac{4\text{ qt}}{1\,\cancel{\text{gal}}} = 28\text{ qt}$

**17.** $17\text{ c} = 17\,\cancel{\text{c}} \times \dfrac{1\,\cancel{\text{pt}}}{2\,\cancel{\text{c}}} \times \dfrac{1\text{ qt}}{2\,\cancel{\text{pt}}} = 4\dfrac{1}{4}\text{ qt}$

## Objective B Exercises

**19.** 4

**21.**

$$\begin{array}{r} 3\text{ gal }2\text{ qt} \\ 4\overline{)14} \\ -12 \\ \hline 2 \end{array}$$

14 qt = 3 gal 2qt

**23.**

$$\begin{array}{l} \quad 3\text{ gal }2\text{ qt} \\ +\,4\text{ gal }3\text{ qt} \\ \hline \quad 7\text{ gal }5\text{ qt} = 8\text{ gal }1\text{ qt} \end{array}$$

**25.**

$$\begin{array}{l} \quad 3\text{ gal }3\text{ qt} \\ +\,1\text{ gal }2\text{ qt} \\ \hline \quad 4\text{ gal }5\text{ qt} = 5\text{ gal }1\text{ qt} \end{array}$$

**27.**

$$\begin{array}{l} \quad 3\text{ gal }\ 1\text{ qt} \\ +\,1\text{ gal }\ 2\text{ qt} \\ \hline \quad 4\text{ gal }\ 3\text{ qt} \end{array}$$

**29.**

$$\begin{array}{l} \quad 3\text{ c }14\text{ fl oz} \\ \quad \cancel{4\text{ c }\ 6\text{ fl oz}} \\ -\,2\text{ c }\ 7\text{ fl oz} \\ \hline \quad 1\text{ c }7\text{ fl oz} \end{array}$$

**31.**

$$\begin{aligned} 4\frac{1}{2}\text{ gal} - 1\frac{3}{4}\text{ gal} &= 4\frac{2}{4}\text{ gal} - 1\frac{3}{4}\text{ gal} \\ &= 3\frac{6}{4}\text{ gal} - 1\frac{3}{4}\text{ gal} \\ &= 2\frac{3}{4}\text{ gal} \end{aligned}$$

**33.** $3\dfrac{1}{2}\text{ pt} \times 5 = \dfrac{7}{2}\text{ pt} \times 5 = \dfrac{35}{2}\text{ pt} = 17\dfrac{1}{2}\text{ pt}$

**35.**

$$\begin{aligned} 3\frac{1}{2}\text{ gal} \div 4 &= 3\frac{1}{2}\text{ gal} \times \frac{1}{4} \\ &= \frac{7}{2}\text{ gal} \times \frac{1}{4} \\ &= \frac{7}{8}\text{ gal} \end{aligned}$$

## Objective C Exercises

**37.** **Strategy** To find how many gallons of coffee should be prepared:

- Find how many cups of coffee should be prepared by multiplying the number of adults attending (60) by the number of cups each adult will drink (2).
- Convert the number of cups to gallons.

**Solution** $2\text{ c} \times 60 = 120\text{ c}$

$$\begin{aligned} 120\,\cancel{\text{c}} \times \frac{1\,\cancel{\text{pt}}}{2\,\cancel{\text{c}}} \times \frac{1\,\cancel{\text{qt}}}{2\,\cancel{\text{pt}}} \times \frac{1\text{ gal}}{4\,\cancel{\text{qt}}} &= \frac{120\text{ gal}}{16} \\ &= 7\frac{1}{2}\text{ gal} \end{aligned}$$

$7\dfrac{1}{2}$ gal of coffee should be prepared.

**39.** **Strategy** To find the more economical purchase:

- Convert 1 qt to ounces.
- Compare the price per ounce of each brand of tomato juice.

© 2013 Cengage Learning. All Rights Reserved. May not be scanned, copied or duplicated, or posted to a publicly accessible website, in whole or in part.

**Solution**

$$1 \text{ qt} = 1 \cancel{\text{qt}} \times \frac{2 \cancel{\text{pt}}}{1 \cancel{\text{qt}}} \times \frac{2 \cancel{\text{c}}}{1 \cancel{\text{pt}}} \times \frac{8 \text{ oz}}{1 \cancel{\text{c}}}$$
$$= 32 \text{ oz}$$

First brand: $32\overline{)1.5900}$ = 0.0497

Second brand: $24\overline{)1.250}$ = 0.052

$0.0497 < 0.052$

The more economical purchase is 1 qt for $1.59 (the first brand).

**41. Strategy** To find the number of cups of bottled water an American drinks per month:

- Convert the number of gallons an American drinks per year (28.3 gal) to cups.
- Divide the result by 12 to find the amount per month.

**Solution**

28.3 gal

$$= 28.3 \cancel{\text{gal}} \times \frac{4 \cancel{\text{qt}}}{1 \cancel{\text{gal}}} \times \frac{2 \cancel{\text{pt}}}{1 \cancel{\text{qt}}} \times \frac{2 \text{ c}}{1 \cancel{\text{pt}}}$$
$$= 452.8 \text{ c}$$

$$\begin{array}{r} 37.73 \\ 12\overline{)452.80} \\ \underline{-36\phantom{.80}} \\ 92\phantom{.80} \\ \underline{-84\phantom{.80}} \\ 88\phantom{0} \\ \underline{-84\phantom{0}} \\ 40 \\ \underline{-36} \\ 4 \end{array}$$

On average, an American drinks 37.7 c of bottled water per month.

**43. Strategy** To find the number of gallons of blood:

- Convert the number of pints to gallons.

**Solution**

$$10 \text{ qt} = 10 \cancel{\text{pt}} \times \frac{1 \cancel{\text{qt}}}{2 \cancel{\text{pt}}} \times \frac{1 \text{ gal}}{4 \cancel{\text{qt}}}$$
$$= 1\frac{1}{4} \text{ gal}$$

There are $1\frac{1}{4}$ gal of blood in the human body.

**45. Strategy** To find the profit the pharmacy makes:

- Divide the number of ounces (500) by 4 to see how many bottles can be made.
- Multiply the number of bottles by $2 to find the total income from the bottles.
- Subtract the cost ($120) from the total income to find the profit.

**Solution**

$$\frac{500 \text{ oz}}{4 \text{ oz}} = 125 \text{ bottles}$$

$125 \times \$2 = \$250$

$250 - 120 = 130$

The pharmacy's profit was $130.

**47.** Number of cups of lemonade in the punch

## Applying the Concepts

**49.** Students may enjoy exercising the creativity required to answer this question. However, they should note that a standard unit of measurement must be developed first. Related units can then be developed using equivalences that allow for conversion of units.

© 2013 Cengage Learning. All Rights Reserved. May not be scanned, copied or duplicated, or posted to a publicly accessible website, in whole or in part.

## Section 8.4

### Objective A Exercises

**1.** Greater than

**3.** Greater than

**5.** $12 \text{ weeks} = 12 \cancel{\text{ weeks}} \times \frac{7 \text{ days}}{1 \cancel{\text{ week}}} = 84 \text{ days}$

**7.** $114 \text{ h} = 114 \cancel{\text{ h}} \times \frac{1 \text{ day}}{24 \cancel{\text{ h}}} = 4\frac{3}{4} \text{ days}$

**9.** $7\frac{3}{4} \text{ h} = 7\frac{3}{4} \cancel{\text{ h}} \times \frac{60 \text{ min}}{1 \cancel{\text{ h}}} = 465 \text{ min}$

**11.** $750 \text{ s} = 750 \cancel{\text{ s}} \times \frac{1 \text{ min}}{60 \cancel{\text{ s}}} = 12\frac{1}{2} \text{min}$

**13.** $15{,}300 \text{ s} = 15{,}300 \cancel{\text{ s}} \times \frac{1 \cancel{\text{ min}}}{60 \cancel{\text{ s}}} \times \frac{1 \text{ h}}{60 \cancel{\text{ min}}}$

$= 4\frac{1}{4} \text{ h}$

**15.** $5\frac{3}{4} \text{ h} = 5\frac{3}{4} \text{ h} \times \frac{60 \cancel{\text{ min}}}{1 \cancel{\text{ h}}} \times \frac{60 \text{ s}}{1 \cancel{\text{ min}}} = 20{,}700 \text{ s}$

**17.** $6840 \text{ min} = 6840 \cancel{\text{ min}} \times \frac{1 \cancel{\text{ h}}}{60 \cancel{\text{ min}}} \times \frac{1 \text{ day}}{24 \cancel{\text{ h}}}$

$= 4\frac{3}{4} \text{ days}$

**19.** $6\frac{1}{4} \text{ days} = 6\frac{1}{4} \cancel{\text{ days}} \times \frac{24 \cancel{\text{ h}}}{1 \cancel{\text{ day}}} \times \frac{60 \text{ min}}{1 \cancel{\text{ h}}}$

$= 9000 \text{ min}$

**21.** $588 \text{ h} = 588 \cancel{\text{ h}} \times \frac{1 \cancel{\text{ day}}}{24 \cancel{\text{ h}}} \times \frac{1 \text{ week}}{7 \cancel{\text{ days}}} = 3\frac{1}{2} \text{ weeks}$

**23.** $5\frac{1}{2} \text{ weeks} = 5\frac{1}{2} \cancel{\text{ weeks}} \times \frac{7 \cancel{\text{ days}}}{1 \cancel{\text{ week}}} \times \frac{24 \text{ h}}{1 \cancel{\text{ day}}}$

$= 924 \text{ h}$

**25.**

$20{,}160 \text{ min} = 20{,}160 \cancel{\text{ min}} \times \frac{1 \cancel{\text{ h}}}{60 \cancel{\text{ min}}} \times \frac{1 \cancel{\text{ day}}}{24 \cancel{\text{ h}}} \times \frac{1 \text{ week}}{7 \cancel{\text{ days}}}$

$= 2 \text{ weeks}$

**27.**

$3 \text{ weeks} = 3 \cancel{\text{ weeks}} \times \frac{7 \cancel{\text{ days}}}{1 \cancel{\text{ week}}} \times \frac{24 \cancel{\text{ h}}}{1 \cancel{\text{ day}}} \times \frac{60 \text{ min}}{1 \cancel{\text{ h}}}$

$= 30{,}240 \text{ min}$

### Applying the Concepts

**29.** **Strategy** To find how long it will take for half, divide the time (3 hr 30 min) by two.

**Solution**

```
    1 hr 45 min
  2)3 hr 30 min
    2
    1 hr = 60 min + 30 min
         = 90
          -90
            0
```

Half will be done in 1 hr 45 min.

## Section 8.5

### Objective A Exercises

**1.** $25 \text{ Btu} = 25 \cancel{\text{ Btu}} \times \frac{778 \text{ ft} \cdot \text{lb}}{1 \cancel{\text{ Btu}}}$

$= 19{,}450 \text{ ft} \cdot \text{lb}$

**3.** $25{,}000 \text{ Btu} = 25{,}000 \cancel{\text{ Btu}} \times \frac{778 \text{ ft} \cdot \text{lb}}{1 \cancel{\text{ Btu}}}$

$= 19{,}450{,}000 \text{ ft} \cdot \text{lb}$

**5.** $\text{Energy} = 150 \text{ lb} \times 10 \text{ ft}$

$= 1500 \text{ ft} \cdot \text{lb}$

**7.** $\text{Energy} = 3300 \text{ lb} \times 9 \text{ ft}$

$= 29{,}700 \text{ ft} \cdot \text{lb}$

**9.** $3 \text{ tons} = 6000 \text{ lb}$

$\text{Energy} = 6000 \text{ lb} \times 5 \text{ ft}$

$= 30{,}000 \text{ ft} \cdot \text{lb}$

© 2013 Cengage Learning. All Rights Reserved. May not be scanned, copied or duplicated, or posted to a publicly accessible website, in whole or in part.

**11.** $850 \times 3 \text{ lb} = 2550 \text{ lb}$
Energy $= 2550 \text{ lb} \times 10 \text{ ft} = 25,500 \text{ ft} \cdot \text{lb}$

**13.** $45,000 \text{ Btu} = 45,000 \cancel{\text{Btu}} \times \dfrac{778 \text{ ft} \cdot \text{lb}}{1 \cancel{\text{Btu}}} = 35,010,000 \text{ ft} \cdot \text{lb}$

**15.** $12,000 \text{ Btu} = 12,000 \cancel{\text{Btu}} \times \dfrac{778 \text{ ft} \cdot \text{lb}}{1 \cancel{\text{Btu}}} = 9,336,000 \text{ ft} \cdot \text{lb}$

**17.** Less than

## Objective B Exercises

**19.** $\dfrac{1100}{550} = 2 \text{ hp}$

**21.** $\dfrac{4400}{550} = 8 \text{ hp}$

**23.** $9 \times 550 \dfrac{\text{ft} \cdot \text{lb}}{\text{s}} = 4950 \dfrac{\text{ft} \cdot \text{lb}}{\text{s}}$

**25.** $7 \times 550 \dfrac{\text{ft} \cdot \text{lb}}{\text{s}} = 3850 \dfrac{\text{ft} \cdot \text{lb}}{\text{s}}$

**27.** Power $= \dfrac{125 \text{ lb} \times 12 \text{ ft}}{3 \text{ s}} = 500 \dfrac{\text{ft} \cdot \text{lb}}{\text{s}}$

**29.** Power $= \dfrac{3000 \text{ lb} \times 40 \text{ ft}}{25 \text{ s}} = 4800 \dfrac{\text{ft} \cdot \text{lb}}{\text{s}}$

**31.** Power $= \dfrac{1200 \text{ lb} \times 18 \text{ ft}}{30 \text{ s}} = 720 \dfrac{\text{ft} \cdot \text{lb}}{\text{s}}$

**33.** $\dfrac{16,500}{550} = 30 \text{ hp}$

## Applying the Concepts

**35.** Students can select from a number of energy sources: natural gas, coal, wood, oil, nuclear power, hydroelectric power, or solar energy. Research will be required to answer the questions concerning sources, possible pollution problems, and future prospects associated with the form of energy.

## Chapter 8 Concept Review

**1.** To convert from feet to inches, use multiplication.

**2.** To convert 5 ft 7 in. to all inches, multiply 5 by 12 and add the product to 7.

**3.** To divide 7 ft 8 in. by 2, first divide 7 ft by 2. The result is 3 ft with 1 ft remaining. Convert the 1 ft remaining to 12 in., and add the 12 in. to 8 in.: 8 in. + 12 in. = 20 in. Divide 20 in. by 2. The result is 10 in. Therefore, 7 ft 8 in. divided by 2 is 3 ft 10 in.

**4.** To convert 5240 lb to tons, use the conversion rate $\dfrac{1 \text{ ton}}{2000 \text{ lb}}$.

**5.** To multiply 6 lb 9 oz by 3, first multiply 9 oz by 3. The result is 27 oz. Multiply 6 lb by 3. The result is 18 lb. 18 lb 27 oz = 19 lb 11 oz. Therefore, 6 lb 9 oz times 3 equals 19 lb 11 oz.

**6.** Five measures of capacity are fluid ounces, cups, pints, quarts, and gallons.

**7.** To convert 7 gal to quarts, use the conversion rate $\dfrac{4 \text{ qt}}{1 \text{ gal}}$.

**8.** To convert 374 min to hours, use the conversion rate $\dfrac{1 \text{ h}}{60 \text{ min}}$.

**9.** A foot-pound of energy is the amount of energy needed to lift 1 lb a distance of 1 ft.

© 2013 Cengage Learning. All Rights Reserved. May not be scanned, copied or duplicated, or posted to a publicly accessible website, in whole or in part.

**10.** To find the power needed to raise 200 lb a distance of 24 ft in 12 s, use multiplication and division. Power $= \dfrac{24\text{ ft} \times 200\text{ lb}}{12\text{ s}} = 400\ \dfrac{\text{ft} \cdot \text{lb}}{\text{s}}$

## Chapter 8 Review Exercises

**1.** $4\text{ ft} = 4\ \cancel{\text{ft}} \times \dfrac{12\text{ in.}}{1\ \cancel{\text{ft}}} = 48\text{ in.}$

**2.**
```
   2 ft  6 in.
3)7 ft  6 in.
 −6 ft
  1 ft = 12 in.
         18 in.
        −18 in.
          0
```

**3.** $53\text{ in} = 53\ \cancel{\text{in}} \times \dfrac{1\text{ ft}}{12\ \cancel{\text{in}}} =$

```
   4 ft 5 in.
12)53
   48
    5
```

**4.** $2\frac{1}{2}\text{ pt} = 2\frac{1}{2}\ \cancel{\text{pt}} \times \dfrac{2\ \cancel{\text{c}}}{1\ \cancel{\text{pt}}} \times \dfrac{8\text{ ft oz}}{1\ \cancel{\text{c}}}$

$= 2\frac{1}{2} \times 16\text{ fl oz}$

$= \frac{5}{2} \times 16\text{ fl oz}$

$= 40\text{ fl oz}$

**5.** $14\text{ ft} = 14\ \cancel{\text{ft}} \times \dfrac{1\text{ yd}}{3\ \cancel{\text{ft}}}$

$= \frac{14}{3}\text{ yd}$

$= 4\frac{2}{3}\text{ oz}$

**6.** $84\text{ oz} = 84\text{ oz} \times \dfrac{1\text{ lb}}{16\text{ oz}} =$

```
   5 lb 4 oz
16)84
   80
    4
```

**7.**
```
  2 lb    7 oz
3)7 lb    5 oz
 −6 lb
  1 lb = 16 oz
         21 oz
        −21 oz
          0
```

**8.** $3\frac{3}{8}\text{ lb} = 3\frac{3}{8}\ \cancel{\text{lb}} \times \dfrac{16\text{ oz}}{1\ \cancel{\text{lb}}}$

$= 3\frac{3}{8} \times 16\text{ oz}$

$= \frac{27}{8} \times 16\text{ oz} = 54\text{ oz}$

**9.**
```
   3 ft   9 in.
 + 5 ft   6 in.
   8 ft  15 in. = 9 ft 3 in.
```

**10.**
```
   2        2500
   3̸ tons  5̸0̸0̸ lb
 −1 ton   1500 lb
  1 ton   1000 lb
```

**11.**
```
   4 c  7 fl oz
 +2 c  3 fl oz
  6 c 10 fl oz = 7 c 2 fl oz
```

**12.**
```
  4     4
  5̸ yd 1̸ ft
 − 3 yd 2 ft
   1 yd 2 ft
```

**13.** $12\ \cancel{\text{c}} \times \dfrac{1\ \cancel{\text{pt}}}{2\ \cancel{\text{c}}} \times \dfrac{1\text{ qt}}{2\ \cancel{\text{pt}}} = \dfrac{12}{4}\text{ qt} = 3\text{ qt}$

**14.** $375\text{ min} \times \dfrac{1\text{ h}}{60\text{ min}} = 6\frac{1}{4}\text{ h}$

**15.** $2.5\text{ hp} \times 550\ \dfrac{\text{ft} \cdot \text{lb}}{\text{s}} = 1375\ \dfrac{\text{ft} \cdot \text{lb}}{\text{s}}$

© 2013 Cengage Learning. All Rights Reserved. May not be scanned, copied or duplicated, or posted to a publicly accessible website, in whole or in part.

**16.**

$$\begin{array}{r} 5 \text{ lb } 8 \text{ oz} \\ \times \quad 8 \\ \hline 40 \text{ lb } 64 \text{ oz} = 44 \text{ lb} \end{array}$$

**17.** **Strategy** To find the patient's height in ft, convert in to ft.

**Solution**
$$67 \text{ in} = 67 \text{ in} \times \frac{1 \text{ ft}}{12 \text{ in}} =$$

$$\begin{array}{r} 5 \text{ ft } 7 \text{ in} \\ 12\overline{)67} \\ \underline{60} \\ 7 \end{array}$$

The patient is 5 ft 7 in.

**18.** **Strategy** To find the weight in pounds, convert ounces to pounds.

**Solution**
$$70 \text{ oz} = 70 \text{ oz} \times \frac{1 \text{ lb}}{16 \text{ oz}} = 4\frac{3}{8} \text{ lb}$$

The baby weighs $4\frac{3}{8}$ lb.

**19.** **Strategy** To find the total amount cut from the roll, add the three lengths (1 ft 3 in., 2 ft 3 in., and 11 in.)

**Solution**
$$\begin{array}{l} 1 \text{ ft } 3 \text{ in} \\ 2 \text{ ft } 3 \text{ in} \\ + \quad 11 \text{ in} \\ \hline 3 \text{ ft } 17 \text{ in} = 4 \text{ ft } 5 \text{ in} \end{array}$$

4 ft 5 in. have been cut from the roll.

**20.** **Strategy** To find the total weight, add the 8 weights (2 lb 8 oz, 2 lb 2 oz, 3 lb 1 oz, 1 lb 12 oz, 2 lb 9 oz, 1 lb 13 oz, and 2 lb 7 oz).

**Solution**
$$\begin{array}{r} 2 \text{ lb} \quad 8 \text{ oz} \\ 2 \text{ lb} \quad 2 \text{ oz} \\ 3 \text{ lb} \quad 1 \text{ oz} \\ 2 \text{ lb} \quad 3 \text{ oz} \\ 1 \text{ lb} \quad 12 \text{ oz} \\ 2 \text{ lb} \quad 9 \text{ oz} \\ 1 \text{ lb} \quad 13 \text{ oz} \\ +2 \text{ lb} \quad 7 \text{ oz} \\ \hline 15 \text{ lb } 55 \text{ oz} = 18 \text{ lb } 7 \text{ oz} \end{array}$$

The total weight of the babies is 18 lb 7 oz.

**21.** **Strategy** To find the number of quarts in a case:

- Find the number of ounces in a case by multiplying the number of ounces in a can (18 fl oz) by the number of cans in a case (24).
- Convert the number of ounces to quarts.

**Solution**
$$\begin{array}{r} 18 \text{ fl oz} \\ \times \quad 24 \\ \hline 432 \text{ fl oz} \end{array}$$

$$432 \text{ fl oz} \times \frac{1 \text{ c}}{8 \text{ fl oz}} \times \frac{1 \text{ pt}}{2 \text{ c}} \times \frac{1 \text{ qt}}{2 \text{ pt}}$$

$$= \frac{432}{32} \text{ qt} = 13\frac{1}{2} \text{ qt}$$

There are $13\frac{1}{2}$ qt in a case.

**22.** **Strategy** To find how many gallons of milk were sold:

- Find the number of cups sold by multiplying the number of cartons (256) by the number of cups per carton (1).
- Convert the number of cups to gallons.

**Solution** 256 cartons × 1 c = 256 c

$$256 \text{ c} = 256 \text{ c} \times \frac{1 \text{ pt}}{2 \text{ c}} \times \frac{1 \text{ qt}}{2 \text{ pt}} \times \frac{1 \text{ gal}}{4 \text{ qt}}$$

$$= \frac{256}{16} \text{ gal} = 16 \text{ gal}$$

16 gal of milk were sold that day.

**23.** $35{,}0000 \text{ Btu} = 35{,}000 \text{ Btu} \times \frac{778 \text{ ft} \cdot \text{lb}}{1 \text{ Btu}}$

$$= 27{,}230{,}000 \text{ ft} \cdot \text{lb}$$

**24.** $\text{Power} = \frac{800 \text{ lb} \times 15 \text{ ft}}{25 \text{ s}} = 480 \frac{\text{ft} \cdot \text{lb}}{\text{s}}$

© 2013 Cengage Learning. All Rights Reserved. May not be scanned, copied or duplicated, or posted to a publicly accessible website, in whole or in part.

# Chapter 8 Test

**1.** $2\frac{1}{2}\text{ ft} = 2\frac{1}{2}\cancel{\text{ft}} \times \frac{12\text{ in.}}{1\cancel{\text{ft}}} = 2\frac{1}{2} \times 12\text{ in.}$

$= \frac{5}{2} \times 12\text{ in.}$

$= 30\text{ in.}$

**2.** $\overset{3}{\cancel{4}}\text{ ft }\overset{14}{\cancel{2}}\text{ in.}$

$-1\text{ ft }9\text{ in.}$

$2\text{ ft }5\text{ in.}$

**3. Strategy** To find the number of pieces:

- Convert the length of the tape (5 yd) to in.
- Divide the number of inches by the length of each piece (10 in.).

**Solution** $5\text{ yd} = 5\cancel{\text{yd}} \times \frac{3\cancel{\text{ft}}}{1\cancel{\text{yd}}} \times \frac{12\text{ in}}{1\cancel{\text{ft}}} = 180\text{ in}$

$180 \div 10 = 18$

18 pieces can be cut.

**4. Strategy** To find Julio's height, add 5 in. to Rodriquez's height (3 ft 9 in.).

**Solution** 3 ft 9 in.

$+$ 5 in.

3 ft 14 in = 4 ft 2 in

Julio is 4 ft 2 in.

**5.** $2\frac{7}{8}\text{ lb} = 2\frac{7}{8}\text{ lb} \times \frac{16\text{ oz}}{1\text{ lb}}$

$= 2\frac{7}{8} \times 16\text{ oz} = \frac{23}{8} \times 16\text{ oz}$

$= 46\text{ oz}$

**6.**

$$\begin{array}{r} 2\text{ lb }8\text{ oz} \\ 16\overline{)40} \\ -32 \\ \hline 8 \end{array}$$

40 oz = 2 lb 8 oz

**7.**

$$\begin{array}{r} 9\text{ lb }\ 6\text{ oz} \\ +\ 7\text{ lb }11\text{ oz} \\ \hline 16\text{ lb }17\text{ oz} = 17\text{ lb }1\text{ oz} \end{array}$$

**8.**

$$\begin{array}{r} 1\text{ lb}\quad 11\text{ oz} \\ 4\overline{)6\text{ lb}\quad 12\text{ oz}} \\ -4\text{ lb}\qquad\qquad \\ 2\text{ lb} = \underline{32\text{ oz}} \\ 44\text{ oz} \\ -44\text{ oz} \\ \hline 0 \end{array}$$

**9. Strategy** To find the total weight of the workbooks in pounds:

- Find the total weight of the workbooks in ounces by multiplying the number of workbooks (1000) by the weight per workbook (12 oz).
- Convert the weight in ounces to pounds.

**Solution** $1000 \times 12\text{ oz} = 12{,}000\text{ oz}$

$12{,}000\text{ oz} = 12{,}000\cancel{\text{oz}} \times \frac{1\text{ lb}}{16\cancel{\text{oz}}}$

$= 750\text{ lb}$

The total weight of the workbooks is 750 lb.

**10. Strategy** To find the amount received for recycling the cans:

- Find the weight in ounces of the cans by solving a proportion.
- Convert the weight in ounces to pounds.
- Multiply the weight in pounds by the price paid per pound.

**Solution** $\frac{4\text{ cans}}{3\text{ oz}} = \frac{800\text{ cans}}{n}$

$4 \times n = 3 \times 800$

$4 \times n = 2400$

$n = 2400 \div 4 = 600$

The cans weigh 600 oz. 600 oz.

© 2013 Cengage Learning. All Rights Reserved. May not be scanned, copied or duplicated, or posted to a publicly accessible website, in whole or in part.

$600 \text{ oz} = 600 \cancel{\text{oz}} \times \frac{1 \text{ lb}}{16 \cancel{\text{oz}}} = 37.5 \text{ lb}$

$37.5 \times 0.75 = 28.13$

The amount the class received for recycling was \$28.13.

**11.** $13 \text{ qt} = 13 \cancel{\text{qt}} \times \frac{1 \text{ gal}}{4 \cancel{\text{qt}}} = \frac{13}{4} \text{ gal} = 3\frac{1}{4} \text{ gal}$

**12.** $3\frac{1}{2} \text{ gal} = 3\frac{1}{2} \cancel{\text{gal}} \times \frac{4 \cancel{\text{qt}}}{1 \cancel{\text{gal}}} \times \frac{2 \text{ pt}}{1 \cancel{\text{qt}}}$

$= 3\frac{1}{2} \times 8 \text{ pt} = 28 \text{ pt}$

**13.** $1\frac{3}{4} \text{ gal} \times 7 = \frac{7}{4} \text{ gal} \times 7 = \frac{49}{4} \text{ gal}$

$= 12\frac{1}{4} \text{ gal}$

**14.**

$$\begin{array}{r} 5 \text{ gal } 2 \text{ qt} \\ +\ 2 \text{ gal } 3 \text{ qt} \\ \hline 7 \text{ gal } 5 \text{ qt} = 8 \text{ gal } 1 \text{ qt} \end{array}$$

**15.** $756 \text{ h} = 756 \cancel{\text{h}} \times \frac{1 \cancel{\text{day}}}{24 \cancel{\text{h}}} \times \frac{1 \text{ week}}{7 \cancel{\text{days}}} = 4\frac{1}{2} \text{ weeks}$

**16.** $3\frac{1}{4} \text{ days} = 3\frac{1}{4} \cancel{\text{days}} \times \frac{24 \cancel{\text{h}}}{1 \cancel{\text{day}}} \times \frac{60 \text{ min}}{1 \cancel{\text{h}}}$

$= 4680 \text{ min}$

**17. Strategy** To find the number of cups of grapefruit juice in a case:

- Find the number of ounces of juice in a case by multiplying the number of cans in a case (24) by the number of ounces in a can (20).
- Convert the number of ounces to cups.

**Solution** $24 \times 20 \text{ oz} = 480 \text{ oz}$

$480 \text{ oz} = 480 \cancel{\text{oz}} \times \frac{1 \text{ c}}{8 \cancel{\text{oz}}} = 60 \text{ c}$

There are 60 c in a case.

**18. Strategy** To find the profit:

- Convert 1 gal to ounces.
- To find the number of bottles, divide the number of ounces by the number of ounces per bottle (8 ounces).
- To find the total income for the sale of the rubbing alcohol, multiply the number of bottles by the sale price per bottle (\$2.75).
- To find the profit, subtract the price the pharmacy pays for the rubbing alcohol (\$25.50) from the total income.

**Solution** 1 gal

$= 1 \cancel{\text{gal}} \times \frac{4 \cancel{\text{qt}}}{1 \cancel{\text{gal}}} \times \frac{2 \cancel{\text{pt}}}{1 \cancel{\text{qt}}} \times \frac{16 \text{ oz}}{1 \cancel{\text{pt}}}$

$= 128 \text{ oz}$

$128 \div 8 = 16$ bottles

$16 \times 2.75 = 44$

$44 - 25.50 = 18.50$

The pharmacy's profit is \$18.50.

**19. Strategy** To find the father's height in ft and in:

- Multiply the boy's height (38in.) by 2.
- Convert the in. to ft and in.

**Solution** $38 \times 2 = 76$

$$\begin{array}{r} 6 \text{ ft } 4 \text{ in.} \\ 12\overline{)76} \\ \underline{72} \\ 4 \end{array}$$

The father's height is 6 ft 4 in.

**20. Strategy** To find the weight gain, subtract the weight at birth (5 lb 12 oz) from the weight at six months (13 lb 5 oz).

© 2013 Cengage Learning. All Rights Reserved. May not be scanned, copied or duplicated, or posted to a publicly accessible website, in whole or in part.

**Solution**

$$\begin{array}{r} 12 \text{ lb } 21 \text{ oz} \\ \not{13} \text{ lb } \ \ 5 \text{ oz} \\ \underline{-5 \text{ lb } 12 \text{ oz}} \\ 7 \text{ lb } \ \ 9 \text{ oz} \end{array}$$

The baby gained 7 lb 9 oz.

**21.** $40{,}000 \text{ Btu} = 40{,}000 \cancel{\text{Btu}} \times \dfrac{778 \text{ ft} \cdot \text{lb}}{1 \cancel{\text{Btu}}}$

$= 31{,}120{,}000 \text{ ft} \cdot \text{lb}$

**22.** $\dfrac{2200}{550} = 4 \text{ hp}$

## Cumulative Review Exercises

**1.**

| | 2 | 3 | 5 |
|---|---|---|---|
| 9 = | | (3 · 3) | |
| 12 = | (2 · 2) | 3 | |
| 15 = | | 3 | (5) |

LCM $= 2 \cdot 2 \cdot 3 \cdot 3 \cdot 5 = 180$

**2.**

$$\frac{43}{8} = 8\overline{)43} \quad \begin{array}{r} 5\frac{3}{8} \\ 8\overline{)43} \\ \underline{-40} \\ 3 \end{array}$$

**3.**

$$\begin{array}{r} 5\dfrac{7}{8} = 5\dfrac{21}{24} \\ -2\dfrac{7}{12} = 2\dfrac{14}{24} \\ \hline 3\dfrac{7}{24} \end{array}$$

**4.** $5\dfrac{1}{3} \div 2\dfrac{2}{3} = \dfrac{16}{3} \div \dfrac{8}{3} = \dfrac{16}{3} \times \dfrac{3}{8} = 2$

**5.**

$\dfrac{5}{8} \div \left(\dfrac{3}{8} - \dfrac{1}{4}\right) - \dfrac{5}{8}$

$= \dfrac{5}{8} \div \left(\dfrac{3}{8} - \dfrac{2}{8}\right) - \dfrac{5}{8}$

$= \dfrac{5}{8} \div \dfrac{1}{8} - \dfrac{5}{8}$

$= \dfrac{5}{8} \times \dfrac{8}{1} - \dfrac{5}{8}$

$= 5 - \dfrac{5}{8}$

$= 4\dfrac{8}{8} - \dfrac{5}{8} = 4\dfrac{3}{8}$

**6.**

2.0972 — Given place value: 9; $7 > 5$

2.10

**7.**

$$\begin{array}{r} 0.0792 \\ \times \quad 0.49 \\ \hline 7128 \\ 3168 \ \\ \hline 0.038808 \end{array}$$

**8.** $\dfrac{n}{12} = \dfrac{44}{60}$

$n \times 60 = 12 \times 44$

$n \times 60 = 528$

$n = 528 \div 60 = 8.8$

**9.** $2\dfrac{1}{2}\% \times 50 = n$

$0.025 \times 50 = n$

$1.25 = n$

**10.** $42\,\% \times n = 18$

$0.42 \times n = 18$

$n = 18 \div 0.42$

$n \approx 42.86$

**11.** $\$37.08 \div 7.2 \text{ lb} = \$5.15/\text{lb}$

© 2013 Cengage Learning. All Rights Reserved. May not be scanned, copied or duplicated, or posted to a publicly accessible website, in whole or in part.

**12.** $$\begin{array}{r} 3\frac{2}{5}\text{ in.} = 3\frac{6}{15}\text{ in.} \\ +5\frac{1}{3}\text{ in.} = 5\frac{5}{15}\text{ in.} \\ \hline 8\frac{11}{15}\text{ in.} \end{array}$$

**13.** $$\begin{array}{r} 1\text{ lb } 8\text{ oz} \\ 16\overline{)24} \\ -16 \\ \hline 8 \end{array} \qquad 24\text{ oz} = 1\text{ lb } 8\text{ oz}$$

**14.** $$\begin{array}{r} 3\text{ lb } 8\text{ oz} \\ \times \quad 9 \\ \hline 27\text{ lb } 72\text{ oz} = 31\text{ lb } 8\text{ oz} \end{array}$$

**15.** $$\begin{array}{r} 4\frac{1}{3}\text{ qt} = 4\frac{2}{6}\text{ qt} = 3\frac{8}{6}\text{ qt} \\ -1\frac{5}{6}\text{ qt} = 1\frac{5}{6}\text{ qt} = 1\frac{5}{6}\text{ qt} \\ \hline 2\frac{3}{6}\text{ qt} = 2\frac{1}{2}\text{ qt} \end{array}$$

**16.** $$\begin{array}{r} \overset{3}{\not 4}\text{ lb } \overset{22}{\not 6}\text{ oz} \\ -2\text{ lb } 10\text{ oz} \\ \hline 1\text{ lb } 12\text{ oz} \end{array}$$

**17.** **Strategy** To find the milligrams of salt, solve a proportion.

**Solution**

$$\frac{2.5\text{ milligrams of salt}}{100\text{ milliliters of solution}} = \frac{x}{250\text{ milliters of solution}}$$

$$100 \times x = 2.5 \times 250$$
$$100x = 625$$
$$x = 625 \div 100$$
$$x = 6.25$$

6.25 milligrams of salt are needed.

**18.** **Strategy** To find Anna's checking balance, subtract the amounts of the checks and add the deposit.

**Solution**

$$\begin{array}{r} 578.56 \\ -216.98 \\ \hline 361.58 \\ -\ 34.12 \\ \hline 327.46 \\ +315.33 \\ \hline 642.79 \end{array}$$

Anna's balance is \$642.79.

**19.** **Strategy** To find the salesman's total monthly income:

- Find the amount of sales over \$25,000 by subtracting \$25,000 from the total sales (\$140,000).
- Find the amount of the commission by solving the basic percent equation for amount. The base is the amount of sales over \$25,000 and the percent is 2%.
- Add the amount of commission to the salary (\$1800).

**Solution**

$$140,000 - 25,000 = 115,000$$
$$\text{Percent} \times \text{base} = \text{amount}$$
$$2\% \times 115,000 = n$$
$$0.02 \times 115,000 = n$$
$$2300 = n$$
$$2300 + 1800 = 4100$$

The saleman's monthly income is \$4100.

**20.** **Strategy** To find the milliliters, solve the proportion.

**Solution**

$$\frac{0.25\text{ milligrams}}{1\text{ milliter}} = \frac{1.5\text{ milligrams}}{x}$$
$$1 \times 1.5 = 0.25x$$
$$1.5 \div 0.25 = x$$
$$6 = x$$

The dose is 6 milliliters.

**21.** **Strategy** To find the percent:

- Find the total number of students who took the final exam

© 2013 Cengage Learning. All Rights Reserved. May not be scanned, copied or duplicated, or posted to a publicly accessible website, in whole or in part.

by reading the histogram and adding the frequencies.

• Find the number of students who received a score between 80% and 90% by reading the histogram.

• Solve the basic percent equation for percent. The base is the total number of students who took the exam and the amount is the number of students with scores between 80% and 90%.

**Solution**

$$\begin{aligned} \text{Score}: 40-50:&\quad 2 \text{ students} \\ 50-60:&\quad 1 \text{ students} \\ 60-70:&\quad 5 \text{ students} \\ 70-80:&\quad 7 \text{ students} \\ 80-90:&\quad 4 \text{ students} \\ 90-100:&\quad \underline{3 \text{ students}} \end{aligned}$$

$\text{total number of students}: 22$

$$\begin{aligned} \text{Percent} \times \text{base} &= \text{amount} \\ n \times 22 &= 4 \\ n &= 4 \div 22 \\ &\approx 0.18 = 18\% \end{aligned}$$

The percent is 18%.

**22. Strategy** To find the selling price:

• Find the amount of the markup by solving the basic percent equation for amount. The base is \$925 and the percent is 40%.

• Add the markup to the cost (\$925).

**Solution**

$$\begin{aligned} \text{Percent} \times \text{base} &= \text{amount} \\ 40\% \times 925 &= n \\ 0.40 \times 925 &= n \\ 370 &= n \\ 925 + 370 &= 1295 \end{aligned}$$

The selling price of the power wheelchair is \$1295.

**23. Strategy** To find the interest paid, multiply the principal (\$200,000) by the annual interest rate (6%) by the time (8 months) in years.

**Solution**

$$200{,}000 \times 0.06 \times \frac{8}{12} = 8000$$

The interest paid on the loan is \$8000.

**24. Strategy** To find how much each student received:

• Convert 1 lb 3 oz to ounces.

• Find the total value of the gold by multiplying the number of ounces by the price per ounce (\$200).

• Divide the total value by the number of students (6).

**Solution**

$$\begin{aligned} &1 \text{ lb } 3 \text{ oz } = 19 \text{ oz} \\ &19 \times 800 = 15{,}200 \quad \text{total value} \\ &15{,}200 \div 6 \approx 2533 \end{aligned}$$

Each student received \$2533.

**25. Strategy** To find the profit:

• Convert 1 gal to ounces to find the total number of ounces.

• Find the number of bottles by dividing the total number of ounces by the number of ounces per bottle (8 oz).

• Find the total income for the sale of the lotion, multiply the number of bottles by the sale price per bottle (\$3.50).

• To find the profit, subtract the price the spa pays for the lotion (\$25.50) from the total income.

© 2013 Cengage Learning. All Rights Reserved. May not be scanned, copied or duplicated, or posted to a publicly accessible website, in whole or in part.

**Solution** 1 gal

$$= 1 \not{gal} \times \frac{4 \not{qt}}{1 \not{gal}} \times \frac{2 \not{pt}}{1 \not{qt}} \times \frac{16 \text{ oz}}{1 \not{pt}}$$

$$= 128 \text{ oz}$$

$128 \div 8 = 16$ bottles

$16 \times 3.50 = 56$

$56 - 32.66 = 23.34$

The spa's profit is \$23.34.

**26. Strategy** To find the better buy:

- Find the unit price for each brand.
- Compare unit prices.

**Solution** \$.79 for 8 oz  \$2.98 for 36 oz

$\frac{0.79}{8} = 0.09875$  $\frac{2.98}{36} \approx 0.08278$

$0.08278 < 0.09875$

The better buy is 36 oz for \$2.98.

**27. Strategy** To calculate the probability:

- Count the number of possible outcomes.
- Count the number of favorable outcomes.
- Use the probability formula.

**Solution** There are 36 possible outcomes.

There are 4 favorable outcomes:

(3, 6), (4, 5), (5, 4), (6, 3).

$$\text{Probability} = \frac{4}{36} = \frac{1}{9}$$

The probability is $\frac{1}{9}$ that the sum of the dots on the two dice is 9.

**28. Strategy** To find the cost, solve the proportion.

$$\frac{9.50}{1000 \text{ units}} = \frac{x}{40{,}000 \text{ units}}$$

$$1000x = 9.5 \times 40{,}000$$

$$1000x = 380{,}000$$

$$x = 380{,}000 \div 1000$$

$$x = 380$$

The cost is \$380 per week.

**29.**

$$70 \text{ in} = 70 \not{in} \times \frac{1 \text{ ft}}{12 \not{in}}$$

$$\begin{array}{r} 5 \text{ ft } 10 \text{ in} \\ 12\overline{)70} \\ \underline{60} \\ 10 \end{array}$$

© 2013 Cengage Learning. All Rights Reserved. May not be scanned, copied or duplicated, or posted to a publicly accessible website, in whole or in part.

# Chapter 9: The Metric System of Measurement

## Prep Test

**1.** $3.732 \times 10{,}000 = 37{,}320$

**2.** $65.9 \times 10^4 = 659{,}000$

**3.** $41.07 \div 1000 = 0.04107$

**4.** $28{,}496 \div 10^3 = 28{,}496 \div 1000 = 28.496$

**5.** $6 - 0.875 = 5.125$

**6.** $5 + 0.96 = 5.96$

**7.** $3.25 \times 0.04 = 0.13$

**8.** $35 \times \frac{1.61}{1} = 35 \times 1.61 = 56.35$

**9.** $1.67 \times \frac{1}{3.34} = 1.67 \div 3.34$

$$3.34\overline{)1.670} = 0.5$$

**10.** $4\frac{1}{2} \times 150 = \frac{9}{2} \times \frac{150}{1}$

$$= \frac{3 \cdot 3 \cdot \cancel{2} \cdot 3 \cdot 5 \cdot 5}{\cancel{2}} = 675$$

## Section 9.1

### Objective A Exercises

**1.** 42 cm = 420 mm

**3.** 81 mm = 8.1 cm

**5.** 6804 m = 6.804 km

**7.** 2.109 km = 2109 m

**9.** 432 cm = 4.32 m

**11.** 0.88 m = 88 cm

**13.** 7038 m = 7.038 km

**15.** 3.5 km = 3500 m

**17.** 260 cm = 2.60 m

**19.** 1.685 m = 168.5 cm

**21.** 14.8 cm = 148 mm

**23.** 62 m 7 cm = 62 m + 0.07 m = 62.07 m

**25.** 31 cm 9 mm = 31 cm + 0.9 cm = 31.9 cm

**27.** 8 km 75m = 8 km + 0.075 km = 8.075 km

**29.** m

### Objective B Exercises

**31.** 11.5 cm = 115 mm

**33.** **Strategy** To find the distance of the walk-a-thon:

- Convert the distances to kilometers.
- Add the three distances.

**Solution**

$$\begin{aligned} 1400 \text{ m} &= 1.4 \text{ km} \\ 1200 \text{ m} &= 1.2 \text{ km} \\ 1800 \text{ m} &= +1.8 \text{ km} \\ &\quad\ 4.4 \text{ km} \end{aligned}$$

The distance of the walk-a-thon was 4.4 km.

**35.** **Strategy** To express the blood pressure in mm, change both measures to mm.

**Solution** 142 mm of mercury to 105 mm of mercury = 14.2 cm of mercury to 10.5 cm of mercury.

**37.** **Strategy** To find the average number of meters adopted by a student nursing club:

- Convert the total length adopted to meters.
- Divide the length in meters by the number of groups.

**Solution** 8502 km = 8,502,000 m

© 2013 Cengage Learning. All Rights Reserved. May not be scanned, copied or duplicated, or posted to a publicly accessible website, in whole or in part.

$$
\begin{array}{r}
2253.9 \\
3772\overline{)8,502,000.0} \\
\underline{-7544} \\
9580 \\
\underline{-7544} \\
20360 \\
\underline{-18860} \\
15000 \\
\underline{-11316} \\
36840 \\
\underline{-33948} \\
2892
\end{array}
$$

Each student nursing club has adopted an average of 2254 m of highway.

**39. Strategy** To find the time for light to travel to Earth from the sun:

- Convert the distance light travels in 1 s (300,000,000 m) to kilometers.
- Divide the distance from the sun to Earth (150,000,000 km) by the distance light travels in 1 s.

**Solution** 300,000,000 m = 300,000 km

150,000,000 km ÷ 300,000 km/s = 500 s

It takes 500 s for light to travel from the sun to Earth.

**41. Strategy** To find the distance that light travels in 1 day:

- Find the number of seconds in 1 day.
- Multiply the distance that light travels in 1 s (300,000 km) by the number of seconds in 1 day.

**Solution** 1 day

$= 1\ \cancel{\text{day}} \times \dfrac{24\ \cancel{\text{h}}}{1\ \cancel{\text{day}}} \times \dfrac{60\ \cancel{\text{min}}}{1\ \cancel{\text{h}}} \times \dfrac{60\ \text{s}}{1\ \cancel{\text{min}}}$

$= 86,400$ s (in 1 day)

$300,000 \times 86,400$

$= 25,920,000,000$ km

Light travels 25,920,000,000 km in 1 day.

# Section 9.2

## Objective A Exercises

**1.** 420 g = 0.420 kg

**3.** 127 mg = 0.127 g

**5.** 4.2 kg = 4200 g

**7.** 0.45 g = 450 mg

**9.** 23 mg = 23,000 μg

**11.** 4057 mg = 4.057 g

**13.** 1.37 kg = 1370 g

**15.** 0.0456 g = 45.6 mg

**17.** 1.5 mg = 1500 μg

**19.** 3 kg 922 g = 3 kg + 0.922 kg = 3.922 kg

**21.** 7 g 891 mg = 7 g + 0.891 g = 7.891 g

**23.** 4 kg 63 g = 4 kg + 0.063 kg = 4.063 kg

**25.** mg

**27.** g

## Objective B Exercises

**29. Strategy** To find the number of tablets to take:

- Convert the amount of the supplement (2 g) to milligrams.
- Divide the amount of the supplement by the amount of

© 2013 Cengage Learning. All Rights Reserved. May not be scanned, copied or duplicated, or posted to a publicly accessible website, in whole or in part.

calcium in one tablet (500 mg).

**Solution** 2 g = 2000 mg

$$500\overline{)2000}^{\,4}$$

The patient should take 4 tablets per day.

**31. Strategy** To find the number of grams of cholesterol in one dozen eggs:

- Convert the amount of cholesterol that one egg contains (274 mg) to grams.
- Multiply the number of grams of cholesterol in one egg by the number of eggs (12).

**Solution** 274 mg = 0.274 g

12 × 0.274 = 3.288 g

There are 3.288 g of cholesterol in 12 eggs.

**33. Strategy** To find the cost of the three packages of ground meat:

- Convert the weight of the three packages to kilograms.

$x = 40 \times 250$

$x = 10,000$

- Add the three weights.
- Multiply the sum by $8.40.

**Solution**

| | |
|---|---|
| 470 g | 0.470 kg |
| 680 g | 0.680 kg |
| 590 g | + 0.590 kg |
| | 1.740 kg |

$1.74 \times 8.40 = 14.616$

The three packages of meat cost $14.62.

**35. Strategy** To find the dose, write and solve a proportion.

**Solution**

$$\frac{10\text{ mg}}{\text{kg}} = \frac{x}{25\text{ kg}}$$
$$x = 10 \times 25$$
$$x = 250$$

The dose is 250 mg.

**37. Strategy** To find the milligrams of solute:

- Write and solve a proportion to find the micrograms.
- Convert micrograms to milligrams.

**Solution**

$$\frac{40\ \mu g}{1\text{ ml}} = \frac{x\ \mu g}{250\text{ ml}}$$
$$x = 40 \times 250$$
$$x = 10,000\mu g$$

10,000 µg = 10 mg

There are 10 mg of solute.

**39. Strategy** To find the amount of drug:

- Convert the injection (200 mcg) to mg.
- Write and solve a proportion.

**Solution** 200 mcg = 0.2 mg

$$\frac{0.1\text{ mg}}{\text{ml}} = \frac{0.2\text{ mg}}{x}$$
$$0.2 = 0.1x$$
$$0.2 \div 0.1 = x$$
$$2 = x$$

The dose is 2 ml.

## Applying the Concepts

**41.** Students might list familiarity among the advantages of the U.S. Customary System and difficulty in converting units among the disadvantages. They might list ease of conversion among the advantages of the metric system, as well as the fact that international trade is based on the metric system.

A disadvantage for Americans is that they are unfamiliar with metric units. Another disadvantage is related to American industry: If forced to change to

© 2013 Cengage Learning. All Rights Reserved. May not be scanned, copied or duplicated, or posted to a publicly accessible website, in whole or in part.

the metric system, companies would face the difficulty and expense of altering the present dimensions of machinery, tools, and products.

## Section 9.3

### Objective A Exercises

**1.** 4200 ml = 4.2 L

**3.** 3.42 L = 3420 ml

**5.** 423 ml = 423 $cm^3$

**7.** 642 $cm^3$ = 642 ml

**9.** 42 $cm^3$ = 42 ml = 0.042 L

**11.** 0.435 L = 4.35 dl

**13.** 4.62 kl = 4620 L

**15.** 1423 L = 1.423 kl

**17.** 1.267 L = 12.67 dl

**19.** 3 L 42 ml = 3 L + 0.042 L = 3.042 L

**21.** 3 kl 4 L = 3 kl + 0.004 kl = 3.004 kl

**23.** 8 L 200 ml = 8 L + 0.200 L = 8.200 L

**25.** L

**27.** L

### Objective B Exercises

**29. Strategy** To find the number of servings:
- Convert the amount of milk (3.78 L) to milliliters.
- Divide the amount of milk by the amount of milk in one serving (230 ml).

**Solution** 3.78 L = 3780 ml

$3780 \div 230 \approx 16.43$

There are 16 servings in the container of milk.

**31. Strategy** To find how many patients can be immunized:
- Convert 3 ml to liters.
- Divide the total number of liters of flu vaccine (12) by the number of liters of vaccine each person receives.

**Solution** 3 ml = 0.003 L

$12 \div 0.003 = 4000$

4000 patients can be immunized.

**33. Strategy** To find when the infusion will be completed:
- Convert 1 liter to ml.
- Multiply the number of ml by $\frac{2}{5}$ to find the number of ml that have been infused.
- Subtract the number of ml that have been infused from the total number of ml to find the ml that are remaining.
- Write and solve a proportion to find the number of hours remaining.
- Add the hours remaining to noon.

**Solution** 1 L = 1000 ml

$$1000 \times \frac{2}{5} = 400$$

$$1000 - 400 = 600$$

$$\frac{60\text{ ml}}{1\text{ hr}} = \frac{600\text{ ml}}{x\text{ hr}}$$

$$1 \times 600 = 60x$$

$$600 \div 60 = x$$

$$10 = x$$

10 hours after noon = 10 P.M.

The infusion will be done at 10 P.M.

© 2013 Cengage Learning. All Rights Reserved. May not be scanned, copied or duplicated, or posted to a publicly accessible website, in whole or in part.

**35.** **Strategy** To determine the better buy:

- Find the unit cost (cost per liter) of the 12 one-liter bottles by dividing the cost ($19.80) by the amount of apple juice (12 L).
- Find the unit cost (cost per liter) of the 24 cans by converting the amount to liters and then dividing $14.50 by the amount of juice.

**Solution** The cost of 12 one-liter bottles:

$19.80 \div 12 = 1.65$

The unit cost is $1.65 per liter.

The cost of 24 cans:

$24 \times 340 \text{ ml} = 8160 \text{ ml} = 8.16 \text{ L}$

$14.50 \div 8.16 \approx 1.78$

The unit cost is $1.78 per liter.

Since $1.65 < $1.78, the 12 one-liter bottles are the better buy.

**37.** **Strategy** To find the profit:

- Convert the volume of 5 L of cough syrup to milliliters.
- Find the number of bottles of cough syrup by dividing the total volume in milliliters by the volume of the 250-ml bottles.
- Find the cost of the bottles by multiplying the number of bottles by the cost per bottle ($.55).
- Add the cost of the bottles to the cost of the 5 L of cough syrup ($195) to find the total cost.
- Multiply the number of bottles by $23.89 to find the total revenue.
- Subtract the total cost from the revenue to find the profit.

**Solution** $5 \text{ L} = 5000 \text{ ml}$

$5000 \div 250 = 20$ (Bottles of cough syrup)

$20 \times 0.55 = 11$ (Cost of the bottles)

$11 + 195 = 206$ (Total cost)

$20 \times 23.89 = 477.80$ (Revenue)

$477.80 - 206 = 271.80$ (Profit)

The profit was $271.80.

**39.** **Strategy** To number of cells in one ml:

- Convert the 1 μl to ml.
- Write and solve a proportion.

**Solution** 1 μl = 1000 ml

$$\frac{5.1 \text{ million cells}}{1\ \mu g} = \frac{x \text{ million cells}}{1000\ \mu g}$$

$$5.1 \text{ million cells} \times 1000 = x$$

$$5100 \text{ million cells} = x$$

$$5.1 \text{ billion cells} = x$$

There are 5.1 bill cells in 1 microliter.

## Applying the Concepts

**41.** $3 \text{ L} - 280 \text{ ml} = 3 \text{ L} - 0.280 \text{ L} = 2.72 \text{ L}$

$2.72 \text{ L} = 2720 \text{ ml}$

$2.72 \text{ L} = 2 \text{ L } 720 \text{ ml}$

# Section 9.4

## Objective A Exercises

**1.** **Strategy** To find the number of Calories that can be omitted from your diet, multiply the number of Calories omitted each day (110) by the number of days (30).

**Solution** $110 \times 30 = 3300$

3300 Calories can be omitted from your diet.

**3a.** **Strategy**

- From the nutrition label find the number of Calories per serving.
- Multiply the number of

© 2013 Cengage Learning. All Rights Reserved. May not be scanned, copied or duplicated, or posted to a publicly accessible website, in whole or in part.

Calories per serving by $1\frac{1}{2}$.

**Solution** There are 60 Calories per serving.

$$60 \times 1\frac{1}{2} = \frac{60}{1} \times \frac{3}{2} = \frac{60 \times 3}{2} = 90$$

There are 90 Calories in $1\frac{1}{2}$ servings.

**b. Strategy** From the nutrition label find the serving size and the number of Calories from fat.

• Determine how many servings are in 6 slices of bread.

• Multiply the number of fat Calories in a serving by the number of servings.

**Solution** 2 slices of bread is one serving.
10 fat Calories are in one serving.
$6 \div 2 = 3$ number of servings
$10 \times 3 = 30$
There are 30 fat Calories in 6 slices of bread.

**5. Strategy** To find how many Calories a 135-pound person would need to maintain body weight, multiply the body weight (135 lb) by the number of Calories per pound needed (15).

**Solution** $135 \times 15 = 2025$
2025 Calories would be needed.

**7. Strategy** To find how many Calories you burn up playing tennis:

• Convert 45 min to hours.

• Find how many hours of tennis are played by multiplying the number of days (30) by the time per day in hours.

• Multiply the number of hours played by the Calories burned per hour (450).

**Solution**

$$45 \text{ min} = 45 \not{\text{min}} \times \frac{1 \text{ h}}{60 \not{\text{min}}} = \frac{3}{4} \text{ h}$$

$$30 \times \frac{3}{4} \text{ h} = \frac{90}{4} \text{ h} = 22.5 \text{ h}$$

450 Calories × 22.5
= 10,125 Calories
You burn 10,125 Calories.

**9. Strategy** To find how many hours you would have to hike:

• Add to find the total number of Calories consumed (375 + 150 + 280).

• Divide the sum by the number of Calories used in 1 h (315).

**Solution**

$$\begin{array}{r} 375 \\ 150 \\ +\,280 \\ \hline 805 \end{array}$$ number of Calories consumed

$805 \div 315 \approx 2.6$

You would have to hike for 2.6 h.

**11. Strategy** To find the energy used, multiply the number of watts (500) by the number of hours $\left(2\frac{1}{2}\right)$.

**Solution**

$$500 \times 2\frac{1}{2} = 1250 \text{ Wh}$$

1250 Wh are used.

**13. Strategy** To find the number of kilowatt-hours used:

• Find the number of watt-hours used in standby mode.

• Find the number of watt-hours used in operation.

• Add the two numbers.

• Convert watt-hours to kilowatt hours.

© 2013 Cengage Learning. All Rights Reserved. May not be scanned, copied or duplicated, or posted to a publicly accessible website, in whole or in part.

**Solution** $30 \times 9 = \quad 351$

$6 \times 36 = +216$

$567$ Wh

$567\ W = 0.567$ kWh

The fax machine used 0.567 kWh.

• Find the number of watt-hours by multiplying the number of watts used (120) by the number of hours.

• Convert watt-hours to kilowatt-hours.

• Multiply the number of kilowatt-hours by the cost per kilowatt-hour (14.4¢).

**Solution** $2\text{ h} \times 14 = 28\text{ h}$

$28\text{ h} \times 120\text{ W} = 3360\text{ Wh}$

$3360\text{ Wh} = 3.360\text{ kWh}$

$3.360 \times 0.144$

$= 0.48384 \approx 0.48$

The cost of listening to the CD player is \$0.48.

**15.** **Strategy** To find the cost:

• Multiply the watts by the number of hours (8) to find the number of watt-hours.

• Convert the watt-hours to kilowatt-hours.

• Multiply the number of kilowatt-hours by the price per kilowatt-hour (\$.12).

**Solution** $2200\text{W} \times 8\text{ h} = 17{,}600\text{ Wh}$

$17{,}600\text{ Wh} = 17.6\text{ kWh}$

$17.6 \times 0.12 = 2.112 \approx 2.11$

The cost of running an air conditioner is \$2.11.

• Multiply the number of kilowatt-hours by the price per kilowatt-hour (11.1¢).

**Solution** $1400\text{ W} \times 3\text{ h} = 4200\text{ Wh}$

$4200\text{ Wh} = 4.2\text{ kWh}$

$4.2 \times 0.111 = 0.4662 \approx 0.47$

The cost of using the heater is \$0.47.

**17a.** **Strategy** To determine if the light output of the Energy Saver Bulb is more or less than half the energy of the Long Life Soft White bulb, compare the light output of each bulb.

**Solution** Energy Saver—400 lumens

Soft White—835 lumens

400 lumens is less than half the output of the Soft White bulb.

**b.** **Strategy** To find the cost for each bulb:

• Find the number of watt-hours by multiplying the number of watts by the number of hours.

• Convert watt-hours to kilowatt-hours.

• Multiply the number of kilowatt-hours by the cost per kilowatt hour.

• Find the difference in cost.

**Solution** Sylvania Long Life Bulb:

$60 \times 150 = 9000\text{ Wh}$

$9000\text{ Wh} = 9\text{ kWh}$

$9 \times 0.108 = 0.972$

Energy Saver Soft White Bulb:

$34 \times 150 = 5100\text{ Wh}$

$5100\text{ Wh} = 5.1\text{ kWh}$

$5.1 \times 0.108 = 0.5508$

$0.972 - 0.5508 = 0.4212$

The energy saver bulb costs \$0.42 less to operate.

**19.** (iii)

© 2013 Cengage Learning. All Rights Reserved. May not be scanned, copied or duplicated, or posted to a publicly accessible website, in whole or in part.

### Applying the Concepts

**20.** $2100 \times 0.049 \text{ W} = 102.9 \text{ W}$

**21.** The energy efficiency of a home can be improved in a number of ways. Students might mention increasing the amount or thickness of insulation, using weather stripping around doors and windows, using window treatments that help to retain heat or cool air in the home, and insulating the hot water heater. Also, repairing a cracked foundation or reproofing an older home can be beneficial.

## Section 9.5

### Objective A Exercises

**1.** $\dfrac{1 \text{ qt}}{4 \text{ c}} \times \dfrac{1 \text{ L}}{1.06 \text{ qt}}$

**3.** $145 \text{ lb} \approx 145 \cancel{\text{lb}} \times \dfrac{1 \text{ kg}}{2.2 \cancel{\text{lb}}} = 65.91 \text{ kg}$

**5.** $2 \text{ c} \approx 2 \cancel{\text{c}} \times \dfrac{1 \cancel{\text{pt}}}{2 \cancel{\text{c}}} \times \dfrac{1 \cancel{\text{qt}}}{2 \cancel{\text{pt}}} \times \dfrac{1 \text{ L}}{1.06 \cancel{\text{qt}}} \approx 0.47 \text{ L}$

**7.** $14.3 \text{ gal} \approx 14.3 \cancel{\text{gal}} \times \dfrac{3.79 \text{ L}}{1 \cancel{\text{gal}}} \approx 54.20 \text{ L}$

**9.** $10 \text{ oz} = 10 \cancel{\text{oz}} \times \dfrac{28.35 \text{ g}}{1 \cancel{\text{oz}}} \approx 283.5 \text{ g}$

$6 \text{ lb} = 6 \cancel{\text{lb}} \times \dfrac{454 \text{ g}}{1 \cancel{\text{lb}}} \approx 2724 \text{ g}$

$283.5 \text{ g} + 2724 \text{ g} = 3007.5 \text{ g}$

**11.** $30 \dfrac{\text{mi}}{\text{h}} \approx 30 \dfrac{\cancel{\text{mi}}}{\text{h}} \times \dfrac{1.61 \text{ km}}{1 \cancel{\text{mi}}} = 48.3 \dfrac{\text{km}}{\text{h}}$

**13.** $\dfrac{\$0.79}{\text{oz}} \approx \dfrac{\$0.79}{\cancel{\text{oz}}} \times \dfrac{1 \cancel{\text{oz}}}{0.02835 \text{ kg}} \approx \$27.87/\text{kg}$

**15.** $\dfrac{\$32.99}{\text{gal}} \approx \dfrac{\$32.99}{\cancel{\text{gal}}} \times \dfrac{1 \cancel{\text{gal}}}{2.79\text{L}} \approx \$8.70/\text{L}$

**17.** $27 \text{ lb} \approx 27 \text{ lb} \times \dfrac{1 \text{ kg}}{2.2 \text{ lb}} \approx 12.27 \text{ kg}$

### Objective B Exercises

**19.** $100 \text{ m} \approx 100 \cancel{\text{m}} \times \dfrac{3.28 \text{ ft}}{1 \cancel{\text{m}}} = 328 \text{ ft}$

**21.** $6 \text{ L} \approx 6 \cancel{\text{L}} \times \dfrac{1 \text{ gal}}{3.79 \cancel{\text{L}}} \approx 1.58 \text{ gal}$

**23.** $1500 \text{ m} \approx 1500 \cancel{\text{m}} \times \dfrac{3.28 \text{ ft}}{1 \cancel{\text{m}}} = 4920 \text{ ft}$

**25.** $3178 \text{ g} \approx 3178 \cancel{\text{g}} \times \dfrac{1 \text{ lb}}{454 \cancel{\text{g}}} \approx 7 \text{ lb}$

**27.** $\dfrac{80 \text{ km}}{\text{h}} \approx \dfrac{80 \cancel{\text{km}}}{\text{h}} \times \dfrac{1 \text{ mi}}{1.61 \cancel{\text{km}}} \approx 49.69 \text{ mph}$

**29.** $\dfrac{\$1.015}{\text{L}} \approx \dfrac{\$1.015}{\cancel{\text{L}}} \times \dfrac{3.79 \cancel{\text{L}}}{\text{gal}} \approx \$3.85/\text{gal}$

**31.** $2.1 \text{ kg} \approx 2.1 \cancel{\text{kg}} \times \dfrac{2.2 \text{ lb}}{\cancel{\text{kg}}} = 4.62 \text{ lb}$

**33.** **Strategy** To find the number of pounds lost:

- Multiply to find the number of hours spent hiking.
- Multiply the number of hours spent hiking by the number of extra Calories used in hiking to find the total number of extra Calories used.
- Multiply the number of extra Calories consumed each day by the number of days.
- Subtract to find the difference between the number of Calories used in hiking and the number of extra Calories consumed.

© 2013 Cengage Learning. All Rights Reserved. May not be scanned, copied or duplicated, or posted to a publicly accessible website, in whole or in part.

• Divide the difference by 3500.

**Solution** $5 \times 5 = 25$

$25 \times 320 = 8000$

$5 \times 900 = 4500$

$8000 - 4500 = 3500$

$\frac{3500}{3500} = 1$

Gary will lose 1 lb.

**35. Strategy** To number of teaspoons per dose:

• Divide the total number of ml (40) by the number of doses (4).

• Convert ml to t.

**Solution** 40 ml $\div 4$ = 10 ml/dose

$10 \text{ ml} \approx 10 \cancel{\text{ml}} \times \frac{1 \text{ t}}{5 \cancel{\text{ml}}}$

$= 2 \text{ t}$

The amount is 2 t per dose.

## Chapter 9 Concept Review

**1.** To convert from millimeters to meters, move the decimal point three places to the left.

**2.** To convert 51 m 2 cm to meters, first convert 2 cm to meters by moving the decimal point two places to the left: 2 cm = 0.02 m. Add 0.02 m to 51 m: 51 m + 0.02 m = 51.02 m.

**3.** On the surface of Earth, mass and weight are the same.

**4.** To convert 4 kg 7 g to kilograms, first convert 7 g to kilograms by moving the decimal point three places to the left: 7 g = 0.007 kg. Add 0.007 kg to 4 kg: 4 kg + 0.007 kg = 4.007 kg.

**5.** One liter is defined as the capacity of a box that is 10 cm long on each side.

**6.** To convert 4 L 27 ml to liters, first convert 27 ml to liters by moving the decimal point three places to the left: 27 ml = 0.027 L. Add 0.027 L to 4 L: 4 L + 0.027 L = 4.027 L.

**7.** To find the cost per week to run a microwave oven rated at 650 W that is used for 30 min per day, at 8.8 cents per kilowatt-hour, use multiplication and conversion. The microwave oven is used $\frac{1}{2} \times 7 = \frac{7}{2}$ hours per week. The microwave uses $\frac{7}{2} \times 650 = 2275 \text{ Wh}$, or 2.275kWh, of energy. The cost is $2.275 \times 8.8 = 20.02$ cents per week.

**8.** To find the Calories from fat for a daily intake of 1800 Calories, multiply 1800 times 30%: $1800 \times 0.30 = 540$ Calories.

**9.** To convert 100 ft to meters, use the conversion rate $\frac{1 \text{ m}}{3.28 \text{ ft}}$.

**10.** To convert the price of gas from \$3.19/gal to a cost per liter, use the conversion rate $\frac{1 \text{ gal}}{3.79 \text{ L}}$.

## Chapter 9 Review Exercises

**1.** 1.25 km = 1250 m

**2.** 0.450 g = 450 mg

**3.** 0.0056 L = 5.6 ml

© 2013 Cengage Learning. All Rights Reserved. May not be scanned, copied or duplicated, or posted to a publicly accessible website, in whole or in part.

**4.** $1000 \text{ m} \approx 1000 \cancel{\text{m}} \times \frac{1.09 \text{ yd}}{1 \cancel{\text{m}}} = 1090 \text{ yd}$

**5.** 79 mm = 7.9 cm

**6.** 5 m 34 cm = 5 m + 0.34 m = 5.34 m

**7.** 900 g = 900,000 mcg

**8.** 2550 ml = 2.550 L

**9.** 4870 m = 4.870 km

**10.** 0.37 cm = 3.7 mm

**11.** 6 g 829 mg = 6 g + 0.829 g = 6.829 g

**12.** 1.2 L = 1200 ml

**13.** 4.050 kg = 4050 g

**14.** 8.7 m = 870 cm

**15.** 192 ml = 192 $\text{cm}^3$

**16.** 356 mg = 0.356 g

**17.** 372 cm = 3.72 m

**18.** 8.3 kl = 8300 L

**19.** 2 L 89 ml = 2 L + 0.089 L = 2.089 L

**20.** 5410 ml = 5.410 L

**21.** 379.2 ml = 3.792 dl

**22.** 468 $\text{cm}^3$ = 468 ml

**23.** **Strategy** To find the amount of the gauze left on the roll:
- Convert the lengths of the three pieces cut from the roll to meters.
- Add the three numbers.
- Subtract the sum from the length of the original roll (3.75 m).

**Solution**

$$\begin{aligned} 24 \text{ cm} &= \phantom{+}0.24 \text{ m} \\ 56 \text{ cm} &= \phantom{+}0.56 \text{ m} \\ 48 \text{ cm} &= \underline{+0.48 \text{ m}} \\ & \phantom{=+}1.28 \text{ m} \end{aligned}$$

$$\begin{array}{r} 3.75 \text{ m} \\ \underline{-1.28 \text{ m}} \\ 2.47 \text{ m} \end{array}$$

There are 2.47 m of gauze left on the roll.

**24.** **Strategy** To find the total cost:
- Convert the weights of the kilograms.
- Add the weights.
- Divide the total weight by the number of babies (3).

**Solution**

$$\begin{aligned} 2100 \text{ g} &= \phantom{+}2.100 \text{ kg} \\ 1650 \text{ g} &= \phantom{+}1.650 \text{ kg} \\ 1725 \text{ g} &= \underline{+\ 1.725 \text{ kg}} \\ & \phantom{=+}5.475 \text{ kg} \end{aligned}$$

$5.475 \div 3 = 1.825 \text{ g}$

The average weight is 1.825 g.

**25.** $\frac{\$104.95}{20 \text{ L}} \approx \frac{\$104.95}{20 \cancel{\text{L}}} \times \frac{3.79 \cancel{\text{L}}}{1 \text{ gal}} = \$19.88/\text{gal}$

**26.** **Strategy** To find how many liters of coffee should be prepared:
- Convert 400 ml to liters.
- Multiply the number of residents (125) by the number of liters per resident.

**Solution** 400 ml = 0.4 L

0.4 L × 125 = 50 L

The amount of coffee that should be prepared is 50 L.

**27.** **Strategy** To find the number of Calories that can be eliminated, multiply the number of Calories in one egg (90) by the number of days it is eliminated (30).

**Solution** 90 Cal × 30 = 2700 Cal

You can eliminate 2700 Calories.

© 2013 Cengage Learning. All Rights Reserved. May not be scanned, copied or duplicated, or posted to a publicly accessible website, in whole or in part.

**28. Strategy** To find the time:

- Convert 1 L to ml.
- Write and solve a proportion.

**Solution** 1 L = 1000 ml

$$\frac{150 \text{ ml}}{\text{hr}} = \frac{1000 \text{ ml}}{x}$$
$$150x = 1000$$
$$x = 1000 \div 150$$
$$6\frac{100}{150} = 6\frac{2}{3} \text{ hr} = 6 \text{ hr } 40 \text{ min}$$

$$\begin{array}{r} 6 \\ 150\overline{)1000} \\ \underline{900} \\ 100 \end{array}$$

The time for the infusion is 6 hr 40 min.

**29.** $38 \text{ lb} = 38 \cancel{\text{lb}} \times \frac{1 \text{ kg}}{2.2 \cancel{\text{lb}}} \approx 17.3 \text{ kg}$

**30. Strategy** To find how many hours of cycling are necessary to lose 1 lb, divide 1 lb (3500 Calories) by the number of Calories cycling burns per hour (400).

**Solution**

$$\begin{array}{r} 8.75 \\ 400\overline{)3500.00} \end{array}$$

8.75 hours of cycling are needed.

**31. Strategy** To find the profit:

- Convert the amount of soap purchased (6 L) to milliliters.
- Divide the volume of one plastic container (150 ml) into the amount of soap purchased to determine the number of containers of soap for sale.
- Multiply the number of containers by the cost per container ($.26) to find the cost of the containers.
- Multiply the number of liters of soap (6) by the cost per liter ($11.40) to find the cost of the soap.
- Add the cost of the soap and the cost of the containers to find the total cost.
- Multiply the number of containers by $3.29 to find the total revenue.
- Subtract the total cost from the total revenue to find the profit.

**Solution** 6 L = 6000 ml amount of soap

6000 ÷ 150 = 40 number of containers

40 × 0.26 = 10.40 cost of containers

6 × 11.40 = 68.40 cost of soap

10.40 + 68.40 = 78.80 total cost

40 × 3.29 = 131.60 revenue

131.60 – 78.80 = 52.80

The profit was $52.80.

**32. Strategy** To find the number of calories burned.

- Multiply the length of each session (45 min) by the number of sessions per week (2) and the number of weeks (4) to get the total number of minutes worked.
- Convert the minutes to hours.
- Write and solve a proportion.

**Solution** 45 × 2 × 4 = 360 min

$$360 \cancel{\text{min}} = \frac{1 \text{ hr}}{60 \cancel{\text{min}}} = 6 \text{ hr}$$

$$\frac{235 \text{ calories}}{\text{hr}} = \frac{x \text{ calories}}{6 \text{ hr}}$$
$$x = 235 \times 6$$
$$x = 1410$$

There are 1410 calories burned

© 2013 Cengage Learning. All Rights Reserved. May not be scanned, copied or duplicated, or posted to a publicly accessible website, in whole or in part.

in one month.

**33.** **Strategy** To find the amount of solute:

• Write and solve a proportion.

• Convert μg to mg.

**Solution** $\frac{75\ \mu g}{\text{ml}} = \frac{x}{500\ \text{ml}}$

$x = 75 \times 500$

$x = 37{,}500\,\mu g$

37,500 μg = 37.5 mg

There are 37.5 mg of solute in 600 ml of solution.

## Chapter 9 Test

**1.** 2.96 km = 2960 m

**2.** 0.378 g = 378 mg

**3.** 0.046 L = 46 ml

**4.** 919 $cm^3$ = 919 ml

**5.** 42.6 mm = 4.26 cm

**6.** 7 m 96 cm = 7 m + 0.96 m = 7.96 m

**7.** 847 g = 0.847 kg

**8.** 3920 ml = 3.920 L

**9.** 588 mcg = 0.588 mg

**10.** 2.12 mg = 2120 μg

**11.** 3 g 89 mg = 3 g + 0.089 g = 3.089 g

**12.** 1.6 L = 1600 ml

**13.** 3.29 kg = 3290 g

**14.** 4.2 m = 420 cm

**15.** 96 ml = 0.96 dl

**16.** 1375 mg = 1.375 g

**17.** 402 cm = 4.02 m

**18.** 0.125 ml = 125 μl

**19.** **Strategy** To find the number of Calories needed to maintain the weight of a 140-pound sedentary person, multiply the weight (140 pounds) by the number of Calories per pound a sedentary person needs (15) to maintain weight.

**Solution** 140 × 15 = 2100

A 140-pound sedentary person should consume 2100 Calories per day to maintain that weight.

**20.** **Strategy** To find amount of drug at the end of the week:

• Multiply the amount of drug (75 mg) by the number of tablets per dose (3) and the number of days (7).

• Convert mg to grams.

**Solution** $75\ \text{mg} \times 3 \times 7 = 1575\ \text{mg}$

1575 mg = 1.575 g

The patient has taken 1.575 g in a week.

**21.** **Strategy** To find the brother's height:

• Convert the difference (16 cm) to m.

• Add the difference to 1.35 m.

**Solution** 16 cm = 0.16 m

1.35 m + 0.16 m = 1.51 m

The brother is 1.51 m.

**22.** **Strategy** To find the grams of medication:

• Write and solve a proportion.

• Convert the mg to g.

• Multiply by the number of hours (2).

© 2013 Cengage Learning. All Rights Reserved. May not be scanned, copied or duplicated, or posted to a publicly accessible website, in whole or in part.

**Solution** $\frac{50 \text{ mg}}{\text{kg}} = \frac{x}{31 \text{ kg}}$

$x = 50 \times 31$

$x = 1550$ mg

1550 mg = 1.55 g

1.55 g × 2 = 3.1 g

The total dose is 3.1 g.

**23. Strategy** To find how many liters of vaccine are needed:

- Multiply the number of people (2600) by the amount of vaccine per flu shot (2 ml).
- Convert the total amount of vaccine to liters.

**Solution**

$$\begin{array}{r} 2600 \\ \times \quad 2 \text{ ml} \\ \hline 5200 \text{ ml} = 5.2 \text{ L} \end{array}$$

The amount of vaccine needed is 5.2 L.

**24.** $35 \text{ mph} \approx \frac{35 \cancel{\text{mi}}}{\text{h}} \times \frac{1.61 \text{ km}}{1 \cancel{\text{mi}}} \approx 56.4 \text{ km/h}$

**25. Strategy** To find the cost per gallon, convert liters to gallons.

**Solution** $\frac{\$7.95}{3.8 \cancel{\text{L}}} \times \frac{3.79 \cancel{\text{L}}}{\text{gal}} = \$7.95/\text{gal}$

The cost is $7.95 per gallon.

**26. Strategy** To number of tests:

- Convert 1 ml to μl.
- Write and solve a proportion.

**Solution** 1 ml = 1000 μl

$\frac{4.0 \ \mu l}{\text{test}} = \frac{1000 \ \mu l}{x}$

$4x = 1000$

$x = 250$

1 ml can be used for 250 tests.

**27. Strategy** To find the cost of the electricity:

- Determine the amount of electricity used by multiplying 1600 W times the hours used per day (4) times the number of days (30).
- Convert the watt-hours to kilowatt-hours.
- Multiply the kilowatt-hours by the cost per kilowatt hour ($.125).

**Solution** 1600 × 4 × 30 = 192,000 Wh

192,000 Wh = 192 kWh

192 × 0.125 = 24.00

The total cost is $24.00.

**28. Strategy** To find how much acid should be ordered:

- Find the amount of acid needed by multiplying the number of classes (3) times the number of students in each class (40) times the amount of acid needed by each student (90).
- Convert the amount to liters.

**Solution** 3 × 40 × 90 = 10,800 ml

10.8 L

The assistant should order 11 L of acid.

**29. Strategy** To find the number of ml:

- Multiply the number of teaspoons per dose (2) by the number of doses (4) and by the number of days (5).
- Convert teaspoons to ml.

**Solution** $2 \text{ t} \times 4 \times 5 = 40 \text{ t}$

$40 \text{ t} = 40 \cancel{\text{t}} \times \frac{5 \text{ ml}}{1 \cancel{\text{t}}} = 200 \text{ ml}$

200 ml are needed for 5 days.

**30. Strategy** Convert ft to m.

**Solution** 5 ft 6 in

$= 5.5 \text{ ft} = 5.5 \cancel{\text{ft}} \times \frac{1 \text{ m}}{3.28 \cancel{\text{ft}}}$

$= 1.68$ m

© 2013 Cengage Learning. All Rights Reserved. May not be scanned, copied or duplicated, or posted to a publicly accessible website, in whole or in part.

The patient is 1.68 m.

## Cumulative Review Exercises

**1.** $12-8\div(6-4)^2\cdot 3=12-8\div 2^2\cdot 3$
$=12-8\div 4\cdot 3$
$=12-2\cdot 3$
$=12-6$
$=6$

**2.**
$$5\frac{3}{4}=5\frac{27}{36}$$
$$1\frac{5}{6}=1\frac{30}{36}$$
$$+4\frac{7}{9}=4\frac{28}{36}$$
$$10\frac{85}{36}=12\frac{13}{36}$$

**3.**
$$4\frac{2}{9}=4\frac{8}{36}=3\frac{44}{36}$$
$$-3\frac{5}{12}=3\frac{15}{36}=3\frac{15}{36}$$
$$\frac{29}{36}$$

**4.** $5\frac{3}{8}\div 1\frac{3}{4}=\frac{43}{8}\div\frac{7}{4}$
$=\frac{43}{8}\times\frac{4}{7}$
$=\frac{43\cdot \overset{1}{\cancel{2}}\cdot \overset{1}{\cancel{2}}}{\underset{1}{\cancel{2}}\cdot \underset{1}{\cancel{2}}\cdot 2\cdot 7}=\frac{43}{14}=3\frac{1}{14}$

**5.** $\left(\frac{2}{3}\right)^4\cdot\left(\frac{9}{4}\right)^2=\left(\frac{2}{3}\cdot\frac{2}{3}\cdot\frac{2}{3}\cdot\frac{2}{3}\right)\left(\frac{9}{4}\cdot\frac{9}{4}\right)$
$=\frac{16}{81}\cdot\frac{81}{16}=1$

**6.**
$$\begin{array}{r}12.0072\\-9.937\\\hline 2.0702\end{array}$$

**7.** $\frac{5}{8}=\frac{n}{50}$
$5\times 50=8\times n$
$250=8\times n$
$250\div 8=n$
$n=31.3$

**8.** $1\frac{3}{4}=\frac{7}{4}\times 100\%=\frac{700}{4}\%=175\%$

**9.** $4.2\%\times n=6.09$
$0.042\times n=6.09$
$n=6.09\div 0.042=145$

**10.** $18\ \cancel{\text{pt}}\times\frac{1\ \cancel{\text{qt}}}{2\ \cancel{\text{pt}}}\times\frac{1\text{ gal}}{4\ \cancel{\text{qt}}}=\frac{18}{8}\text{ gal}=2.25\text{ gal}$

**11.** 875 cm = 8.75 m

**12.** 3420 m = 3.420 km

**13.** 5.05 kg = 5050 g

**14.** 3 g 672 mg = 3 g + 0.672 g = 3.672 g

**15.** 6 L = 6000 ml

**16.** 2.4 kl = 2400 L

**17.** **Strategy** To find how much money is left after the rent is paid:
- Find the amount that is paid in rent by multiplying $\frac{1}{4}$ by the total monthly income ($5244).
- Subtract the amount paid in rent from the total monthly income.

**Solution** $\frac{1}{4}\times 5244=\frac{5244}{4}=1311$

$$\begin{array}{r}5244\\-1311\\\hline 3933\end{array}$$

$3933 is left after the rent is paid.

© 2013 Cengage Learning. All Rights Reserved. May not be scanned, copied or duplicated, or posted to a publicly accessible website, in whole or in part.

**18. Strategy** To find the amount of income tax paid:

- Find the amount of income tax paid on the profit by multiplying 0.08 by the profit ($82,340).
- Add $620 to the amount of income tax paid on the profit.

**Solution** $0.08 \times 82,340 = 6587.20$

$$\begin{array}{r} 6587.20 \\ +\ 620.00 \\ \hline 7207.20 \end{array}$$

The medical practice paid $7207.20 in income tax.

**19. Strategy** To find the number of males:

- Solve a proportion to find the number of females.
- Subtract the number of females from the total number of nurses (615).

**Solution**

$$\begin{aligned} \frac{4 \text{ female}}{5 \text{ nurses}} &= \frac{n}{615 \text{ nurses}} \\ 5n &= 4 \times 615 \\ 5n &= 2460 \\ n &= 2460 \div 5 \\ n &= 492 \end{aligned}$$

$615 - 492 = 123$

There are 123 male nurses.

**20. Strategy** To find the wage:

- Solve percent equation for amount. The base is $31.50 and the rate is 2%.
- Add the raise to the base to get the new wage.

**Solution**

$$\begin{aligned} \text{Percent} \times \text{base} &= \text{amount} \\ 2\% \times 31.50 &= n \\ 0.02 \times 31.50 &= n \\ 0.63 &= n \end{aligned}$$

$31.50 + 0.63 = 32.13$

The new wage is $32.13 per h.

**21. Strategy** To find the amount of water:

- Find the percent of alcohol, solve the basic percent equation for percent. The base is 500 ml and the amount is 75 ml.
- Subtract the percent of alcohol from 100%.

**Solution**

$$\begin{aligned} \text{Percent} \times \text{base} &= \text{amount} \\ n \times 500 &= 75 \\ n &= 75 \div 500 \\ n &= 0.15 = 15\% \end{aligned}$$

$100\% - 15\% = 85\%$

The percent of water is 85%.

**22. Strategy** To find your mean grade, find the sum of the grades and divide the sum by the number of grades (5).

**Solution**

$$\begin{array}{r} 78 \\ 92 \\ 45 \\ 80 \\ +85 \\ \hline 380 \end{array} \text{ sum of grades}$$

$$5\overline{)380} = 76$$

Your average grade is 76.

**23. Strategy** To find what the salary will be next year, find the amount of the increase by solving the basic percent equation for amount. The base is $22,500 and the percent is 12%.

**Solution**

$$\begin{aligned} \text{Percent} \times \text{base} &= \text{amount} \\ 12\% \times 22,500 &= n \\ 0.12 \times 22,500 &= n \\ 2700 &= n \end{aligned}$$

$$\begin{array}{r} 22,500 \\ +\ 2,700 \\ \hline 25,200 \end{array}$$

Karla's salary next year will be $25,200.

**24. Strategy** To find the discount rate:

- Find the amount of the

© 2013 Cengage Learning. All Rights Reserved. May not be scanned, copied or duplicated, or posted to a publicly accessible website, in whole or in part.

discount by subtracting the sale price ($140.40) from the original price ($180).

• Solve the basic percent equation for percent. The base is the original price ($180) and the amount is the amount of the discount.

**Solution**

$$\begin{array}{r} 180.00 \\ -\ 140.40 \\ \hline 39.60 \end{array}$$

$$\begin{aligned} \text{Percent} \times \text{base} &= \text{amount} \\ n \times 180 &= 39.60 \\ n &= 39.60 \div 180 \\ n &= 0.22 = 22\% \end{aligned}$$

The discount rate is 22%.

**25. Strategy** To find amount below the minimum, subtract 3 in from 4 ft 2 in.

**Solution**

3 ft 14 in.
~~4~~ ft 2 in.
− 3 in.
3 ft 11 in

The boy is 3 ft 11 in.

**26. Strategy** To find ml:

• Convert 2.5 g to mg.

• Solve a proportion.

• Convert to t.

**Solution** 2.5 g = 2500 mg

$$\begin{aligned} \frac{1250 \text{ mg}}{5 \text{ ml}} &= \frac{2500 \text{ mg}}{x} \\ 5 \times 2500 &= 1250x \\ 12{,}500 &= 1250x \\ 12{,}500 \div 1250 &= x \\ 10 \text{ ml} &= x \end{aligned}$$

The dose is ml.

$$10 \text{ ml} \approx 10 \cancel{\text{ml}} \times \frac{1 \text{ t}}{5 \cancel{\text{ml}}} = 2 \text{ t}$$

The dose is 2 t.

**27. Strategy** To find the profit:

• Convert the amount of nasal solution to ounces.

• Find the number of bottles by dividing the number of ounces by the number of ounces per bottle (1.5 ounces).

• Find the revenue by multiplying the number of bottles by the selling price per bottle ($3.75).

• Subtract the cost ($150) from the revenue.

**Solution** 1 gal

$$= 1 \cancel{\text{gal}} \times \frac{4 \cancel{\text{qt}}}{1 \cancel{\text{gal}}} \times \frac{2 \cancel{\text{pt}}}{1 \cancel{\text{qt}}} \times \frac{16 \text{ oz}}{1 \cancel{\text{pt}}}$$

$$= 128 \text{ oz}$$

$$\frac{128 \text{ oz}}{1.5 \text{ oz}} = 85.3 = 85 \text{ bottles}$$

$85 \times 3.75 = 318.75$ revenue

$318.75 - 150 = 168.75$ profit

The profit was $168.75.

**28. Strategy** To find the time:

• Convert 1 liter to ml.

• Multiply the ml by $\frac{3}{4}$ to find the number of ml that have been infused.

• Subtract the ml that have been infused from the number of milliliters.

• Solve a proportion to find the time remaining.

• Add the time remaining to 8 A.M. to find the time.

1 L = 1000 ml

$$1000 \text{ ml} \times \frac{3}{4} = 750 \text{ ml}$$

$1000 \text{ ml} - 750 \text{ ml} = 250 \text{ ml}$

© 2013 Cengage Learning. All Rights Reserved. May not be scanned, copied or duplicated, or posted to a publicly accessible website, in whole or in part.

$$\frac{50\text{ ml}}{\text{hr}} = \frac{250\text{ ml}}{x}$$
$$50x = 250$$
$$x = 250 \div 50$$
$$x = 5\text{ hr}$$

8 A.M. + 5 hr = 1 P.M.

The infusion will be complete at 1 P.M.

**29.** **Strategy** To find the weight after six months:

• Solve a basic percent problem to find the amount lost. The base is 275 and the percent is 12%.

• Subtract the amount lost from the original weight (275 lb).

**Solution** interest × base = amount

$$12\% \times 275 = n$$
$$0.12 \times 275 = n$$
$$33 = n$$

275 – 33 = 242

The patient's weight at the end of six months is 242 lb.

**30.** **Strategy** To find the total intake, add the three amounts $\left(1\frac{1}{2}\text{ cup, } \frac{3}{4}\text{ cup, and } 1\frac{1}{4}\text{ cup}\right)$.

**Solution**

$$1\frac{1}{2} = 1\frac{2}{4}$$
$$\frac{3}{4} = \frac{3}{4}$$
$$+1\frac{1}{4} = 1\frac{1}{4}$$
$$2\frac{6}{4} = 3\frac{1}{2}$$

The total intake was $3\frac{1}{2}$ cups.

© 2013 Cengage Learning. All Rights Reserved. May not be scanned, copied or duplicated, or posted to a publicly accessible website, in whole or in part.

# Chapter 10: Rational Numbers

## Prep Test

**1.** $54 > 45$

**2.** 4 units

**3.** $7654 + 8193 = 15{,}847$

**4.** $6097 - 2318 = 3779$

**5.** $472 \times 56 = 26{,}432$

**6.** $$\frac{144}{24} = \frac{2 \cdot \cancel{2} \cdot \cancel{2} \cdot \cancel{2} \cdot 3 \cdot \cancel{3}}{\cancel{2} \cdot \cancel{2} \cdot \cancel{2} \cdot \cancel{3}} = 6$$

**7.** $$\frac{2}{3} + \frac{3}{5} = \frac{10}{15} + \frac{9}{15} = \frac{19}{15} = 1\frac{4}{15}$$

**8.** $$\frac{3}{4} - \frac{5}{16} = \frac{12}{16} - \frac{5}{16} = \frac{7}{16}$$

**9.** $0.75 + 3.9 + 6.408 = 11.058$

**10.** $5.4 - 1.619 = 3.781$

**11.** $$\frac{3}{4} \times \frac{8}{15} = \frac{\cancel{3} \cdot \cancel{2} \cdot \cancel{2} \cdot 2}{\cancel{2} \cdot \cancel{2} \cdot \cancel{3} \cdot 5} = \frac{2}{5}$$

**12.** $$\frac{5}{12} \div \frac{3}{4} = \frac{5}{12} \cdot \frac{4}{3} = \frac{5 \cdot \cancel{2} \cdot \cancel{2}}{\cancel{2} \cdot \cancel{2} \cdot 3 \cdot 3} = \frac{5}{9}$$

**13.** $23.5 \times 0.4 = 9.4$

**14.** $$\begin{array}{r} 0.4 \\ 2.4\overline{)0.96} \end{array}$$

**15.** $$\begin{aligned}(8-6)^2 + 12 \div 4 \cdot 3^2 &= 2^2 + 12 \div 4 \cdot 9 \\ &= 4 + 3 \cdot 9 \\ &= 4 + 27 \\ &= 31\end{aligned}$$

## Section 10.1

### Objective A Exercises

**1.** –120 ft

**3.** –324 dollars

**5.**

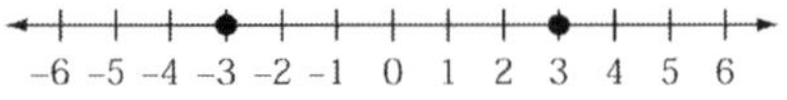


**7.**

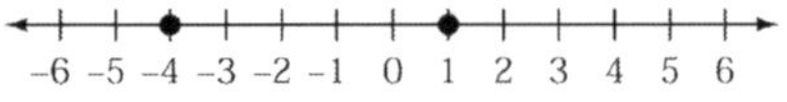


**9.** 1

**11.** –1

**13.** 3

**15.**

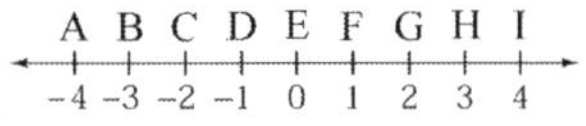


**a.** *A* is –4.

**b.** *C* is –2.

**a.** *B* is –4.

**b.** *D* is –2.

**17.**

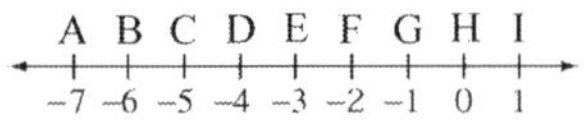


**a.** *A* is –7.

**b.** *D* is –4.

**19.** $-2 > -5$

**21.** $-16 < 1$

**23.** $3 > -7$

**25.** $-11 < -8$

**27.** $35 > 28$

**29.** $-42 < 27$

**31.** $21 > -34$

**33.** $-27 > -39$

**35.** $-87 < 63$

© 2013 Cengage Learning. All Rights Reserved. May not be scanned, copied or duplicated, or posted to a publicly accessible website, in whole or in part.

**37.** $86 > -79$

**39.** $-62 > -84$

**41.** $-131 < 101$

**43.** $-7, -2, 0, 3$

**45.** $-5, -3, 1, 4$

**47.** $-4, 0, 5, 9$

**49.** $-10, -7, -5, 4, 12$

**51.** $-11, -7, -2, 5, 10$

**53.** Always true

**55.** Sometimes true

### Objective B Exercises

**57.** $-16$

**59.** 3

**61.** $-45$

**63.** 59

**65.** 88

**67.** 4

**69.** 9

**71.** 11

**73.** 12

**75.** $|-2| = 2$

**77.** $|6| = 6$

**79.** $|5| = 5$

**81.** $|-1| = 1$

**83.** $-|-5| = -5$

**85.** $|16| = 16$

**87.** $|-12| = 12$

**89.** $-|29| = -29$

**91.** $-|-14| = -14$

**93.** $|-15| = 15$

**95.** $-|33| = -33$

**97.** $|32| = 32$

**99.** $-|-42| = -42$

**101.** $|-61| = 61$

**103.** $-|52| = -52$

**105.** $|-12| = 12, |8| = 8; |-12| > |8|$

**107.** $|6| = 6, |13| = 13; |6| < |13|$

**109.** $|-1| = 1, |-17| = 17; |-1| < |-17|$

**111.** $|17| = 17, |-17| = 17; |17| = |-17|$

**113.** $-|6| = -6, |-7| = 7;$

$-9, -|6|, -4, |-7|$

**115.** $-|-7| = -7, |4| = 4;$

$-9, -|-7|, |4|, 5$

**117.** $-|-8| = -8, |5| = 5, -|10| = -10$

$-|10|, -|-8|, -3, |5|$

**119.** Positive integers

**121.** Negative integers

## Applying the Concepts

**123a.** 8 and $-2$ are 5 units from 3.

**b.** 2 and $-4$ are 3 units from $-1$.

**125.** $-12$ min and counting is closer to blastoff.

**127.** The weight lose was greater in January.

## Section 10.2

### Objective A Exercises

**1.** $-14, -364$

**3.** $3 + (-5) = -2$

© 2013 Cengage Learning. All Rights Reserved. May not be scanned, copied or duplicated, or posted to a publicly accessible website, in whole or in part.

**4.** $-4 + 2 = -2$

**5.** $8 + 12 = 20$

**7.** $-3 + (-8) = -11$

**9.** $-4 + (-5) = -9$

**11.** $6 + (-9) = -3$

**13.** $-6 + 7 = 1$

**15.** $2 + (-3) + (-4) = -1 + (-4) = -5$

**17.** $-3 + (-12) + (-15) = -15 + (-15) = -30$

**19.** $-17 + (-3) + 29 = -20 + 29 = 9$

**21.** $-3 + (-8) + 12 = -11 + 12 = 1$

**23.** $13 + (-22) + 4 + (-5) = -9 + 4 + (-5)$
$= -5 + (-5) = -10$

**25.** $-22 + 10 + 2 + (-18) = -12 + 2 + (-18)$
$= -10 + (-18) = -28$

**27.** $-16 + (-17) + (-18) + 10 = -33 + (-18) + 10$
$= -51 + 10 = -41$

**29.** $-126 + (-247) + (-358) + 339$
$= -373 + (-358) + 339$
$= -731 + 339$
$= -392$

**31.** $-12 + (-8) = -20$

**33.** $-7 + (-16) = -23$

**35.** $-4 + 2 = -2$

**37.** $-2 + 8 + (-12) = 6 + (-12) = -6$

**39.** $2 + (-3) + 8 + (-13) = -1 + 8 + (-13)$
$= 7 + (-13) = -6$

**41.** Always true

**43.** Sometimes true

## Objective B Exercises

**45.** Negative six minus positive four

**47.** Positive six minus negative four

**49.** $9 + 5$

**51.** $1 + (-8)$

**53.** $16 - 8 = 16 + (-8) = 8$

**55.** $7 - 14 = 7 + (-14) = -7$

**57.** $-7 - 2 = -7 + (-2) = -9$

**59.** $7 - (-29) = 7 + 29 = 36$

**61.** $-6 - (-3) = -6 + 3 = -3$

**63.** $6 - (-12) = 6 + 12 = 18$

**65.** $-4 - 3 - 2 = -4 + (-3) + (-2)$
$= -7 + (-2) = -9$

**67.** $12 - (-7) - 8 = 12 + 7 + (-8)$
$= 19 + (-8) = 11$

**69.** $4 - 12 - (-8) = 4 + (-12) + 8$
$= -8 + 8 = 0$

**71.** $-6 - (-8) - (-9) = -6 + 8 + 9$
$= 2 + 9 = 11$

**73.** $-30 - (-65) - 29 - 4$
$= -30 + 65 + (-29) + (-4)$
$= 35 + (-29) + (-4)$
$= 6 + (-4) = 2$

**75.** $-16 - 47 - 63 - 12$
$= -16 + (-47) + (-63) + (-12)$
$= -63 + (-63) + (-12)$
$= -126 + (-12)$
$= -138$

**77.** $47 - (-67) - 13 - 15$
$= 47 + 67 + (-13) + (-15)$
$= 114 + (-13) + (-15)$
$= 101 + (-15) = 86$

© 2013 Cengage Learning. All Rights Reserved. May not be scanned, copied or duplicated, or posted to a publicly accessible website, in whole or in part.

**79.** $167 - 432 - (-287) - 359$
$= 167 + (-432) + 287 + (-359)$
$= -265 + 287 + (-359)$
$= 22 + (-359)$
$= -337$

**81.** $-4 - (-8) = -4 + 8 = 4$

**83.** $-8 - 4 = -8 + (-4) = -12$

**85.** $-4 - 8 = -4 + (-8) = -12$

**87.** $1 - (-2) = 1 + 2 = 3$

**89.** Never true

**91.** Sometimes true

## Objective C Exercises

**93.** **Strategy** To find the difference between the temperatures, subtract the smaller number (–51°C) from the larger number (–40°C).

**Solution** $-40 - (-51) = -40 + 51 = 11$

The difference in the temperatures is 11°C.

**95.** **Strategy** To find the temperature, add the increase (7°C) to the previous temperature (–8°C).

**Solution** $-8 + 7 = -1$

The temperature is –1°C.

**97.** Above

**99.** −19° F, 30 min

**101.** **Strategy** To find the difference, subtract the wind chill temperature at 30 mph (−26° F) from the wind chill temperature at15 mph (−19° F).

**Solution** $-19 - (-26) = -19 + 26 = 7$

The difference in the wind chill temperature is 7° F.

**103.** **Strategy** To find the total, add the five changes (−5 lb, −2 lb, +1 lb, −4 lb, −3 lb).

**Solution** $-5 + (-2) + 1 + (-4) + (-3) =$
$-7 + 1 + (-4) + (-3) =$
$-6 + (-4) + (-3) = -10 + (-3) =$
$-13$

The patient's weight change was −13 pounds.

**105.** **Strategy** To find the difference in elevation, subtract the elevation of Lake Assal (–156 m) from the elevation of Mt. Kilimanjaro (5895 m).

**Solution** $5895 - (-156) = 5895 + 156$
$= 6051$

The difference in elevation is 6051 m.

**107.** **Strategy** To find in which continent the difference in elevation is greatest:

- Find the difference in elevation for each continent.
- Determine the greatest difference in elevation.

**Solution** Africa:
$5895 - (-156) = 5895 + 156$
$= 6051$

Asia:
$8850 - (-411) = 8850 + 411$
$= 9261$

North America:
$5642 - (-28) = 5642 + 28$
$= 5670$

South America:
$6960 - (-86) = 6960 + 86$
$= 7046$

The greatest difference in elevation is found in Asia.

**109.** **Strategy** To find the difference between the highest and lowest temperatures in South America, subtract the lowest

© 2013 Cengage Learning. All Rights Reserved. May not be scanned, copied or duplicated, or posted to a publicly accessible website, in whole or in part.

temperature (–33°C) from the highest temperature (49°C).

**Solution** 49 – (–33) = 49 + 33 = 82

The difference is 82°C.

### Applying the Concepts

**111.** The largest difference: 13 – (–9) = 22

The smallest positive difference: –7 – (–9) = 2 or

–5 – (–7) = –5 + 7 = 2

**113.** There are 4 possibilities:

$$-7+(-1)=-8$$
$$-6+(-2)=-8$$
$$-5+(-3)=-8$$
$$-4+(-4)=-8$$

## Section 10.3

### Objective A Exercises

**1.** Subtraction

**3.** Multiplication

**5.** 14 × 3 = 42

**7.** –4 · 6 = –24

**9.** –2 · (–3) = 6

**11.** (9)(2) = 18

**13.** 5 (–4) = –20

**15.** –8(2) = –16

**17.** (–5) (–5) = 25

**19.** (–7) (0) = 0

**21.** –24 × 3 = –72

**23.** 6 (–17) = –102

**25.** –4 (–35) = 140

**27.** –6 · (38) = –228

**29.** 8 (–40) = –320

**31.** –4 (39) = –156

**33.** 5 × 7 × (–2) = 35 × (–2) = –70

**35.** (–9) (–9) (2) = 81 (2) = 162

**37.** –5 (8) (–3) = –40 (–3) = 120

**39.** –1 (4) (–9) = –4 (–9) = 36

**41.** 4 (–4) · 6 (–2) = –16 · 6 (–2) = –96 (–2) = 192

**43.** –9 (4) · 3 (1) = –36 · 3 (1) = –108 (1) = –108

**45.**
$$\begin{aligned}(-6)\cdot 7\cdot(-10)(-5) &= -42\cdot(-10)(-5)\\ &= 420(-5)\\ &= -2100\end{aligned}$$

**47.** –5 (–4) = 20

**49.** –8 (6) = –48

**51.** –4 (7) (–5) = –28 (–5) = 140

**53.** Negative

**54.** Positive

**55.** Zero

### Objective B Exercises

**57.** 3 (–12) = –36

**59.** –5 (11) = –55

**61.** 12 ÷ (–6) = –2

**63.** (–72) ÷ (–9) = 8

**65.** 0 ÷ (–6) = 0

**67.** 45 ÷ (–5) = –9

**69.** –36 ÷ 4 = –9

**71.** –81 ÷ (–9) = 9

**73.** 72 ÷ (–3) = –24

**75.** (–60) ÷ 5 = –12

**77.** –93 ÷ (–3) = 31

© 2013 Cengage Learning. All Rights Reserved. May not be scanned, copied or duplicated, or posted to a publicly accessible website, in whole or in part.

**79.** $(-85) \div (-5) = 17$

**81.** $120 \div 8 = 15$

**83.** $78 \div (-6) = -13$

**85.** $-72 \div 4 = -18$

**87.** $-114 \div (-6) = 19$

**89.** $-104 \div (-8) = 13$

**91.** $57 \div (-3) = -19$

**93.** $-136 \div (-8) = 17$

**95.** $-130 \div (-5) = 26$

**97.** $(-92) \div (-4) = 23$

**99.** $-150 \div (-6) = 25$

**101.** $204 \div (-6) = -34$

**102.** $165 \div (-5) = -33$

**103.** $-132 \div (-12) = 11$

**105.** $-182 \div 14 = -13$

**107.** $143 \div 11 = 13$

**109.** $-180 \div (-15) = 12$

**111.** $154 \div (-11) = -14$

**113.** $\dfrac{182}{-13} = -14$

**115.** $\dfrac{144}{-24} = -6$

**117.** $\dfrac{-88}{22} = -4$

**119.** Never true

**121.** Always true

## Objective C Exercises

**123.** **Strategy** To find the average daily high temperature:

- Add the seven temperature readings.
- Divide by 7.

**Solution**

$$\begin{aligned}&-6+(-11)+1+5+(-3)+(-9)+(-5)\\&=-17+1+5+(-3)+(-9)+(-5)\\&=-16+5+(-3)+(-9)+(-5)\\&=-11+(-3)+(-9)+(-5)\\&=-14+(-9)+(-5)\\&=-23+(-5)\\&=-28\end{aligned}$$

$$-28 \div 7 = -4$$

The average high temperature was –4°F.

**125.** False

**127.** **Strategy** To find the average weight loss, divide the losses (–24) by the number of patients (8).

**Solution** $-24 \div 8 = -3$

The average weight lose was –3 lb.

**129.** **Strategy** To find loss, multiply the loss for one employee (–$1685) by the number of employees (50).

**Solution** $-1685 \times 50 = -84{,}250$

The total loss was –$84,250.

**131.** **Strategy** To find the wind chill factor, multiply the wind chill factor at 10°F with a 20 mph wind (–9°F) by 5.

**Solution** $-9 \times 5 = -45$

The wind chill factor is –45°F.

## Applying the Concepts

**133a.** The greatest possible product is that of (–5) and (–5). (–5) (–5) = 25

All other contributions, (–1) and (–9), (–2) and (–8), (–3) and (–7), and (–4) and (–6) have a product less than 25.

© 2013 Cengage Learning. All Rights Reserved. May not be scanned, copied or duplicated, or posted to a publicly accessible website, in whole or in part.

**b.** The least possible sum is –17.

(–1) + (–16) = –17 (the sum) –1 (–16) = 16

(the product)

Other combinations are (–2) and (–8), and (–4) and

(–4), which have a product of 16 and a sum greater

than –17.

**135a.** True **b.** True

# Section 10.4

## Objective A Exercises

**1.** $\frac{5}{8}-\frac{5}{6}=\frac{15}{24}-\frac{20}{24}$
$=\frac{15}{24}+\frac{(-20)}{24}$
$=\frac{15+(-20)}{24}$
$=-\frac{5}{24}$

**3.** $-\frac{5}{12}-\frac{3}{8}=\frac{-10}{24}-\frac{9}{24}$
$=\frac{-10}{24}+\frac{(-9)}{24}$
$=\frac{-10+(-9)}{24}=\frac{-19}{24}=-\frac{19}{24}$

**5.** $-\frac{6}{13}+\frac{17}{26}=\frac{-12}{26}+\frac{17}{26}$
$=\frac{-12+17}{26}=\frac{5}{26}$

**7.** $-\frac{5}{8}-\left(-\frac{11}{12}\right)=\frac{-15}{24}-\left(\frac{-22}{24}\right)$
$=\frac{-15}{24}+\frac{22}{24}=\frac{-15+22}{24}=\frac{7}{24}$

**9.** $\frac{5}{12}-\frac{11}{15}=\frac{25}{60}-\frac{44}{60}$
$=\frac{25}{60}+\frac{(-44)}{60}=\frac{25+(-44)}{60}$
$=\frac{-19}{60}=-\frac{19}{60}$

**11.** $-\frac{3}{4}-\frac{5}{8}=\frac{-6}{8}-\frac{5}{8}$
$=\frac{-6}{8}+\frac{(-5)}{8}$
$=\frac{-6+(-5)}{8}=\frac{-11}{8}=-1\frac{3}{8}$

**13.** $-\frac{5}{2}-\left(-\frac{13}{4}\right)=\frac{-10}{4}-\left(\frac{-13}{4}\right)$
$=\frac{-10}{4}+\frac{13}{4}=\frac{-10+13}{4}=\frac{3}{4}$

**15.** $-\frac{3}{8}-\frac{5}{12}-\frac{3}{16}=\frac{-18}{48}-\frac{20}{48}-\frac{9}{48}$
$=\frac{-18}{48}+\frac{(-20)}{48}+\frac{(-9)}{48}$
$=\frac{-18+(-20)+(-9)}{48}$
$=\frac{-47}{48}=-\frac{47}{48}$

**17.** $\frac{1}{2}-\frac{3}{8}-\left(-\frac{1}{4}\right)=\frac{4}{8}-\frac{3}{8}-\left(\frac{-2}{8}\right)$
$=\frac{4}{8}+\frac{(-3)}{8}+\frac{2}{8}$
$=\frac{4+(-3)+2}{8}=\frac{3}{8}$

**19.** $\frac{1}{3}-\frac{1}{4}-\frac{1}{5}=\frac{20}{60}-\frac{15}{60}-\frac{12}{60}$
$=\frac{20}{60}+\frac{(-15)}{60}+\frac{(-12)}{60}$
$=\frac{20+(-15)+(-12)}{60}$
$=\frac{-7}{60}=-\frac{7}{60}$

© 2013 Cengage Learning. All Rights Reserved. May not be scanned, copied or duplicated, or posted to a publicly accessible website, in whole or in part.

**21.** $\frac{1}{2}+\left(-\frac{3}{8}\right)+\frac{5}{12}=\frac{12}{24}+\frac{(-9)}{24}+\frac{10}{24}$
$=\frac{12+(-9)+10}{24}=\frac{13}{24}$

**23.** $3.4+(-6.8)=-3.4$

**25.** $-8.32+(-0.57)=-8.89$

**27.** $-4.8+(-3.2)=-8.0$

**29.** $-4.6+3.92=-0.68$

**31.** $-45.71+(-135.8)=-181.51$

**33.** $4.2+(-6.8)+5.3=-2.6+5.3=2.7$

**35.** $-4.5+3.2+(-19.4)=-1.3+(-19.4)=-20.7$

**37.** $-18.39+4.9-23.7$
$=-18.39+4.9+(-23.7)$
$=-13.49+(-23.7)$
$=-37.19$

**38.** $19-(-3.72)-82.75=19+3.72+(-82.75)$
$=22.72+(-82.75)$
$=-60.03$

**39.** $-3.09-4.6-27.3$
$=-3.09+(-4.6)+(-27.3)$
$=-7.69+(-27.3)$
$=-34.99$

**41.** $-4.02+6.809-(-3.57)-(-0.419)$
$=-4.02+6.809+3.57+0.419$
$=2.789+3.57+0.419$
$=6.359+0.419=6.778$

**43.** $0.27+(-3.5)-(-0.27)+(-5.44)$
$=0.27+(-3.5)+0.27+(-5.44)$
$=-3.23+0.27+(-5.44)$
$=-2.96+(-5.44)$
$=-8.4$

**45.** Negative

## Objective B Exercises

**47.** $-\frac{2}{9}\times\left(-\frac{3}{14}\right)=\frac{2\cdot 3}{9\cdot 14}=\frac{1}{21}$

**49.** $\left(-\frac{3}{4}\right)\left(-\frac{8}{27}\right)=\frac{3\cdot 8}{4\cdot 27}=\frac{2}{9}$

**51.** $\frac{5}{12}\times\left(-\frac{8}{15}\right)=-\left(\frac{5\cdot 8}{12\cdot 15}\right)=-\frac{2}{9}$

**53.** $\left(\frac{3}{8}\right)\left(-\frac{15}{41}\right)=-\left(\frac{3\cdot 15}{8\cdot 41}\right)=-\frac{45}{328}$

**55.** $\left(-\frac{5}{7}\right)\left(-\frac{14}{15}\right)=\frac{5\cdot 14}{7\cdot 15}=\frac{2}{3}$

**57.** $\left(\frac{1}{2}\right)\left(-\frac{3}{4}\right)\left(-\frac{5}{8}\right)=\frac{1\cdot 3\cdot 5}{2\cdot 4\cdot 8}=\frac{15}{64}$

**59.** $-\frac{3}{8}\div\frac{7}{8}=-\frac{3}{8}\times\frac{8}{7}=-\frac{3}{7}$

**61.** $\frac{5}{6}\div\left(-\frac{3}{4}\right)=\frac{5}{6}\times\left(-\frac{4}{3}\right)$
$=-\left(\frac{5\cdot 4}{6\cdot 3}\right)=-\frac{10}{9}=-1\frac{1}{9}$

**63.** $-\frac{5}{16}\div\left(-\frac{3}{8}\right)=-\frac{5}{16}\times-\frac{8}{3}=\frac{5\cdot 8}{16\cdot 3}=\frac{5}{6}$

**65.** $-\frac{8}{19}\div\frac{7}{38}=-\frac{8}{19}\times\frac{38}{7}$
$=-\left(\frac{8\cdot 38}{19\cdot 7}\right)=-\frac{16}{7}=-2\frac{2}{7}$

**67.** $-6\div\frac{4}{9}=-\frac{6}{1}\times\frac{9}{4}$
$=-\left(\frac{6\cdot 9}{1\cdot 4}\right)=-\frac{27}{2}=-13\frac{1}{2}$

**69.**
```
   8.9
 × 3.5
   445
  267
 -----
 31.15
```
$-8.9\times(-3.5)=8.9\times 3.5=31.15$

© 2013 Cengage Learning. All Rights Reserved. May not be scanned, copied or duplicated, or posted to a publicly accessible website, in whole or in part.

**71.**

$$\begin{array}{r} 14.3 \\ \times\ 7.9 \\ \hline 1287 \\ 1001\ \\ \hline 112.97 \end{array}$$

$-14.3 \times 7.9 = -(14.3 \times 7.9) = -112.97$

**73.**

$$\begin{array}{r} 1.21 \\ \times\ 0.03 \\ \hline 0.0363 \end{array}$$

$(-1.21)(-0.03) = (1.21)(0.03) = 0.0363$

**75.**

$$\begin{array}{r} 97. \\ 0.8\overline{)77.6} \\ \underline{72}\ \ \\ 56 \\ \underline{-56} \\ 0 \end{array}$$

$-77.6 \div (-0.8) = 77.6 \div 0.8 = 97$

**77.**

$$\begin{array}{r} 2.2 \\ 3.2\overline{)7.04} \\ \underline{-64}\ \\ 64 \\ \underline{-64} \\ 0 \end{array}$$

$(-7.04) \div (-3.2) = 7.04 \div 3.2 = 2.2$

**79.**

$$\begin{array}{r} 4.14 \\ 0.8\overline{)3.312} \\ \underline{-32}\ \ \\ 11\ \\ \underline{-8}\ \\ 32 \\ \underline{-32} \\ 0 \end{array}$$

$-3.312 \div (0.8) = -(3.312 \div 0.8) = -4.14$

**81.**

$$\begin{array}{r} 3.8 \\ 6.9\overline{)26.23} \\ \underline{-207}\ \\ 552 \\ \underline{-552} \\ 0 \end{array}$$

$26.22 \div (-6.9) = -(26.22 \div 6.9) = -3.8$

**83.** $21.792 \div (-0.96) = -(21.792 \div 0.96) = -22.70$

**85.** $-3.171 \div (-45.3) = 3.171 \div 45.3 = 0.07$

**87.** $(-13.97) \div (-25.4) = 13.97 \div 25.4 = 0.55$

**89.** False

## Objective C Exercises

**91.** **Strategy** To determine is the patient is suffering from hypothermia
- Find the patient's temperature by adding $-3.4°$ to the normal body temperature (98.6°).
- Compare the patient's temperature to 95°.

**Solution** $98.6 + (-3.4) = 95.2$

$95.2° > 95°$

No, the patient is not suffering from hypothermia.

**93.** Greater than

**95.** **Strategy** To find the difference, subtract the melting point of nitrogen (–209.86°C) from its boiling point (–195.8°C).

**Solution**

$$\begin{aligned} &-195.8 - (-209.86) \\ &= -195.8 + 209.86 \\ &= 14.06 \end{aligned}$$

The difference between the boiling point of nitrogen and its melting point is 14.06°C.

**97a.** **Strategy** To find the closing price on the previous day, subtract the change in price (+$.21) from the closing price on September 4, 2008 ($66.93).

**Solution** $66.93 - 0.21 = 66.72$

The closing price the previous day for General Mills was $66.72.

**b.** **Strategy** To find the closing price on the previous day, subtract the change in price (–$.07) from the closing price on September 4, 2008 ($35.39).

© 2013 Cengage Learning. All Rights Reserved. May not be scanned, copied or duplicated, or posted to a publicly accessible website, in whole or in part.

**Solution** 35.39 – (–0.07)
= 35.39 + 0.07 = 35.46
The closing price the previous day for Hormel Foods was $35.46.

**99.** Betelguese, Polaris, Vega, Sirius, Sun

**101. Strategy** To find the distance modulus for Polaris, find its apparent magnitude (1.99) minus its absolute magnitude (–3.2).

**Solution** $1.99-(-3.2)=1.99+3.2=5.19$
The distance modulus for Polaris is 5.19.

**103. Strategy** To determine which of the stars is farthest from Earth:
• Find the distance modulus for each star.
• Compare the results and determine the largest distance modulus.

**Solution** Sun: $-26.8-4.83=-31.63$
Sirius: $-1.47-1.41=-2.88$
Betelguese:
$0.41-(-5.6)=0.41+5.6=6.01$
Vega: $0.04-0.5=-4.5$
Polaris:
$1.99-(-3.2)=1.99+3.2=5.19$
The star that is the farthest from Earth is Betelguese.

## Applying the Concepts

**105.** Answers will vary. For example, $-\frac{17}{24}$.

**107.** Given any two different rational numbers, it is always possible to find a rational number between them. One method is to add the two numbers and divide by 2. Another method is to add the numerators and add the denominators. For example, given the fractions $\frac{2}{5}$ and $\frac{3}{4}, \frac{2+3}{5+4}=\frac{5}{9}$ and $\frac{2}{5}<\frac{5}{9}<\frac{3}{4}$.

# Section 10.5

## Objective A Exercises

**1.** Less than 1

**3.** Since the number is greater than 10, move the decimal point 6 places to the left. The exponent on 10 is 6.

$2{,}370{,}000 = 2.37 \times 10^6$

$75{,}000 = 7.5 \times 10^4$

**5.** Since the number is less than 1, move the decimal point 4 places to the right. The exponent on 10 is –4.

$0.00045 = 4.5 \times 10^{-4}$

**7.** Since the number is greater than 10, move the decimal point 5 places to the left. The exponent on 10 is 5.

$309{,}000 = 3.09 \times 10^5$

$819{,}000{,}000 = 8.19 \times 10^8$

**9.** Since the number is less than 1, move the decimal point 7 places to the right. The exponent on 10 is –7.

$0.000000601 = 6.01 \times 10^{-7}$

**11.** Since the number is greater than 10, move the decimal point 10 places to the left. The exponent on 10 is 10.

$57{,}000{,}000{,}000 = 5.7 \times 10^{10}$

© 2013 Cengage Learning. All Rights Reserved. May not be scanned, copied or duplicated, or posted to a publicly accessible website, in whole or in part.

**13.** Since the number is less than 1, move the decimal point 8 places to the right. The exponent on 10 is –8.

$0.000000017 = 1.7 \times 10^{-8}$

**15.** The exponent on 10 is positive. Move the decimal point 5 places to the right.

$7.1 \times 10^5 = 710{,}000$

**17.** The exponent on 10 is negative. Move the decimal point 5 places to the left.

$4.3 \times 10^{-5} = 0.000043$

**19.** The exponent on 10 is positive. Move the decimal point 8 places to the right.

$6.71 \times 10^8 = 671{,}000{,}000$

**21.** The exponent on 10 is negative. Move the decimal point 6 places to the left.

$7.13 \times 10^{-6} = 0.00000713$

**23.** The exponent on 10 is positive. Move the decimal point 12 places to the right.

$5 \times 10^{12} = 5{,}000{,}000{,}000{,}000$

**25.** The exponent on 10 is negative. Move the decimal point 3 places to the left.

$8.01 \times 10^{-3} = 0.00801$

**27.** The number is greater than 10. Move the decimal point 10 places to the left. The exponent on 10 is 10.

$16{,}000{,}000{,}000 \text{ mi} = 1.6 \times 10^{10} \text{ mi}$

**29.** The number is greater than 10. Move the decimal three places to the left. The exponent on 10 is 3.

$4000 = 4.0 \times 10^3$

The number is greater than 10. Move the decimal four places to the left. The exponent on 10 is 4.

$11{,}000 = 1.1 \times 10^4$

The range is $4.0 \times 10^3$ cells/μl to $1.1 \times 10^4$ cells/μl.

**31.** The number is greater than 10. Move the decimal point 6 places to the left. The exponent on 10 is 6.

$$2{,}700{,}000 = 2.7\times10^6 \text{ cells}/\mu l$$
$$2.7\times10^6 < 3.6\times10^6$$

Yes, the patient is anemic.

**33.** The number is less than 1. Move the decimal point 19 places to the right. The exponent on 10 is –19.

$0.00000000000000000016$ coulomb

$= 1.6 \times 10^{-19}$ coulomb

**35.** The number is less than 1. Move the decimal point 12 places to the right. The exponent on 10 is –12.

$0.000000000001 = 1 \times 10^{-12}$

## Objective B Exercises

**37.** $8 \div 4 + 2 = 2 + 2 = 4$

**39.** $4 + (-7) + 3 = -3 + 3 = 0$

**41.** $4^2 - 4 = 16 - 4 = 16 + (-4) = 12$

**43.**
$$\begin{aligned} 2 \times (3 - 5) - 2 &= 2 \times [3+(-5)]-2 \\ &= 2 \times (-2) - 2 \\ &= 4 - 2 \\ &= -4 + (-2) = -6 \end{aligned}$$

**45.** $4 - (-3)^2 = 4 - 9 = 4 + (-9) = -5$

**47.**
$$\begin{aligned} 4 - (-3) - 5 &= 4 + 3 + (-5) \\ &= 7 + (-5) = 2 \end{aligned}$$

**49.**
$$\begin{aligned} 4-(-2)^2+(-3) &= 4-4+(-3) \\ &= 4+(-4)+(-3) \\ &= 0+(-3) = -3 \end{aligned}$$

© 2013 Cengage Learning. All Rights Reserved. May not be scanned, copied or duplicated, or posted to a publicly accessible website, in whole or in part.

**51.** $3^2 - 4\times 2 = 9 - 4\times 2$
$= 9 - 8 = 9 + (-8) = 1$

**53.** $3\times(6-2)\div 6 = 3\times[6+(-2)]\div 6$
$= 3\times 4\div 6 = 12\div 6 = 2$

**55.** $2^2 - (-3)^2 + 2 = 4 - 9 + 2$
$= 4 + (-9) + 2$
$= -5 + 2 = -3$

**57.** $6 - 2\times(1-5) = 6 - 2\times[1+(-5)]$
$= 6 - 2\times(-4)$
$= 6 - (-8) = 6 + 8 = 14$

**59.** $(-2)^2 - (-3)^2 + 1 = 4 - 9 + 1$
$= 4 + (-9) + 1$
$= -5 + 1 = -4$

**61.** $6 - (-3)\times(-3)^2 = 6 - (-3)\times 9$
$= 6 - (-27) = 6 + 27 = 33$

**63.** $4\times 2 - 3\times 7 = 8 - 3\times 7$
$= 8 - 21 = 8 + (-21) = -13$

**65.** $(-2)^2 - 5\times 3 - 1 = 4 - 5\times 3 - 1$
$= 4 - 15 - 1$
$= 4 + (-15) + (-1)$
$= -11 + (-1) = -12$

**67.** $7\times 6 - 5\times 6 + 3\times 2 - 2 + 1$
$= 42 - 5\times 6 + 3\times 2 - 2 + 1$
$= 42 - 30 + 3\times 2 - 2 + 1$
$= 42 - 30 + 6 - 2 + 1$
$= 42 + (-30) + 6 + (-2) + 1$
$= 12 + 6 + (-2) + 1$
$= 18 + (-2) + 1$
$= 16 + 1 = 17$

**69.** $-4\times 3\times(-2) + 12\times(3-4) + (-12)$
$= -4\times 3\times(-2) + 12\times[3+(-4)] + (-12)$
$= -4\times 3\times(-2) + 12\times(-1) + (-12)$
$= -12\times(-2) + 12\times(-1) + (-12)$
$= 24 + 12\times(-1) + (-12)$
$= 24 + (-12) + (-12)$
$= 12 + (-12) = 0$

**71.** $-12\times(6-8) + 1^2\times 3^2\times 2 - 6\times 2$
$= -12\times[6+(-8)] + 1^2\times 3^2\times 2 - 6\times 2$
$= -12\times(-2) + 1^2\times 3^2\times 2 - 6\times 2$
$= -12\times(-2) + 1\times 9\times 2 - 6\times 2$
$= 24 + 1\times 9\times 2 - 6\times 2$
$= 24 + 18 - 6\times 2$
$= 24 + 18 - 2$
$= 24 + 18 + (-12)$
$= 42 + (-12) = 30$

**73.** $10\times 9 - (8+7)\div 5 + 6 - 7 + 8$
$= 10\times 9 - 15\div 5 + 6 - 7 + 8$
$= 90 - 15\div 5 + 6 - 7 + 8$
$= 90 - 3 + 6 - 7 + 8$
$= 90 + (-3) + 6 + (-7) + 8$
$= 87 + 6 + (-7) + 8$
$= 93 + (-7) + 8$
$= 86 + 8 = 94$

**75.** $3^2\times(4-7)\div 9 + 6 - 3 - 4\times 2$
$= 3^2\times[4+(-7)]\div 9 + 6 - 3 - 4\times 2$
$= 3^2\times(-3)\div 9 + 6 - 3 - 4\times 2$
$= 9\times(-3)\div 9 + 6 - 3 - 4\times 2$

© 2013 Cengage Learning. All Rights Reserved. May not be scanned, copied or duplicated, or posted to a publicly accessible website, in whole or in part.

$= -27 \div 9 + 6 - 3 - 4 \times 2$

$= -3 + 6 - 3 - 4 \times 2$

$= -3 + 6 - 3 - 8$

$= -3 + 6 + (-3) + (-8)$

$= 3 + (-3) + (-8)$

$= 0 + (-8) = -8$

**77.** $(-3)^2 \times (5-7)^2 - (-9) \div 3$
$= (-3)^2 \times [5 + (-7)]^2 - (-9) \div 3$
$= (-3)^2 \times (-2)^2 - (-9) \div 3$
$= 9 \times 4 - (-9) \div 3$
$= 36 - (-9 \div 3)$
$= 36 - (-3)$
$= 36 + 3 = 39$

**79.** $4 - 6(2-5)^3 \div (17-8)$
$= 4 - 6[2 + (-5)]^3 \div [17 + (-8)]$
$= 4 - 6(-3)^3 \div 9$
$= 4 - 6(-27) \div 9$
$= 4 - (-162) \div 9$
$= 4 - (-18) = 4 + 8 = 22$

**81.** $(1.2)^2 - 4.1 \times 0.3 = 1.44 - 4.1 \times 0.3$
$= 1.44 - 1.23$
$= 1.44 + (-1.23) = 0.21$

**83.** $1.6 - (-1.6)^2 = 1.6 - 2.56$
$= 1.6 + (-2.56) = -0.96$

**85.** $(4.1 - 3.9) - 0.7^2 = [4.1 + (-3.9)] - 0.7^2$
$= 0.2 - 0.7^2$
$= 0.2 - 0.49$
$= 0.2 + (-0.49) = -0.29$

**87.** $(-0.4)^2 \times 1.5 - 2 = 0.16 \times 1.5 - 2$
$= 0.24 - 2$
$= 0.24 + (-2) = -1.76$

**89.** $4.2 - (-3.9) - 6 = 4.2 + 3.9 + (-6)$
$= 8.1 + (-6) = 2.1$

**91.** $\left(\frac{3}{4}\right)^2 - \frac{3}{8} = \frac{9}{16} - \frac{3}{8}$
$= \frac{9}{16} - \frac{6}{16} = \frac{3}{16}$

**93.** $\frac{5}{16} - \frac{3}{8} + \frac{1}{2} = \frac{5}{16} - \frac{6}{16} + \frac{1}{2}$
$= \frac{5}{16} + \left(-\frac{6}{16}\right) + \frac{1}{2}$
$= -\frac{1}{16} + \frac{1}{2} = -\frac{1}{16} + \frac{8}{16} = \frac{7}{16}$

**95.** $\frac{1}{2} \times \frac{1}{4} \times \frac{1}{2} - \frac{3}{8} = \frac{1}{8} \times \frac{1}{2} - \frac{3}{8}$
$= \frac{1}{16} - \frac{3}{8}$
$= \frac{1}{16} + \left(-\frac{3}{8}\right)$
$= \frac{1}{16} + \left(-\frac{6}{16}\right) = -\frac{5}{16}$

**97.** $\frac{1}{2} - \left(\frac{3}{4} - \frac{3}{8}\right) \div \frac{1}{3} = \frac{1}{2} - \left(\frac{6}{8} - \frac{3}{8}\right) \div \frac{1}{3}$
$= \frac{1}{2} - \frac{3}{8} \div \frac{1}{3} = \frac{1}{2} - \frac{3}{8} \times \frac{3}{1}$
$= \frac{1}{2} - \frac{9}{8} = \frac{4}{8} + \left(-\frac{9}{8}\right) = -\frac{5}{8}$

**99.** (i)

## Applying the Concepts

**101a.** $3.45 \times 10^{-14} > 3.45 \times 10^{-15}$

**b.** $5.23 \times 10^{18} > 5.23 \times 10^{17}$

**c.** $3.12 \times 10^{12} > 3.12 \times 10^{11}$

© 2013 Cengage Learning. All Rights Reserved. May not be scanned, copied or duplicated, or posted to a publicly accessible website, in whole or in part.

**103a.** $1^3 + 2^3 + 3^3 + 4^3 = 1 + 8 + 27 + 64 = 100$

**b.** $(-1)^3 + (-2)^3 + (-3)^3 + (-4)^3$
$= -1 + (-8) + (-27) + (-64)$
$= -100$

**c.** $1^3 + 2^3 + 3^3 + 4^3 + 5^3$
$= 1 + 8 + 27 + 64 + 125$
$= 225$

**d.** $(-1)^3 + (-2)^3 + (-3)^3 + (-4)^3 + (-5)^3 = -225$

**105.** Because the first statement is false (it was either Becky or Diana), neither Becky nor Diana could have done it. Therefore, it was either Abdul or Carl. Because the second statement is false, (it was neither Becky nor Carl), either Becky or Carl did it. Because the first statement ensured that it was Abdul or Carl, it must have been Carl.

**107a.** $1.99 \times 10^{30}$ kg

**b.** $1.67 \times 10^{-27}$ kg

## Chapter 10 Concept Review

**1.** To find two numbers that are 6 units from 4, move 6 units to the right of 4 and 6 units to the left of 4. The two numbers are 10 and $-2$.

**2.** The absolute value of $-6$ is the distance from 0 to $-6$ on the number line. The absolute value of $-6$ is 6.

**3.** Rule for adding two integers:

- To add numbers with the same sign, add the absolute values of the numbers. Then attach the sign of the addends.
- To add numbers with different signs, find the difference between the absolute values of the numbers. Then attach the sign of the addend with the greater absolute value.

**4.** The rule for subtracting two integers is to add the opposite of the second number to the first number.

**5.** To find the change in temperature from $-5°C$ to $-14°C$, use subtraction.

**6.** $4 - 9 = 4 + (-9)$. To show this addition on the number line, start at 4 on the number line. Draw an arrow 9 units long pointing to the left, with its tail at 4. The head of the arrow is at $-5$. $4 + (-9) = -5$.

**7.** If you multiply two nonzero numbers with different signs, the product is negative.

**8.** If you divide two nonzero numbers with the same sign, the quotient is positive.

**9.** When a number is divided by zero, the result is undefined because division by zero is undefined.

**10.** A terminating decimal is one that ends. For example, 0.75 is a terminating decimal.

**11.** The steps in the Order of Operations Agreement are:

1. Do all operations inside parentheses.
2. Simplify any number expressions containing exponents.
3. Do multiplication and division as they occur from left to right.

© 2013 Cengage Learning. All Rights Reserved. May not be scanned, copied or duplicated, or posted to a publicly accessible website, in whole or in part.

4. Rewrite subtraction as addition of the opposite. Then do additions as they occur from left to right.

**12.** To write the number 0.000754 in scientific notation, move the decimal point to the right of the 7. Because we move the decimal 4 places to the right, the exponent on 10 is $-4$. 0.000754 written in scientific notation is $7.54\times10^{-4}$.

## Chapter 10 Review Exercises

**1.** –22

**2.** $$\begin{aligned}-8-(-2)-(-10)-3&=-8+2+10-3\\&=-6+10-3\\&=4-3=1\end{aligned}$$

**3.** $$\begin{aligned}\frac{5}{8}-\frac{5}{6}&=\frac{15}{24}-\frac{20}{24}\\&=\frac{15}{24}+\frac{(-20)}{24}=\frac{15+(-20)}{24}=\frac{-5}{24}=-\frac{5}{24}\end{aligned}$$

**4.** $$\begin{aligned}-0.33+1.98-1.44&=-0.33+1.98+(-1.44)\\&=1.65+(-1.44)=0.21\end{aligned}$$

**5.** $$\left(-\frac{2}{3}\right)\left(\frac{6}{11}\right)\left(-\frac{22}{25}\right)=\frac{2\cdot6\cdot22}{3\cdot11\cdot25}=\frac{8}{25}$$

**6.** $$\begin{array}{r}16\\ \times\ .08\\ \hline 1.28\end{array}$$

$$-0.08\times16=-(0.08\times16)=-1.28$$

**7.** 12 – 6 ÷ 3 = 12 – 2 = 12 + (–2) = 10

**8.** $$\begin{aligned}\left(\frac{2}{3}\right)^2-\frac{5}{6}&=\left(\frac{2}{3}\cdot\frac{2}{3}\right)-\frac{5}{6}\\&=\frac{4}{9}-\frac{5}{6}=\frac{8}{18}-\frac{15}{18}\\&=\frac{8}{18}+\left(-\frac{15}{18}\right)=\frac{8+(-15)}{18}=-\frac{7}{18}\end{aligned}$$

**9.** 4

**10.** $0>-3$

**11.** $-|-6|=-6$

**12.** –18 ÷ (–3) = 18 ÷ 3 = 6

**13.** $$\begin{aligned}-\frac{3}{8}+\frac{5}{12}+\frac{2}{3}&=\frac{-9}{24}+\frac{10}{24}+\frac{16}{24}\\&=\frac{-9+10+16}{24}=\frac{17}{24}\end{aligned}$$

**14.** $$\frac{1}{3}\times\left(-\frac{3}{4}\right)=-\left(\frac{1}{3}\times\frac{3}{4}\right)=-\frac{1}{4}$$

**15.** $$\begin{aligned}-\frac{7}{12}\div\left(-\frac{14}{39}\right)&=-\frac{7}{12}\times\left(-\frac{39}{14}\right)\\&=\frac{7\cdot39}{12\cdot14}=\frac{13}{8}=1\frac{5}{8}\end{aligned}$$

**16.** $$\begin{aligned}16\div4(8-2)&=16\div4[8+(-2)]\\&=16\div4(6)=4(6)=24\end{aligned}$$

**17.** –22 + 14 + (–18) = –8 + (–18) = –26

**18.** $$\begin{aligned}3^2-9+2&=9-9+2\\&=9+(-9)+2\\&=0+2=2\end{aligned}$$

**19.** The number is less than 1. Move the decimal point 5 places to the right. The exponent on 10 is –5.

$0.0000397 = 3.97\times10^{-5}$

**20.**

$$\begin{array}{r}0.08\\ 18.3.\overline{)1.4.64}\\ -1464\\ \hline 0\end{array}$$

$-1.464\div18.3=-(1.464\div18.3)=-0.08$

**21.** $$\begin{aligned}-\frac{5}{12}+\frac{7}{9}-\frac{1}{3}&=\frac{-15}{36}+\frac{28}{36}-\frac{12}{36}\\&=\frac{-15}{36}+\frac{28}{36}+\frac{(-12)}{36}\\&=\frac{-15+28+(-12)}{36}=\frac{1}{36}\end{aligned}$$

© 2013 Cengage Learning. All Rights Reserved. May not be scanned, copied or duplicated, or posted to a publicly accessible website, in whole or in part.

**22.** $\frac{6}{34} \times \frac{17}{40} = \frac{6 \cdot 17}{34 \cdot 40} = \frac{3}{40}$

**23.**
$$\begin{array}{r} 0.035 \\ \underline{\times \;\; 1.2} \\ 70 \\ \underline{35 \;\;} \\ 0.042 \end{array}$$

$1.2 \times (-0.035) = -(1.2 \times 0.035) = -0.042$

**24.** $-\frac{1}{2} + \frac{3}{8} : \frac{9}{20} = \frac{1}{2} + \frac{3}{8} \times \frac{20}{9}$

$= -\frac{1}{2} + \frac{3 \cdot 20}{8 \cdot 9}$

$= -\frac{1}{2} + \frac{5}{6} = -\frac{3}{6} + \frac{5}{6} = \frac{2}{6} = \frac{1}{3}$

**25.** $|-5| = 5$

**26.** $-2 > -40$

**27.** $2 \times (-13) = -(2 \times 13) = -26$

**28.** $-0.4 \times 5 - (-3.33) = -2 - (-3.33)$

$= -2 + 3.33 = 1.33$

**29.** $\frac{5}{12} + \left(-\frac{2}{3}\right) = \frac{5}{12} + \frac{(-8)}{12}$

$= \frac{5 + (-8)}{12} = \frac{-3}{12} = \frac{-1}{4} = -\frac{1}{4}$

**30.** $-33.4 + 9.8 - (-16.2) = -33.4 + 9.8 + 16.2$

$= -23.6 + 16.2 = -7.4$

**31.** $\left(-\frac{3}{8}\right) \div \left(-\frac{4}{5}\right) = -\frac{3}{8} \times \left(-\frac{5}{4}\right) = \frac{3 \cdot 5}{8 \cdot 4} = \frac{15}{32}$

**32.** The exponent on 10 is positive. Move the decimal point 5 places to the right.

$2.4 \times 10^5 = 240{,}000$

**33.** **Strategy** To find the total change, add the changes (−6 lb, −4 lb, + 2 lb, +1 lb, and −3 lb).

**Solution** $(-6) + (-4) + 2 + 1 + (-3)$

$= -10 + 2 + 1 + (-3)$

$= -8 + 1 + (-3)$

$= -7 + (-3) = -10$

The total change was −10 lb.

**34.** **Strategy** To find the student's score:

- Multiply the number of questions answered correctly (38) by 3.
- Multiply the number of questions left blank (8) by −1.
- Multiply the number of questions answered incorrectly (4) by −2.
- Add the three products.

**Solution** $38 \times 3 = 114$

$8 \times (-1) = -8$

$4 \times (-2) = -8$

$114 + (-8) + (-8)$

$= 106 + (-8) = 98$

The student's score was 98.

**35.** **Strategy** To find the difference between the boiling point and the melting point of mercury, subtract the melting point (−38.87°C) from the boiling point (356.58°C).

**Solution** 356.58 − (−38.87)

= 356.58 + 38.87 = 395.45

The difference between the boiling and melting points is 395.45°C.

# Chapter 10 Test

**1.** $-5 - (-8) = -5 + 8 = 3$

**2.** $-|-2| = -2$

© 2013 Cengage Learning. All Rights Reserved. May not be scanned, copied or duplicated, or posted to a publicly accessible website, in whole or in part.

**3.** $-\frac{2}{5}+\frac{7}{15}=\frac{-6}{15}+\frac{7}{15}=\frac{-6+7}{15}=\frac{1}{15}$

**4.**
$$\begin{array}{r} 0.032 \\ \times 1.9 \\ \hline 288 \\ 32\phantom{0} \\ \hline 0.0608 \end{array}$$

$0.032\times(-1.9)=-(0.032\times 1.9)=-0.0608$

**5.** $-8>-10$

**6.** $1.22+(-3.1)=-1.88$

**7.** $4\times(4-7)\div(-2)-4\times 8$
$=4\times[4+(-7)]\div(-2)-4\times 8$
$=4\times(-3)\div(-2)-4\times 8$
$=-12\div(-2)-4\times 8$
$=6-4\times 8$
$=6-32$
$=6+(-32)=-26$

**8.** $-5\times(-6)\times 3=30\times 3=90$

**9.** $-1.004-3.01=-1.004+(-3.01)=-4.014$

**10.** $-72\div 8=-(72\div 8)=-9$

**11.** $-2+3+(-8)=1+(-8)=-7$

**12.** $-\frac{3}{8}+\frac{2}{3}=\frac{-9}{24}+\frac{16}{24}=\frac{-9+16}{24}=\frac{7}{24}$

**13.** The number is greater than 10. Move the decimal point 10 places to the left. The exponent on 10 is 10.

$87{,}600{,}000{,}000=8.76\times 10^{10}$

**14.** $-4\times 12=-(4\times 12)=-48$

**15.** $\frac{0}{-17}=0$

**16.** $16-4-(-5)-7=16+(-4)+5+(-7)$
$=12+5+(-7)$
$=17+(-7)=10$

**17.** $-\frac{2}{3}\div\frac{5}{6}=-\frac{2}{3}\times\frac{6}{5}=-\left(\frac{2\cdot 6}{3\cdot 5}\right)=-\frac{4}{5}$

**18.** $0>-4$

**19.** $16+(-10)+(-20)=6+(-20)=-14$

**20.** $(-2)^2-(-3)^2\div(1-4)^2\times 2-6$
$=(-2)^2-(-3)^2\div[1+(-4)]^2\times 2-6$
$=(-2)^2-(-3)^2\div(-3)^2\times 2-6$
$=4-9\div 9\times 2-6$
$=4-1\times 2-6$
$=4-2-6$
$=4+(-2)+(-6)$
$=2+(-6)=-4$

**21.** $-\frac{2}{5}-\left(\frac{-7}{10}\right)=\frac{-4}{10}-\left(-\frac{7}{10}\right)$
$=\frac{-4}{10}+\frac{7}{10}=\frac{-4+7}{10}=\frac{3}{10}$

**22.** The exponent on 10 is negative. Move the decimal point 8 places to the left.

$9.601\times 10^{-8}=0.00000009601$

**23.**
$$\begin{array}{r} 3.4 \\ 4.6\,\overline{)15.64} \\ -138\phantom{0} \\ \hline 184 \\ -184 \\ \hline 0 \end{array}$$

$-15.64\div(-4.6)=(15.64\div 4.6)=3.4$

**24.** $-\frac{1}{2}+\frac{1}{3}+\frac{1}{4}=\frac{-6}{12}+\frac{4}{12}+\frac{3}{12}$
$=\frac{-6+4+3}{12}=\frac{1}{12}$

**25.** $\frac{3}{8}\times\left(-\frac{5}{6}\right)\times\left(-\frac{4}{15}\right)=\frac{3}{8}\times\frac{5}{6}\times\frac{4}{15}$
$=\frac{3\cdot 5\cdot 4}{8\cdot 6\cdot 15}=\frac{1}{12}$

**26.** $2.113-(-1.1)=2.113+1.1=3.213$

© 2013 Cengage Learning. All Rights Reserved. May not be scanned, copied or duplicated, or posted to a publicly accessible website, in whole or in part.

**27. Strategy** To find the temperature, add the increase (11°C) to the previous temperature (–4°C).

**Solution** $-4 + 11 = 7$

The temperature is 7°C.

**28. Strategy** To find the melting point of oxygen, multiply the melting point of radon (–71°C) by 3.

**Solution** $-71 \times 3 = -213$

The melting point of oxygen is –213°C.

**29. Strategy** To find the patient's temperature at 4 P.M., add the changes (+0.5° and −1.9°) to the temperature at noon (101.9° F).

**Solution** $101.9 + 0.5 + (-1.9)$

$= 102.4 + (-1.9) = 100.5$

The temperature at 4 P.M. was 100.5° F.

**30. Strategy** To find the average daily low temperature:

- Add the three temperature readings.
- Divide by 3.

**Solution** $-7+9+(-8)=2+(-8)=-6$

$-6 \div 3 = -2$

The average low temperature was –2°F.

## Cumulative Review Exercises

**1.** $16-4\cdot(3-2)^2\cdot 4 = 16-4\cdot(1)^2\cdot 4$

$= 16-4\cdot(1)\cdot 4 = 16-16 = 0$

**2.**
$$\begin{array}{r} 8\frac{1}{2} = 8\frac{7}{14} = 7\frac{21}{14} \\ -3\frac{4}{7} = 3\frac{8}{14} = 3\frac{8}{14} \\ \hline 4\frac{13}{14} \end{array}$$

**3.** $3\frac{7}{8} \div 1\frac{1}{2} = \frac{31}{8} \div \frac{3}{2}$

$= \frac{31}{8} \times \frac{2}{3}$

$= \frac{31}{12} = 2\frac{7}{12}$

**4.**

$\frac{3}{8} \div \left(\frac{3}{8}-\frac{1}{4}\right) \div \frac{7}{3} = \frac{3}{8} \div \left(\frac{3}{8}-\frac{2}{8}\right) \div \frac{7}{3}$

$= \frac{3}{8} \div \left(\frac{1}{8}\right) \div \frac{7}{3}$

$= \frac{3}{8} \times \frac{8}{1} \div \frac{7}{3}$

$= 3 \div \frac{7}{3} = 3 \times \frac{3}{7} = \frac{3\cdot 3}{7}$

$= \frac{9}{7} = 1\frac{2}{7}$

**5.**
$$\begin{array}{r} 2.90700 \\ -1.09761 \\ \hline 1.80939 \end{array}$$

**6.** $\frac{7}{12} = \frac{n}{32}$

$7\cdot 32 = 12 \times n$

$224 = 12 \times n$

$224 \div 12 = n$

$18.67 \approx n$

**7.** $160\% \times n = 22$

$1.6 \times n = 22$

$n = 22 \div 1.6$

$n = 13.75$

**8.** 1 gal 3 qt

$$\begin{array}{r} 4\overline{)7} \\ -4 \\ \hline 3 \end{array}$$

**9.** 6692 ml = 6.692 L

**10.** $4.2\text{ ft} = 4.2\text{ ft} \times \frac{1\text{ m}}{3.28\text{ ft}}$

$= \frac{4.2}{3.28}\text{m} \approx 1.28\text{ m}$

© 2013 Cengage Learning. All Rights Reserved. May not be scanned, copied or duplicated, or posted to a publicly accessible website, in whole or in part.

**11.** Percent × base = amount

$$0.32 \times 180 = n$$
$$57.6 = n$$

**12.** $3\frac{2}{5} \times 100\% = \frac{1700}{5}\% = 340\%$

**13.** $-8 + 5 = -3$

**14.** $3\frac{1}{4} + \left(-6\frac{5}{8}\right) = \frac{13}{4} + \left(\frac{-53}{8}\right) = \frac{26}{8} + \frac{(-53)}{8}$
$= \frac{26 + (-53)}{8} = \frac{-27}{8} = -3\frac{3}{8}$

**15.**

$$-6\frac{1}{8} - 4\frac{5}{12} = \frac{-49}{8} - \frac{-53}{12}$$
$$= \frac{-147}{24} - \frac{106}{24} = \frac{-147}{24} + \frac{(-106)}{24}$$
$$= \frac{-147 + (-106)}{24} = \frac{-253}{24} = -10\frac{13}{24}$$

**16.** $-12 - (-7) - 3(-8) = -12 + 7 + 24 = -5 + 24 = 19$

**17.**
```
  1.09
 ×3.2
  218
 327
 3.488
```
$-3.2 \times -1.09 = 3.2 \times 1.09 = 3.488$

**18.** $-6 \times 7 \times \left(-\frac{3}{4}\right) = 6 \times 7 \times \frac{3}{4}$
$= \frac{6 \cdot 7 \cdot 3}{4} = \frac{126}{4} = \frac{63}{2} = 31\frac{1}{2}$

**19.** $42 \div (-6) = -(42 \div 6) = -7$

**20.** $-2\frac{1}{7} \div \left(3\frac{3}{5}\right) = \frac{15}{7} \div \left(\frac{18}{5}\right)$
$= \frac{15}{7} \times \left(\frac{5}{18}\right) = \frac{25}{42}$

**21.** $3 \times (3 - 7) \div 6 - 2 = 3 \times [3 + (-7)] \div 6 - 2$
$= 3 \times (-4) \div 6 - 2$
$= -12 \div 6 - 2$
$= -2 + (-2) = -4$

**22.** $4 - (-2)^2 \div (1 - 2)^2 \times 3 + 4$
$= 4 - (-2)^2 \div [1 + (2 - 2)]^2 \times 3 + 4$
$= 4 - (-2)^2 \div (-1)^2 \times 3 + 4$
$= 4 - 4 \div 1 \times 3 + 4$
$= 4 - 4 \times 3 + 4$
$= 4 - 12 + 4$
$= 4 + (-12) + 4$
$= -8 + 4 = -4$

**23. Strategy** To find the gauze remaining, subtract the amount cut off $\left(3\frac{2}{3}\text{ in}\right)$ from the amount on the roll (10 in).

**Solution**

$$10 \text{ in.} = 9\frac{3}{3} \text{ in.}$$
$$-3\frac{2}{3} \text{ in.} = 3\frac{2}{3} \text{ in.}$$
$$6\frac{1}{3} \text{ in.}$$

The length remaining is $6\frac{1}{3}$ in.

**24. Strategy** To find Nimisha's new balance:

- Subtract the amounts of the checks written.
- Add the amount of the deposit.

**Solution**
```
  763.56
– 135.88
  627.68
  –47.81
  579.87
+ 223.44
  803.31
```
Nimisha's new balance is $803.31.

**25. Strategy** To find the discount:

- Subtract the sale price ($28) from the original price ($35) to find the amount of the decrease.
- Solve the basic percent equation for percent. The base is $35 and the amount is the amount of the

© 2013 Cengage Learning. All Rights Reserved. May not be scanned, copied or duplicated, or posted to a publicly accessible website, in whole or in part.

decrease.

**Solution** $35 - 28 = 7$

$$\begin{aligned} \text{Percent} \times \text{base} &= \text{amount} \\ n \times 35 &= 7 \\ n &= 7 \div 35 \\ n = 0.20 &= 20\% \end{aligned}$$

The discount is 20%.

**26. Strategy** To find how many gallons liquid was consumed, convert 40 cups to gallons.

**Solution** 40 c

$$= 40\,\cancel{c} \times \frac{1\,\cancel{pt}}{2\,\cancel{c}} \times \frac{1\,\cancel{qt}}{2\,\cancel{pt}} \times \frac{1\text{ gal}}{4\,\cancel{qt}}$$
$$= \frac{40}{16}\text{ gal} = 2\frac{1}{2}\text{ gal}$$

$2\frac{1}{2}$ gal of liquid were consumed.

**27. Strategy** To find the markup rate:

- Find the markup by subtracting the cost ($550) from the sale price ($797.50)
- Solve the basic percent equation for percent. The base amount is $550 and the amount is the markup.

**Solution** $797.50 - 550.00 = 247.50$

$$\begin{aligned} n \times 550 &= 247.50 \\ n &= 247.50 - 550 \\ n &= 0.45 = 45\% \end{aligned}$$

The markup rate is 45%.

**28a. Strategy** To find the number of households:

- Locate the sector of the graph that represents once a week and read the percent.
- Write and solve the basic percent equation using $n$ to represent the number of households that have a family night once a week. The percent is from the graph and the base is 114 million.

**Solution** The percent is 6%.

$$\begin{aligned} \text{Percent} \times \text{base} &= \text{amount} \\ 6\% \times 114{,}000{,}000 &= n \\ 0.06 \times 114{,}000{,}000 &= n \\ 6{,}840{,}000 &= n \end{aligned}$$

6.84 million households have a family night once a week.

**b. Strategy** To find the fraction of U.S. households:

- Locate the sector of the graph that represents rarely or never and read the percent.
- Convert the percent to a fraction.

**Solution** The percent is 24%.

$$\begin{aligned} 24\% &= 24 \times \frac{1}{100} \\ &= \frac{24}{1} \times \frac{1}{100} \\ &= \frac{24}{100} = \frac{6}{25} \end{aligned}$$

$\frac{6}{25}$ of U.S. households rarely or never have a family night.

**c. Strategy** To determine if the number is more or less:

- Locate the sectors of the graph that represent once a month and once a week and read the percents.
- Multiply the percent that represents once a week by 3. Compare the result to the percent that represents once a month.

**Solution** Once a month: 21%

Once a week: 6%

$6\% \times 3 = 18\%$

$21\% > 18\%$

The number of households that

© 2013 Cengage Learning. All Rights Reserved. May not be scanned, copied or duplicated, or posted to a publicly accessible website, in whole or in part.

have a family night only once a month is more than three times the number of households that have family night once a week.

**29.** **Strategy** To time, write and solve a proportion.

**Solution**

$$\frac{150\text{ ml}}{1\text{ h}} = \frac{500\text{ ml}}{x\text{ hr}}$$

$$1 \times 500 = 150 \times x$$

$$500 \div 150 = x$$

$$3\frac{1}{3} = x$$

The infusion will take $3\frac{1}{3}$ h.

**30.** **Strategy** To find the average:

- Add the readings (−19°, −7°, 1°, and 9°).
- Divide by the number of readings (4).

**Solution**

$$-19 + (-7) + 1 + 9 = -16$$

$$-16 \div 4 = -4$$

The average reading is −4° F.

© 2013 Cengage Learning. All Rights Reserved. May not be scanned, copied or duplicated, or posted to a publicly accessible website, in whole or in part.

# Chapter 11: Introduction to Algebra

## Prep Test

**1.** $2-9=-7$

**2.** $-5(4)=-20$

**3.** $-16+16=0$

**4.** $\dfrac{-7}{-7}=1$

**5.** $-\dfrac{3}{8}\left(-\dfrac{8}{3}\right)=1$

**6.** $\left(\dfrac{3}{5}\right)^3\cdot\left(\dfrac{5}{9}\right)^2=\dfrac{3}{5}\cdot\dfrac{3}{5}\cdot\dfrac{3}{5}\cdot\dfrac{5}{9}\cdot\dfrac{5}{9}$
$=\dfrac{\overset{1}{\cancel{3}}\cdot\overset{1}{\cancel{3}}\cdot\overset{1}{\cancel{3}}\cdot\overset{1}{\cancel{5}}\cdot\overset{1}{\cancel{5}}}{\underset{1}{\cancel{5}}\cdot\underset{1}{\cancel{5}}\cdot 5\cdot\underset{1}{\cancel{3}}\cdot\underset{1}{\cancel{3}}\cdot\underset{1}{\cancel{3}}\cdot 3}$
$=\dfrac{1}{15}$

**7.** $\dfrac{2}{3}+\left(\dfrac{3}{4}\right)^2\cdot\dfrac{2}{9}=\dfrac{2}{3}+\dfrac{9}{16}\cdot\dfrac{2}{9}$
$=\dfrac{2}{3}+\dfrac{1}{8}$
$=\dfrac{16}{24}+\dfrac{3}{24}$
$=\dfrac{19}{24}$

**8.** $-8\div(-2)^2+6=-8\div 4+6$
$=-2+6$
$=4$

**9.** $4+5(2-7)^2\div(-8+3)$
$=4+5(-5)^2\div(-5)$
$=4+5(25)\div(-5)$
$=4+125\div(-5)$
$=4+(-25)=-21$

## Section 11.1

### Objective A Exercises

**1.** $5a-3b=5(-3)-3(6)$
$=-15-18$
$=-15+(-18)$
$=-33$

**3.** $2a+3c=2(-3)+3(-2)$
$=-6+(-6)=-12$

**5.** $-c^2=-(-2)^2=-4$

**7.** $b-a^2=6-(-3)^2=6-9=6+(-9)=-3$

**9.** $ab-c^2=(-3)(6)-(-2)^2$
$=-18-4$
$=-18+(-4)=-22$

**11.** $2ab-c^2=2(-3)6-(-2)^2$
$=-36-4$
$=-36+(-4)=-40$

**13.** $a-(b\div a)=-3-[6\div(-3)]$
$=-3-(-2)$
$=-3+2=-1$

**15.** $2ac-(b\div a)=2(-3)(-2)-[6\div(-3)]$
$=12-(-2)$
$=12+2=14$

**17.** $b^2-c^2=(6)^2-(-2)^2$
$=36-4$
$=36+(-4)=32$

**19.** $b^2\div(ac)=(6)^2\div(-3)(-2)$
$=36\div 6=6$

**21.** $c^2-(b\div c)=(-2)^2-[6\div(-2)]$
$=4-(-3)$
$=4+3=7$

© 2013 Cengage Learning. All Rights Reserved. May not be scanned, copied or duplicated, or posted to a publicly accessible website, in whole or in part.

**23.** $$\begin{aligned} a^2+b^2+c^2 &= (-3)^2+6^2+(-2)^2 \\ &= 9+36+4 \\ &= 45+4=49 \end{aligned}$$

**25.** $$\begin{aligned} ac+bc+ab &= (-3)(-2)+6(-2)+(-3)(6) \\ &= 6+(-12)+(-18) \\ &= -6+(-18)=-24 \end{aligned}$$

**27.** $$\begin{aligned} a^2+b^2-ab &= (-3)^2+6^2-(-3)(6) \\ &= 9+36-(-3)(6) \\ &= 9+36-(-18) \\ &= 9+36+18 \\ &= 45+18=63 \end{aligned}$$

**29.** $$\begin{aligned} 2b-(3c+a^2) &= 2(6)-\left[3(-2)+(-3)^2\right] \\ &= 2(6)-\left[3(-2)+9\right] \\ &= 2(6)-(-6+9) \\ &= 2(6)-3 \\ &= 12-3 \\ &= 12+(-3)=9 \end{aligned}$$

**31.** $$\begin{aligned} &\frac{1}{3}a+\left(\frac{1}{2}b-\frac{2}{3}a\right) \\ &= \frac{1}{3}(-3)+\left[\frac{1}{2}\cdot 6-\frac{2}{3}(-3)\right] \\ &= \frac{1}{3}(-3)+\left[3-(-2)\right] \\ &= \frac{1}{3}(-3)+(3+2)=-1+5=4 \end{aligned}$$

**33.** $$\begin{aligned} \frac{1}{6}b+\frac{1}{3}(c+a) &= \frac{1}{6}\cdot 6+\frac{1}{3}\left[-2+(-3)\right] \\ &= \frac{1}{6}\cdot 6+\frac{1}{3}(-5) \\ &= 1+\left(-\frac{5}{3}\right)=\frac{3}{3}+\left(-\frac{5}{3}\right)=-\frac{2}{3} \end{aligned}$$

**35.** $$\begin{aligned} 4a+(3b-c) &= 4\left(-\frac{1}{2}\right)+\left[3\left(\frac{3}{4}\right)-\frac{1}{4}\right] \\ &= 4\left(-\frac{1}{2}\right)+\left[\frac{9}{4}-\frac{1}{4}\right] \\ &= 4\left(-\frac{1}{2}\right)+\frac{8}{4} \\ &= -2+2=0 \end{aligned}$$

**37.** $$\begin{aligned} 2a-b^2\div c &= 2\left(-\frac{1}{2}\right)-\left(\frac{3}{4}\right)^2\div\frac{1}{4} \\ &= 2\left(-\frac{1}{2}\right)-\frac{9}{16}\div\frac{1}{4} \\ &= -1-\frac{9}{16}\div\frac{1}{4} \\ &= -1-\frac{9}{16}\times\frac{4}{1} \\ &= -1-\frac{9}{4} \\ &= -1+\left(-\frac{9}{4}\right)=-3\frac{1}{4} \end{aligned}$$

**39.** $$\begin{aligned} a^2-b^2 &= (3.48)^2-(-2.31)^2 \\ &= 12.1104-5.3361=6.7743 \end{aligned}$$

**41.** $$\begin{aligned} &3ac-(a\div c) \\ &= 3(3.48)(-1.74)-(3.48\div -1.74) \\ &\approx -16.1656 \end{aligned}$$

**43.** Positive

**45.** Positive

## Objective B Exercises

**47.** $2x^2$, $3x$, $\underline{-4}$

**49.** $3a^2$, $-4a$, $\underline{8}$

**51.** $\underline{3}x^2$, $\underline{-4}x$

**53.** $\underline{1}y^2$, $\underline{6}a$

**55.** (ii), (iii)

**57.** $7z+9z=16z$

**59.** $12m-3m=12m+(-3)m=9m$

**61.** $5at+7at=12at$

**63.** $-4yt+7yt=3yt$

**65.** $-3x-12y$; Unlike terms

**67.** $3t^2-5t^2=3t^2+(-5)t^2=-2t^2$

**69.** $6c-5+7c=6c+7c-5=13c-5$

**71.** $2t+3t-7t=2t+3t+(-7)t=5t+(-7)t=-2t$

© 2013 Cengage Learning. All Rights Reserved. May not be scanned, copied or duplicated, or posted to a publicly accessible website, in whole or in part.

**73.** $7y^2 - 2 - 4y^2 = 7y^2 + (-2) + (-4)y^2$
$= 7y^2 + (-4)y^2 + (-2)$
$= 3y^2 - 2$

**75.** $6w - 8u + 8w = 6w + (-8)u + 8w$
$= 6w + 8w + (-8)u$
$= 14w - 8u$

**77.** $10 - 11xy - 12xy = 10 + (-11)xy + (-12)xy$
$= 10 + (-23)xy$
$= 10 - 23xy = -23xy + 10$

**79.** $3v^2 - 6v^2 - 8v^2 = 3v^2 + (-6)v^2 + (-8)v^2$
$= -3v^2 + (-8)v^2$
$= -11v^2$

**81.** $-10ab - 3a + 2ab = -10ab + 2ab - 3a$
$= -8ab - 3a$

**83.** $-3y^2 - y + 7y^2 = -3y^2 + 7y^2 - y$
$= 4y^2 - y$

**85.** $2a - 3b^2 - 5a + b^2$
$= 2a + (-3)b^2 + (-5)a + b^2$
$= 2a + (-5)a + (-3)b^2 + b^2$
$= -3a - 2b^2$

**87.** $3x^2 - 7x + 4x^2 - x$
$= 3x^2 + (-7)x + 4x^2 + (-1)x$
$= 3x^2 + 4x^2 + (-7)x + (-1)x$
$= 7x^2 - 8x$

**89.** $6s - t - 9s + 7t = 6s + (-1)t + (-9)s + 7t$
$= 6s + (-9)s + (-1)t + 7t$
$= -3s + 6t$

**91.** $4m + 8n - 7m + 2n = 4m + 8n + (-7)m + 2n$
$= 4m + (-7)m + 8n + 2n$
$= -3m + 10n$

**93.** $-5ab + 7ac + 10ab - 3ac$
$= -5ab + 7ac + 10ab + (-3)ac$
$= -5ab + 10ab + 7ac + (-3)ac$
$= 5ab + 4ac$

**95.** $\frac{4}{9}a^2 - \frac{1}{5}b^2 + \frac{2}{9}a^2 + \frac{4}{5}b^2$

$= \frac{4}{9}a^2 + \left(-\frac{1}{5}\right)b^2 + \frac{2}{9}a^2 + \frac{4}{5}b^2$

$= \frac{4}{9}a^2 + \frac{2}{9}a^2 + \left(-\frac{1}{5}\right)b^2 + \frac{4}{5}b^2$

$= \frac{6}{9}a^2 + \frac{3}{5}b^2$

$= \frac{2}{3}a^2 + \frac{3}{5}b^2$

**97.** $7.81m + 3.42n - 6.25m - 7.19n$
$= 7.81m + 3.42n + (-6.25)m + (-7.19)n$
$= 7.81m + (-6.25)m + 3.42n + (-7.19)n$
$= 1.56m - 3.77n$

## Objective C Exercises

**99.** (ii), (iii)

**101.** $5(x + 4) = 5x + 5 \cdot 4 = 5x + 20$

**103.** $(y - 3)4 = [y + (-3)]4$
$= y \cdot 4 + (-3)4$
$= 4y + (-12)$
$= 4y - 12$

**105.** $-2(a + 4) = -2(a) + (-2)(4)$
$= -2a + (-8)$
$= -2a - 8$

**107.** $3(5x + 10) = 3(5x) + 3(10) = 15x + 30$

**109.** $5(3c - 5) = 5[3c + (-5)]$
$= 5(3c) + 5(-5)$
$= 15c + (-25)$
$= 15c - 25$

**111.** $-3(y - 6) = -3[y + (-6)]$
$= -3y + (-3)(-6)$
$= -3y + 18$

**113.** $5x + 2(x + 7) = 5x + 2x + 2(7) = 7x + 14$

© 2013 Cengage Learning. All Rights Reserved. May not be scanned, copied or duplicated, or posted to a publicly accessible website, in whole or in part.

**115.** $8y - 4(y + 2) = 8y + (-4)(y + 2)$
$= 8y + (-4)y + (-4)(2)$
$= 8y + (-4y) + (-8)$
$= 4y - 8$

**117.** $9x - 4(x - 6) = 9x + (-4)[x + (-6)]$
$= 9x + (-4)(x) + (-4)(-6)$
$= 9x + (-4)x + 24$
$= 5x + 24$

**119.** $-2y + 3(y - 2) = -2y + 3[y + (-2)]$
$= -2y + 3y + 3(-2)$
$= -2y + 3y + (-6)$
$= y - 6$

**121.** $4n + 2(n + 1) - 5 = 4n + 2(n + 1) + (-5)$
$= 4n + 2n + 2(1) + (-5)$
$= 4n + 2n + 2 + (-5)$
$= 6n - 3$

**123.** $9y - 3(y - 4) + 8$
$= 9y + (-3)[y + (-4)] + 8$
$= 9y + (-3)(y) + (-3)(-4) + 8$
$= 9y + (-3)y + 12 + 8$
$= 6y + 20$

**125.** $3x + 2(x + 2) + 5x = 3x + 2x + 2(2) + 5x$
$= 3x + 2x + 4 + 5x$
$= 3x + 2x + 5x + 4$
$= 5x + 5x + 4$
$= 10x + 4$

**127.** $-7t + 2(t - 3) - t = -7t + 2[t + (-3)] + (-1)t$
$= -7t + 2t + 2(-3) + (-1)t$
$= -7t + 2t + (-6) + (-1)t$
$= -7t + 2t + (-1)t + (-6)$
$= -5t + (-1)t + (-6)$
$= -6t - 6$

**129.** $z - 2(1 - z) - 2z$
$= z + (-2)[1 + (-z)] + (-2)z$
$= z + (-2)(1) + (-2)(-z) + (-2)z$
$= z + (-2) + 2z + (-2)z$
$= z + 2z + (-2)z + (-2)$
$= 3z + (-2)z + (-2)$
$= z - 2$

**131.** $3(y - 2) - 2(y - 6)$
$= 3[y + (-2)] + (-2)[y + (-6)]$
$= 3y + 3(-2) + (-2)y + (-2)(-6)$
$= 3y + (-6) + (-2)y + 12$
$= 3y + (-2)y + (-6) + 12$
$= y + 6$

**133.** $2(t - 3) + 7(t + 3) = 2[t + (-3)] + 7(t + 3)$
$= 2t + 2(-3) + 7t + 7(3)$
$= 2t + (-6) + 7t + 21$
$= 2t + 7t + (-6) + 21$
$= 9t + 15$

**135.** $3t - 6(t - 4) + 8t$
$= 3t + (-6)[t + (-4)] + 8t$
$= 3t + (-6)(t) + (-6)(-4) + 8t$
$= 3t + (-6)t + 24 + 8t$
$= 3t + (-6)t + 8t + 24$
$= -3t + 8t + 24$
$= 5t + 24$

## Applying the Concepts

**137a.** $2 + 3x$

| | | | | |
|---|---|---|---|---|
| 1 | 1 | $x$ | $x$ | $x$ |

**b.** $5x$

| | | | | |
|---|---|---|---|---|
| $x$ | $x$ | $x$ | $x$ | $x$ |

**c.** No. $2 + 3x \neq 5x$. Because 2 and $3x$ are *not* like terms, 2 and $3x$ cannot be combined.

| | | | | | | | | | |
|---|---|---|---|---|---|---|---|---|---|
| $x$ | $x$ | $x$ | $x$ | 1 | 1 | 1 | 1 | 1 | 1 |

© 2013 Cengage Learning. All Rights Reserved. May not be scanned, copied or duplicated, or posted to a publicly accessible website, in whole or in part.

**d.** No, $2(2x + 3)$ does not equal $4x + 3$. $2(2x + 3) = 4x + 6$. This equivalence shows that the Distributive Property preserves the quantity. $2(2x + 3)$ and $4x + 6$ differ in arrangement only.

## Section 11.2

### Objective A Exercises

**1.**
$$\begin{array}{r|l} \multicolumn{2}{c}{2x+9=3} \\ \hline 2(-3)+9 & 3 \\ -6+9 & 3 \\ \multicolumn{2}{c}{3=3} \end{array}$$

Yes, –3 is a solution.

**3.**
$$\begin{array}{r|l} \multicolumn{2}{c}{4-2x=8} \\ \hline 4-2(2) & 8 \\ 4-4 & 8 \\ \multicolumn{2}{c}{0\neq 8} \end{array}$$

No, 2 is not a solution.

**5.**
$$\begin{array}{r|l} \multicolumn{2}{c}{3x-2=x+4} \\ \hline 3(3)-2 & 3+4 \\ 9-2 & 7 \\ \multicolumn{2}{c}{7=7} \end{array}$$

Yes, 3 is a solution.

**7.**
$$\begin{array}{r|l} \multicolumn{2}{c}{x^2-5x+1=10-5x} \\ \hline 3^2-5(3)+1 & 10-5(3) \\ 9-15+1 & 10-15 \\ \multicolumn{2}{c}{-5=-5} \end{array}$$

Yes, 3 is a solution.

**9.**
$$\begin{array}{r|l} \multicolumn{2}{c}{2x(x-1)=3-x} \\ \hline 2(-1)(-1-1) & 3-(-1) \\ -2(-2) & 3+1 \\ \multicolumn{2}{c}{4=4} \end{array}$$

Yes, –1 is a solution.

**11.**
$$\begin{array}{r|l} \multicolumn{2}{c}{x(x-2)=x^2-4} \\ \hline 2(2-2) & 2^2-4 \\ 2(0) & 4-4 \\ \multicolumn{2}{c}{0=0} \end{array}$$

Yes, 2 is a solution.

**13.**
$$\begin{array}{r|l} \multicolumn{2}{c}{3x+6=4} \\ \hline 3(-\frac{2}{3})+6 & 4 \\ -2+6 & 4 \\ \multicolumn{2}{c}{4=4} \end{array}$$

Yes, $-\frac{2}{3}$ is a solution.

**15.**
$$\begin{array}{r|l} \multicolumn{2}{c}{2x-3=1-14x} \\ \hline 2\left(\frac{1}{4}\right)-3 & 1-14\left(\frac{1}{4}\right) \\ \frac{2}{4}-3 & 1-\frac{14}{4} \\ \frac{1}{2}-3 & 1-\frac{7}{2} \end{array}$$

$$-2\frac{1}{2}=-2\frac{1}{2}$$

Yes, $\frac{1}{4}$ is a solution.

**17.**
$$\begin{array}{r|l} \multicolumn{2}{c}{x^2-3x=x+3.8} \\ \hline (-1.9)^2-3(-1.9) & -1.9+3.8 \\ 3.61+5.7 & 1.9 \\ \multicolumn{2}{c}{9.31\neq 1.9} \end{array}$$

No, –1.9 is not a solution.

**19.** True

### Objective B Exercises

**21.**
$$\begin{aligned} y-6&=16 \\ y-6+6&=16+6 \\ y+0&=22 \\ y&=22 \end{aligned}$$

The solution is 22.

**23.**
$$\begin{aligned} 3+n&=4 \\ 3-3+n&=4-3 \\ 0+n&=1 \\ n&=1 \end{aligned}$$

The solution is 1.

© 2013 Cengage Learning. All Rights Reserved. May not be scanned, copied or duplicated, or posted to a publicly accessible website, in whole or in part.

**25.**
$$\begin{aligned} z+7&=2 \\ z+7-7&=2-7 \\ z+0&=-5 \\ z&=-5 \end{aligned}$$

The solution is $-5$.

**27.**
$$\begin{aligned} x-3&=-7 \\ x-3+3&=-7+3 \\ x+0&=-4 \\ x&=-4 \end{aligned}$$

The solution is $-4$.

**29.**
$$\begin{aligned} y+6&=6 \\ y+6-6&=6-6 \\ y+0&=0 \\ y&=0 \end{aligned}$$

The solution is 0.

**31.**
$$\begin{aligned} v-7&=-4 \\ v-7+7&=-4+7 \\ v+0&=3 \\ v&=3 \end{aligned}$$

The solution is 3.

**33.**
$$\begin{aligned} 1+x&=0 \\ 1-1+x&=0-1 \\ 0+x&=0+(-1) \\ 0+x&=-1 \\ x&=-1 \end{aligned}$$

The solution is $-1$.

**35.**
$$\begin{aligned} x-10&=5 \\ x-10+10&=5+10 \\ x+0&=15 \\ x&=15 \end{aligned}$$

The solution is 15.

**37.**
$$\begin{aligned} x+4&=-7 \\ x+4-4&=-7-4 \\ x+0&=-7+(-4) \\ x+0&=-11 \\ x&=-11 \end{aligned}$$

The solution is $-11$.

**39.**
$$\begin{aligned} w+5&=-5 \\ w+5-5&=-5-5 \\ w+0&=-5+(-5) \\ w+0&=-10 \\ w&=-10 \end{aligned}$$

The solution is $-10$.

**41.**
$$\begin{aligned} x+\frac{1}{2}&=-\frac{1}{2} \\ x+\frac{1}{2}-\frac{1}{2}&=-\frac{1}{2}-\frac{1}{2} \\ x+0&=-\frac{1}{2}+\left(-\frac{1}{2}\right) \\ x&=-1 \end{aligned}$$

The solution is $-1$.

**43.**
$$\begin{aligned} \frac{2}{5}+x&=-\frac{3}{5} \\ \frac{2}{5}-\frac{2}{5}+x&=-\frac{3}{5}-\frac{2}{5} \\ 0+x&=-\frac{3}{5}+\left(-\frac{2}{5}\right) \\ x&=-\frac{5}{5} \\ x&=-1 \end{aligned}$$

The solution is $-1$.

**45.**
$$\begin{aligned} x+\frac{1}{2}&=-\frac{1}{3} \\ x+\frac{1}{2}-\frac{1}{2}&=-\frac{1}{3}-\frac{1}{2} \\ x+0&=-\frac{1}{3}+\left(-\frac{1}{2}\right) \\ x&=-\frac{5}{6} \end{aligned}$$

The solution is $-\frac{5}{6}$.

© 2013 Cengage Learning. All Rights Reserved. May not be scanned, copied or duplicated, or posted to a publicly accessible website, in whole or in part.

**47.** $$t+\frac{1}{4}=-\frac{1}{2}$$
$$t+\frac{1}{4}-\frac{1}{4}=-\frac{1}{2}-\frac{1}{4}$$
$$t+0=-\frac{1}{2}+\left(-\frac{1}{4}\right)$$
$$t=-\frac{3}{4}$$

The solution is $-\frac{3}{4}$.

**49.** Must be negative

**51.** Must be positive

## Objective C Exercises

**53.** $3y=12$
$$\frac{3y}{3}=\frac{12}{3}$$
$$1y=4$$
$$y=4$$

The solution is 4.

**55.** $5z=-20$
$$\frac{5z}{5}=\frac{-20}{5}$$
$$1z=-4$$
$$z=-4$$

The solution is $-4$.

**57.** $-2x=6$
$$\frac{-2x}{-2}=\frac{6}{-2}$$
$$1x=-3$$
$$x=-3$$

The solution is $-3$.

**59.** $-5x=-40$
$$\frac{-5x}{-5}=\frac{-40}{-5}$$
$$1x=8$$
$$x=8$$

The solution is 8.

**61.** $40=8x$
$$\frac{40}{8}=\frac{8x}{8}$$
$$5=1x$$
$$5=x$$

The solution is 5.

**63.** $-24=4x$
$$\frac{-24}{4}=\frac{4x}{4}$$
$$-6x=1x$$
$$-6=x$$

The solution is $-6$.

**65.** $$\frac{x}{3}=5$$
$$\frac{1}{3}x=5$$
$$3\left(\frac{1}{3}x\right)=3(5)$$
$$1x=15$$
$$x=15$$

The solution is 15.

**67.** $$\frac{n}{4}=-2$$
$$\frac{1}{4}n=-2$$
$$4\left(\frac{1}{4}n\right)=4(-2)$$
$$1n=-8$$
$$n=-8$$

The solution is $-8$.

**69.** $$-\frac{x}{4}=1$$
$$-\frac{1}{4}x=1$$
$$-4\left(-\frac{1}{4}x\right)=-4(1)$$
$$1x=-4$$
$$x=-4$$

The solution is $-4$.

© 2013 Cengage Learning. All Rights Reserved. May not be scanned, copied or duplicated, or posted to a publicly accessible website, in whole or in part.

**71.** $\frac{2}{3}w = 4$

$$\frac{3}{2}\left(\frac{2}{3}w\right) = \frac{3}{2}(4)$$
$$1w = 6$$
$$w = 6$$

The solution is 6.

**73.** $\frac{3}{4}v = -3$

$$\frac{4}{3}\left(\frac{3}{4}v\right) = \frac{4}{3}(-3)$$
$$1v = -4$$
$$v = -4$$

The solution is $-4$.

**75.** $-\frac{1}{3}x = -2$

$$-3\left(-\frac{1}{3}x\right) = -3(-2)$$
$$1x = 6$$
$$x = 6$$

The solution is 6.

**77.** $-4 = -\frac{2}{3}z$

$$-\frac{3}{2}(-4) = -\frac{3}{2}\left(-\frac{2}{3}z\right)$$
$$6 = 1z$$
$$6 = z$$

The solution is 6.

**79.** $\frac{2}{3}x = -\frac{2}{7}$

$$\frac{3}{2}\left(\frac{2}{3}x\right) = \frac{3}{2}\left(-\frac{2}{7}\right)$$
$$1x = -\frac{3}{7}$$
$$x = -\frac{3}{7}$$

The solution is $-\frac{3}{7}$.

**81.** $4x - 2x = 7$

$$2x = 7$$
$$\frac{2x}{2} = \frac{7}{2}$$
$$1x = \frac{7}{2}$$
$$x = 3\frac{1}{2}$$

The solution is $3\frac{1}{2}$.

**83.** $\frac{4}{5}m - \frac{1}{5}m = 9$

$$\frac{3}{5}m = 9$$
$$\frac{5}{3}\left(\frac{3}{5}m\right) = \frac{5}{3}(9)$$
$$1m = 15$$
$$m = 15$$

The solution is 15.

**85.** True

**87.** False

© 2013 Cengage Learning. All Rights Reserved. May not be scanned, copied or duplicated, or posted to a publicly accessible website, in whole or in part.

## Objective D Exercises

**89. Strategy** To find the number of gallons of gasoline used, replace the variables $D$ and $M$ in the formula by the given values and solve for $G$.

**Solution**

$$D = M \cdot G$$
$$621 = 28 \cdot G$$
$$\frac{621}{28} = \frac{28G}{28}$$
$$22.2 \approx G$$

22.2 gal of gasoline was used.

**91. Strategy** To find the number of miles per gallon, replace the variables $D$ and $G$ in the formula by the given values and solve for $M$.

**Solution**

$$D = M \cdot G$$
$$560 = M \cdot 15$$
$$\frac{560}{15} = \frac{15M}{15}$$
$$37.3 \approx M$$

The car gets 37.3 mi/gal.

**93. Strategy** To find the amount of the original investment, replace the variables $A$ and $I$ by the given values and solve for $P$.

**Solution**

$$A = P + I$$
$$17,700 = P + 2700$$
$$17,700 - 2700 = P + 2700 - 2700$$
$$17,700 + (-2700) = P + 0$$
$$15,000 = P$$

The original investment was $15,000.

**95. Strategy** To find the increase in value of the investment, replace the variables $A$ and $P$ in the formula by the given values and solve for $I$.

**Solution**

$$A = P + I$$
$$11,420 = 8000 + I$$
$$11,420 - 8000 = 8000 - 8000 + I$$
$$11,420 + (-8000) = 0 + I$$
$$3420 = I$$

The increase is $3420.

**97. Strategy** To find the cost, replace the variables $S$ and $M$ in the formula by the given values and solve for $C$.

© 2013 Cengage Learning. All Rights Reserved. May not be scanned, copied or duplicated, or posted to a publicly accessible website, in whole or in part.

**Solution**

$$S = C + M$$
$$2240 = C + 420$$
$$2240 - 420 = C + 420 - 420$$
$$2240 + (-420) = C + 0$$
$$1820 = C$$

The cost of the power wheelchair is $1820.

**99. Strategy** To find the cost of the medical equipment, replace the variables $S$ and $R$ in the formula by the given values and solve for $C$.

**Solution**

$$S = C + RC$$
$$179 = C + 0.25C$$
$$179 = 1.25C$$
$$\frac{179}{1.25} = \frac{1.25C}{1.25}$$
$$143.20 = C$$

The medical equipment costs $143.20.

## Applying the Concepts

**101.** $x - 3 = -5$

$x - 3 + 3 = -5 + 3$ Addition Property of Equations

$x + 0 = -2$

$x = -2$ Addition Property of Zero

**103.** Answers will vary. For example, $x + 5 = 1$.

# Section 11.3

## Objective A Exercises

**1.**

$$3x + 5 = 14$$
$$3x + 5 - 5 = 14 - 5$$
$$3x = 9$$
$$\frac{3x}{3} = \frac{9}{3}$$
$$x = 3$$

The solution is 3.

**3.**

$$2n - 3 = 7$$
$$2n - 3 + 3 = 7 + 3$$
$$2n = 10$$
$$\frac{2n}{2} = \frac{10}{2}$$
$$n = 5$$

The solution is 5.

**5.**

$$5w + 8 = 3$$
$$5w + 8 - 8 = 3 - 8$$
$$5w = -5$$
$$\frac{5w}{5} = \frac{-5}{5}$$
$$w = -1$$

The solution is $-1$.

**7.**

$$3z - 4 = -16$$
$$3z - 4 + 4 = -16 + 4$$
$$3z = -12$$
$$\frac{3z}{3} = \frac{-12}{3}$$
$$z = -4$$

The solution is $-4$.

© 2013 Cengage Learning. All Rights Reserved. May not be scanned, copied or duplicated, or posted to a publicly accessible website, in whole or in part.

**9.**
$$\begin{aligned} 5 + 2x &= 7 \\ 5 - 5 + 2x &= 7 - 5 \\ 2x &= 2 \\ \frac{2x}{2} &= \frac{2}{2} \\ x &= 1 \end{aligned}$$

The solution is 1.

**11.**
$$\begin{aligned} 6 - x &= 3 \\ 6 + (-1)x &= 3 \\ 6 - 6 + (-1)x &= 3 - 6 \\ (-1)x &= -3 \\ (-1)(-1)x &= (-1)(-3) \\ x &= 3 \end{aligned}$$

The solution is 3.

**13.**
$$\begin{aligned} 3 - 4x &= 11 \\ 3 - 3 - 4x &= 11 - 3 \\ -4x &= 8 \\ \frac{-4x}{-4} &= \frac{8}{-4} \\ x &= -2 \end{aligned}$$

The solution is $-2$.

**15.**
$$\begin{aligned} 5 - 4x &= 17 \\ 5 - 5 - 4x &= 17 - 5 \\ -4x &= 12 \\ \frac{-4x}{-4} &= \frac{12}{-4} \\ x &= -3 \end{aligned}$$

The solution is $-3$.

**17.**
$$\begin{aligned} 3x + 6 &= 0 \\ 3x + 6 - 6 &= 0 - 6 \\ 3x &= -6 \\ \frac{3x}{3} &= \frac{-6}{3} \\ x &= -2 \end{aligned}$$

The solution is $-2$.

**19.**
$$\begin{aligned} -3x - 4 &= -1 \\ -3x - 4 + 4 &= -1 + 4 \\ -3x &= 3 \\ \frac{-3x}{-3} &= \frac{3}{-3} \\ x &= -1 \end{aligned}$$

The solution is $-1$.

**21.**
$$\begin{aligned} 12y - 30 &= 6 \\ 12y - 30 + 30 &= 6 + 30 \\ 12y &= 36 \\ \frac{12y}{12} &= \frac{36}{12} \\ y &= 3 \end{aligned}$$

The solution is 3.

**23.**
$$\begin{aligned} 3c + 7 &= 4 \\ 3c + 7 - 7 &= 4 - 7 \\ 3c &= -3 \\ \frac{3c}{3} &= \frac{-3}{3} \\ c &= -1 \end{aligned}$$

The solution is $-1$.

**25.**
$$\begin{aligned} -2x + 11 &= -3 \\ -2x + 11 - 11 &= -3 - 11 \\ -2x &= -14 \\ \frac{-2x}{-2} &= \frac{-14}{-2} \\ x &= 7 \end{aligned}$$

The solution is 7.

**27.**
$$\begin{aligned} 14 - 5x &= 4 \\ 14 - 14 - 5x &= 4 - 14 \\ -5x &= -10 \\ \frac{-5x}{-5} &= \frac{-10}{-5} \\ x &= 2 \end{aligned}$$

The solution is 2.

**29.**
$$\begin{aligned} -8x + 7 &= -9 \\ -8x + 7 - 7 &= -9 - 7 \\ -8x &= -16 \\ \frac{-8x}{-8} &= \frac{-16}{-8} \\ x &= 2 \end{aligned}$$

The solution is 2.

**31.**
$$\begin{aligned} 9x + 13 &= 13 \\ 9x + 13 - 13 &= 13 - 13 \\ 9x &= 0 \\ \frac{9x}{9} &= \frac{0}{9} \\ x &= 0 \end{aligned}$$

The solution is 0.

**33.**
$$\begin{aligned} 7d - 14 &= 0 \\ 7d - 14 + 14 &= 0 + 14 \\ 7d &= 14 \\ \frac{7d}{7} &= \frac{14}{7} \\ d &= 2 \end{aligned}$$

The solution is 2.

**35.**
$$\begin{aligned} 4n - 4 &= -4 \\ 4n - 4 + 4 &= -4 + 4 \\ 4n &= 0 \\ \frac{4n}{4} &= \frac{0}{4} \\ n &= 0 \end{aligned}$$

The solution is 0.

**37.**
$$\begin{aligned} 3x + 5 &= 7 \\ 3x + 5 - 5 &= 7 - 5 \\ 3x &= 2 \\ \frac{3x}{3} &= \frac{2}{3} \\ x &= \frac{2}{3} \end{aligned}$$

The solution is $\frac{2}{3}$.

© 2013 Cengage Learning. All Rights Reserved. May not be scanned, copied or duplicated, or posted to a publicly accessible website, in whole or in part.

**39.**
$$\begin{aligned} 6x - 1 &= 16 \\ 6x - 1 + 1 &= 16 + 1 \\ 6x &= 17 \\ \frac{6x}{6} &= \frac{17}{6} \\ x &= 2\frac{5}{6} \end{aligned}$$

The solution is $2\frac{5}{6}$.

**41.**
$$\begin{aligned} 2x - 3 &= -8 \\ 2x - 3 + 3 &= -8 + 3 \\ 2x &= -5 \\ \frac{2x}{2} &= \frac{-5}{2} \\ x &= -2\frac{1}{2} \end{aligned}$$

The solution is $-2\frac{1}{2}$.

**43.**
$$\begin{aligned} -6x + 2 &= -7 \\ -6x + 2 - 2 &= -7 - 2 \\ -6x &= -9 \\ \frac{-6x}{-6} &= \frac{-9}{-6} \\ x &= 1\frac{1}{2} \end{aligned}$$

The solution is $1\frac{1}{2}$.

**45.**
$$\begin{aligned} -2x - 3 &= -7 \\ -2x - 3 + 3 &= -7 + 3 \\ -2x &= -4 \\ \frac{-2x}{-2} &= \frac{-4}{-2} \\ x &= 2 \end{aligned}$$

The solution is 2.

**47.**
$$\begin{aligned} 3x + 8 &= 2 \\ 3x + 8 - 8 &= 2 - 8 \\ 3x &= -6 \\ \frac{3x}{3} &= \frac{-6}{3} \\ x &= -2 \end{aligned}$$

The solution is $-2$.

**49.**
$$\begin{aligned} 3w - 7 &= 0 \\ 3w - 7 + 7 &= 0 + 7 \\ 3w &= 7 \\ \frac{3w}{3} &= \frac{7}{3} \\ w &= 2\frac{1}{3} \end{aligned}$$

The solution is $2\frac{1}{3}$.

**51.**
$$\begin{aligned} -2d + 9 &= 12 \\ -2d + 9 - 9 &= 12 - 9 \\ -2d &= 3 \\ \frac{-2d}{-2} &= \frac{3}{-2} \\ d &= -1\frac{1}{2} \end{aligned}$$

The solution is $-1\frac{1}{2}$.

**53.**
$$\begin{aligned} \frac{1}{2}x - 2 &= 3 \\ \frac{1}{2}x - 2 + 2 &= 3 + 2 \\ \frac{1}{2}x &= 5 \\ 2\left(\frac{1}{2}x\right) &= 5 \cdot 2 \\ x &= 10 \end{aligned}$$

The solution is 10.

**55.**
$$\begin{aligned} \frac{3}{5}w - 1 &= 2 \\ \frac{3}{5}w - 1 + 1 &= 2 + 1 \\ \frac{3}{5}w &= 3 \\ \frac{5}{3} \cdot \frac{3}{5}w &= 3 \cdot \frac{5}{3} \\ w &= 5 \end{aligned}$$

The solution is 5.

**57.**
$$\begin{aligned} \frac{2}{9}t - 3 &= 5 \\ \frac{2}{9}t - 3 + 3 &= 5 + 3 \\ \frac{2}{9}t &= 8 \\ \frac{9}{2} \cdot \frac{2}{9}t &= 8 \cdot \frac{9}{2} \\ t &= 36 \end{aligned}$$

The solution is 36.

**59.**
$$\begin{aligned} \frac{y}{3} - 6 &= -8 \\ \frac{y}{3} - 6 + 6 &= -8 + 6 \\ \frac{y}{3} &= -2 \\ 3 \cdot \frac{y}{3} &= 3(-2) \\ y &= -6 \end{aligned}$$

The solution is $-6$.

**61.**
$$\begin{aligned} \frac{x}{3} - 2 &= -5 \\ \frac{x}{3} - 2 + 2 &= -5 + 2 \\ \frac{x}{3} &= -3 \\ 3 \cdot \frac{x}{3} &= 3(-3) \\ x &= -9 \end{aligned}$$

The solution is $-9$.

**63.**
$$\begin{aligned} \frac{5}{8}v + 6 &= 3 \\ \frac{5}{8}v + 6 - 6 &= 3 - 6 \\ \frac{5}{8}v &= -3 \\ \frac{8}{5} \cdot \frac{5}{8}v &= \frac{8}{5} \cdot (-3) \\ v &= -\frac{24}{5} = -4\frac{4}{5} \end{aligned}$$

The solution is $-4\frac{4}{5}$.

© 2013 Cengage Learning. All Rights Reserved. May not be scanned, copied or duplicated, or posted to a publicly accessible website, in whole or in part.

**65.**
$$\begin{aligned}\frac{4}{7}z+10&=5\\ \frac{4}{7}z+10-10&=5-10\\ \frac{4}{7}z&=-5\\ \frac{7}{4}\cdot\frac{4}{7}z&=\frac{7}{4}\cdot(-5)\\ z&=-\frac{35}{4}=-8\frac{3}{4}\end{aligned}$$

The solution is $-8\frac{3}{4}$.

**67.**
$$\begin{aligned}\frac{2}{9}x-3&=5\\ \frac{2}{9}x-3+3&=5+3\\ \frac{2}{9}x&=8\\ \frac{9}{2}\cdot\frac{2}{9}x&=\frac{9}{2}\cdot 8\\ x&=36\end{aligned}$$

The solution is 36.

**69.**
$$\begin{aligned}\frac{3}{4}x-5&=-4\\ \frac{3}{4}x-5+5&=-4+5\\ \frac{3}{4}x&=1\\ \frac{4}{3}\cdot\frac{3}{4}x&=\frac{4}{3}\cdot 1\\ x&=\frac{4}{3}=1\frac{1}{3}\end{aligned}$$

The solution is $1\frac{1}{3}$.

**71.**
$$\begin{aligned}1.5x-0.5&=2.5\\ 1.5x-0.5x+0.5&=2.5+0.5\\ 1.5x&=3\\ \frac{1.5x}{1.5}&=\frac{3}{1.5}\\ x&=2\end{aligned}$$

The solution is 2.

**73.**
$$\begin{aligned}0.8t+1.1&=4.3\\ 0.8t+1.1-1.1&=4.3-1.1\\ 0.8t&=3.2\\ \frac{0.8t}{0.8}&=\frac{3.2}{0.8}\\ t&=4\end{aligned}$$

The solution is 4.

**75.**
$$\begin{aligned}0.4x-2.3&=1.3\\ 0.4x-2.3+2.3&=1.3+2.3\\ 0.4x&=3.6\\ \frac{0.4x}{0.4}&=\frac{3.6}{0.4}\\ x&=9\end{aligned}$$

The solution is 9.

**77.**
$$\begin{aligned}3.5y-3.5&=10.5\\ 3.5y-3.5+3.5&=10.5+3.5\\ 3.5y&=14\\ \frac{3.5y}{3.5}&=\frac{14}{3.5}\\ y&=4\end{aligned}$$

The solution is 4.

**79.**
$$\begin{aligned}0.32x+4.2&=3.2\\ 0.32x+4.2-4.2&=3.2-4.2\\ 0.32x&=-1\\ \frac{0.32x}{0.32}&=\frac{-1}{0.32}\\ x&=-3.125\end{aligned}$$

The solution is $-3.125$.

**81.**
$$\begin{aligned}6m+2m-2&=5\\ 8m-3&=5\\ 8m-3+3&=5+3\\ 8m&=8\\ \frac{8m}{8}&=\frac{8}{8}\\ m&=1\end{aligned}$$

The solution is 1.

© 2013 Cengage Learning. All Rights Reserved. May not be scanned, copied or duplicated, or posted to a publicly accessible website, in whole or in part.

**83.** $3y - 8y - 9 = 6$
$$-5y - 9 = 6$$
$$-5y - 9 + 9 = 6 + 9$$
$$-5y = 15$$
$$\frac{-5y}{-5} = \frac{15}{-5}$$
$$y = -3$$

The solution is $-3$.

**85.** $-2y + y - 3 = 6$
$$-y - 3 = 6$$
$$-y - 3 + 3 = 6 + 3$$
$$-y = 9$$
$$(-1)(-y) = (-1)9$$
$$y = -9$$

The solution is $-9$.

**87.** Must be negative

**89.** Must be positive

## Objective B Exercises

**91.** **Strategy** To find the Celsius temperature, replace the variable $F$ in the formula by the given value and solve for $C$.

**Solution**
$$F = 1.8C + 32$$
$$-40 = 1.8C + 32$$
$$-40 - 32 = 1.8C + 32 - 32$$
$$-72 = 1.8C$$
$$\frac{-72}{1.8} = \frac{1.8C}{1.8}$$
$$-40 = C$$

The temperature is –40°C.

**93.** **Strategy** To find the time required, replace the variables $V$ and $V_0$ in the formula by the given values and solve for $t$.

**Solution**
$$V = V_0 + 32t$$
$$472 = 8 + 32t$$
$$472 - 8 = 8 - 8 + 32t$$
$$464 = 32t$$
$$\frac{464}{32} = \frac{32t}{32}$$
$$14.5 = t$$

The time is 14.5 s.

**95.** **Strategy** To find the height, replace the variable $L$ in the formula with the length (20 in.) and solve for $H$.

**Solution**
$$H = 1.9L + 32$$
$$H = 1.9(20) + 32$$
$$H = 38 + 32$$
$$H = 70$$

The victim's height is 70 in.

**97.** **Strategy** To find the length of the femur, replace the variable $H$ in the formula with the height (71 in.) and solve for $L$.

**Solution**
$$H = 1.9L + 32$$
$$71 = 1.9L + 32$$
$$71 - 32 = 1.9L + 32 - 32$$
$$39 = 1.9L$$
$$\frac{39}{1.9} = \frac{1.9L}{1.9}$$
$$20.5 \approx L$$

The length of the femur is 20.5 in.

**99.** **Strategy** To find the total sales, replace the variables $M$, $R$, and $B$ in the formula by the given values and solve for $S$.

© 2013 Cengage Learning. All Rights Reserved. May not be scanned, copied or duplicated, or posted to a publicly accessible website, in whole or in part.

**Solution**
$$\begin{aligned} M &= S \cdot R + B \\ 3480 &= S \cdot 0.09 + 600 \\ 3480 - 600 &= 0.09S + 600 - 600 \\ 2880 &= 0.09S \\ \frac{2880}{0.09} &= \frac{0.09S}{0.09} \\ 32{,}000 &= S \end{aligned}$$
The total sales were \$32,000.

**101. Strategy** To find the commission rate, replace the variables $M$, $S$, and $B$ in the formula by the given values and solve for $R$.

**Solution**
$$\begin{aligned} M &= S \cdot R + B \\ 2640 &= 42{,}000R + 750 \\ 2640 - 750 &= 42{,}000R + 750 - 750 \\ 1890 &= 42{,}000R \\ \frac{1890}{42{,}000} &= \frac{42{,}000R}{42{,}000} \\ 0.045 &= R \\ 4.5\% &= R \end{aligned}$$
Miguel's commission rate was 4.5%.

## Applying the Concepts

**103.** $\frac{2}{3}x - 4 = 10$

$\frac{2}{3}x - 4 + 4 = 10 + 4$ Addition Property of Equations

$\frac{2}{3}x + 0 = 14$ Addition Property of Zero

$\frac{2}{3}x = 14$

$\frac{3}{2}\left(\frac{2}{3}x\right) = \frac{3}{2}(14)$ Multiplication Property of Equations

$1x = 21$ Multiplication Property of Reciprocals

$x = 21$ Multiplication Property of One

**105.** No, the sentence "Solve $3x + 4(x - 3)$" does not make sense because $3x + 4(x - 3)$ is an expression, and you cannot solve an expression. You can solve an equation.

# Section 11.4

## Objective A Exercises

**1.**
$$\begin{aligned} 6x + 3 &= 2x + 5 \\ 6x - 2x + 3 &= 2x - 2x + 5 \\ 4x + 3 &= 5 \\ 4x + 3 - 3 &= 5 - 3 \\ 4x &= 2 \\ \frac{4x}{4} &= \frac{2}{4} \\ x &= \frac{1}{2} \end{aligned}$$

The solution is $\frac{1}{2}$.

**3.**
$$\begin{aligned} 3x + 3 &= 2x + 2 \\ 3x - 2x + 3 &= 2x - 2x + 2 \\ x + 3 &= 2 \\ x + 3 - 3 &= 2 - 3 \\ x &= -1 \end{aligned}$$

The solution is $-1$.

**5.**
$$\begin{aligned} 5x + 4 &= x - 12 \\ 5x - x + 4 &= x - x - 12 \\ 4x + 4 &= -12 \\ 4x + 4 - 4 &= -12 - 4 \\ 4x &= -16 \\ \frac{4x}{4} &= \frac{-16}{4} \\ x &= -4 \end{aligned}$$

The solution is $-4$.

© 2013 Cengage Learning. All Rights Reserved. May not be scanned, copied or duplicated, or posted to a publicly accessible website, in whole or in part.

**7.**
$$\begin{aligned} 7b-2&=3b-6\\ 7b-3b-2&=3b-3b-6\\ 4b-2&=-6\\ 4b-2+2&=-6+2\\ 4b&=-4\\ \frac{4b}{4}&=\frac{-4}{4}\\ b&=-1 \end{aligned}$$

The solution is $-1$.

**9.**
$$\begin{aligned} 9n-4&=5n-20\\ 9n-5n-4&=5n-5n-20\\ 4n-4&=-20\\ 4n-4+4&=-20+4\\ 4n&=-16\\ \frac{4n}{4}&=\frac{-16}{4}\\ n&=-4 \end{aligned}$$

The solution is $-4$.

**11.**
$$\begin{aligned} 2x+1&=16-3x\\ 2x+3x+1&=16-3x+3x\\ 5x+1&=16\\ 5x+1-1&=16-1\\ 5x&=15\\ \frac{5x}{5}&=\frac{15}{5}\\ x&=3 \end{aligned}$$

**13.**
$$\begin{aligned} 5x-2&=-10-3x\\ 5x+3x-2&=-10-3x+3x\\ 8x-2&=-10\\ 8x-2+2&=-10+2\\ 8x&=-8\\ \frac{8x}{8}&=\frac{-8}{8}\\ x&=-1 \end{aligned}$$

The solution is $-1$.

**15.**
$$\begin{aligned} 2x+7&=4x+3\\ 2x-4x+7&=4x-4x+3\\ -2x+7&=3\\ -2x+7-7&=3-7\\ -2x&=-4\\ \frac{-2x}{-2}&=\frac{-4}{-2}\\ x&=2 \end{aligned}$$

The solution is 2.

**17.**
$$\begin{aligned} c+4&=6c-11\\ c-6c+4&=6c-6c-11\\ -5c+4&=-11\\ -5c+4-4&=-11-4\\ -5c&=-15\\ \frac{-5c}{-5}&=\frac{-15}{-5}\\ c&=3 \end{aligned}$$

The solution is 3.

**19.**
$$\begin{aligned} 3x-7&=x-7\\ 3x-x-7&=x-x-7\\ 2x-7&=-7\\ 2x-7+7&=-7+7\\ 2x&=0\\ \frac{2x}{2}&=\frac{0}{2}\\ x&=0 \end{aligned}$$

The solution is 0.

**21.**
$$\begin{aligned} 3-4x&=5-3x\\ 3-4x+3x&=5-3x+3x\\ 3-x&=5\\ 3-3-x&=5-3\\ -x&=2\\ (-1)(-x)&=(-1)2\\ x&=-2 \end{aligned}$$

The solution is $-2$.

**23.**
$$\begin{aligned} 7+3x&=9+5x\\ 7+3x-5x&=9+5x-5x\\ 7-2x&=9\\ 7-7-2x&=9-7\\ -2x&=2\\ \frac{-2x}{-2}&=\frac{2}{-2}\\ x&=-1 \end{aligned}$$

The solution is $-1$.

**25.**
$$\begin{aligned} 5+2y&=7+5y\\ 5+2y-5y&=7+5y-5y\\ 5-3y&=7\\ 5-5-3y&=7-5\\ -3y&=2\\ \frac{-3y}{-3}&=\frac{2}{-3}\\ y&=-\frac{2}{3} \end{aligned}$$

The solution is $-\frac{2}{3}$.

**27.**
$$\begin{aligned} 8-5w&=4-6w\\ 8-5w+6w&=4-6w+6w\\ 8+w&=4\\ 8-8+w&=4-8\\ w&=-4 \end{aligned}$$

The solution is $-4$.

**29.**
$$\begin{aligned} 6x+1&=3x+2\\ 6x-3x+1&=3x-3x+2\\ 3x+1&=2\\ 3x+1-1&=2-1\\ 3x&=1\\ \frac{3x}{3}&=\frac{1}{3}\\ x&=\frac{1}{3} \end{aligned}$$

The solution is $\frac{1}{3}$.

© 2013 Cengage Learning. All Rights Reserved. May not be scanned, copied or duplicated, or posted to a publicly accessible website, in whole or in part.

**31.**
$$\begin{aligned}
5x + 8 &= x + 5\\
5x - x + 8 &= x - x + 5\\
4x + 8 &= 5\\
4x + 8 - 8 &= 5 - 8\\
4x &= -3\\
\frac{4x}{4} &= \frac{-3}{4}\\
x &= -\frac{3}{4}
\end{aligned}$$

The solution is $-\frac{3}{4}$.

**33.**
$$\begin{aligned}
2x - 3 &= 6x - 4\\
2x - 6x - 3 &= 6x - 6x - 4\\
-4x - 3 &= -4\\
-4x - 3 + 3 &= -4 + 3\\
-4x &= -1\\
\frac{-4x}{-4} &= \frac{-1}{-4}\\
x &= \frac{1}{4}
\end{aligned}$$

The solution is $\frac{1}{4}$.

**35.**
$$\begin{aligned}
6 - 3x &= 6 - 5x\\
6 - 3x + 5x &= 6 - 5x + 5x\\
6 + 2x &= 6\\
6 - 6 + 2x &= 6 - 6\\
2x &= 0\\
\frac{2x}{2} &= \frac{0}{2}\\
x &= 0
\end{aligned}$$

The solution is 0.

**37.**
$$\begin{aligned}
6x - 2 &= 2x - 9\\
6x - 2x - 2 &= 2x - 2x - 9\\
4x - 2 &= -9\\
4x - 2 + 2 &= -9 + 2\\
4x &= -7\\
\frac{4x}{4} &= \frac{-7}{4}\\
x &= -\frac{7}{4}\\
x &= -1\frac{3}{4}
\end{aligned}$$

The solution is $-1\frac{3}{4}$.

**39.**
$$\begin{aligned}
6x - 3 &= -5x + 8\\
6x + 5x - 3 &= -5x + 5x + 8\\
11x - 3 &= 8\\
11x - 3 + 3 &= 8 + 3\\
11x &= 11\\
\frac{11x}{11} &= \frac{11}{11}\\
x &= 1
\end{aligned}$$

The solution is 1.

**41.**
$$\begin{aligned}
-6t - 2 &= -8t - 4\\
-6t + 8t - 2 &= -8t + 8t - 4\\
2t - 2 &= -4\\
2t - 2 + 2 &= -4 + 2\\
2t &= -2\\
\frac{2t}{2} &= \frac{-2}{2}\\
t &= -1
\end{aligned}$$

The solution is $-1$.

**43.**
$$\begin{aligned}
-3 - 4x &= 7 - 2x\\
-3 - 4x + 2x &= 7 - 2x + 2x\\
-3 - 2x &= 7\\
-3 + 3 - 2x &= 7 + 3\\
-2x &= 10\\
\frac{-2x}{-2} &= \frac{10}{-2}\\
x &= -5
\end{aligned}$$

The solution is $-5$.

**45.**
$$\begin{aligned}
3 - 7x &= -2 + 5x\\
3 - 7x - 5x &= -2 + 5x - 5x\\
3 - 12x &= -2\\
3 - 3 - 12x &= -2 - 3\\
-12x &= -5\\
\frac{-12x}{-12} &= \frac{-5}{-12}\\
x &= \frac{5}{12}
\end{aligned}$$

The solution is $\frac{5}{12}$.

**47.**
$$\begin{aligned}
5x + 8 &= 4 - 2x\\
5x + 2x + 8 &= 4 - 2x + 2x\\
7x + 8 &= 4\\
7x + 8 - 8 &= 4 - 8\\
7x &= -4\\
\frac{7x}{7} &= \frac{-4}{7}\\
x &= -\frac{4}{7}
\end{aligned}$$

The solution is $-\frac{4}{7}$.

**49.**
$$\begin{aligned}
12z - 9 &= 3z + 12\\
12z - 3z - 9 &= 3z - 3z + 12\\
9z - 9 &= 12\\
9z - 9 + 9 &= 12 + 9\\
9z &= 21\\
\frac{9z}{9} &= \frac{21}{9}\\
z &= \frac{7}{3}\\
z &= 2\frac{1}{3}
\end{aligned}$$

The solution is $2\frac{1}{3}$.

© 2013 Cengage Learning. All Rights Reserved. May not be scanned, copied or duplicated, or posted to a publicly accessible website, in whole or in part.

**51.** $\frac{5}{7}m - 3 = \frac{2}{7}m + 6$

$\frac{5}{7}m - \frac{2}{7}m - 3 = \frac{2}{7}m - \frac{2}{7}m + 6$

$\frac{3}{7}m - 3 = 6$

$\frac{3}{7}m - 3 + 3 = 6 + 3$

$\frac{3}{7}m = 9$

$\frac{7}{3} \cdot \frac{3}{7}m = \frac{7}{3} \cdot 9$

$m = 21$

The solution is 21.

**53.** $\frac{3}{7}x + 5 = \frac{5}{7}x - 7$

$\frac{3}{7}x - \frac{5}{7}x + 5 = \frac{5}{7}x - \frac{5}{7}x - 1$

$\frac{-2}{7}x + 5 = -1$

$\frac{-2}{7}x + 5 - 5 = -1 - 5$

$\frac{-2}{7}x = -6$

$\left(\frac{-7}{2}\right)\left(\frac{-2}{7}x\right) = \left(\frac{-7}{2}\right)(-6)$

$x = 21$

The solution is 21.

**55.** Positive

## Objective B Exercises

**57.** (iv)

**59.** $6x + 2(x - 1) = 14$

$6x + 2x - 2 = 14$

$8x - 2 = 14$

$8x - 2 + 2 = 14 + 2$

$8x = 16$

$\frac{8x}{8} = \frac{16}{8}$

$x = 2$

The solution is 2.

**61.** $-3 + 4(x + 3) = 5$

$-3 + 4x + 12 = 5$

$4x + 9 = 5$

$4x + 9 - 9 = 5 - 9$

$4x = -4$

$\frac{4x}{4} = \frac{-4}{4}$

$x = -1$

The solution is $-1$.

**63.** $6 - 2(d + 4) = 6$

$6 - 2d - 8 = 6$

$-2d - 2 = 6$

$-2d - 2 + 2 = 6 + 2$

$-2d = 8$

$\frac{-2d}{-2} = \frac{8}{-2}$

$d = -4$

The solution is $-4$.

**65.** $5 + 7(x + 3) = 20$

$5 + 7x + 21 = 20$

$7x + 26 = 20$

$7x + 26 - 26 = 20 - 26$

$7x = -6$

$\frac{7x}{7} = \frac{-6}{7}$

$x = -\frac{6}{7}$

The solution is $-\frac{6}{7}$.

**67.** $2x + 3(x - 5) = 10$

$2x + 3x - 15 = 10$

$5x - 15 = 10$

$5x - 15 + 15 = 10 + 15$

$5x = 25$

$\frac{5x}{5} = \frac{25}{5}$

$x = 5$

The solution is 5.

**69.** $3(x - 4) + 2x = 3$

$3x - 12 + 2x = 3$

$5x - 12 = 3$

$5x - 12 + 12 = 3 + 12$

$5x = 15$

$\frac{5x}{5} = \frac{15}{5}$

$x = 3$

The solution is 3.

**71.** $2x - 3(x - 4) = 12$

$2x - 3x + 12 = 12$

$-x + 12 = 12$

$-x + 12 - 12 = 12 - 12$

$-x = 0$

$(-1)(-x) = (-1)0$

$x = 0$

The solution is 0.

**73.** $2x + 3(x + 4) = 7$

$2x + 3x + 12 = 7$

$5x + 12 = 7$

$5x + 12 - 12 = 7 - 12$

$5x = -5$

$\frac{5x}{5} = \frac{-5}{5}$

$x = -1$

The solution is $-1$.

© 2013 Cengage Learning. All Rights Reserved. May not be scanned, copied or duplicated, or posted to a publicly accessible website, in whole or in part.

**75.** $3(x-2)+5=5$

$$3x-6+5=5$$
$$3x-1=5$$
$$3x-1+1=5+1$$
$$3x=6$$
$$\frac{3x}{3}=\frac{6}{3}$$
$$x=2$$

The solution is 2.

**77.** $3y+7(y-2)=5$

$$3y+7y-14=5$$
$$10y-14=5$$
$$10y-14+14=5+14$$
$$10y=19$$
$$\frac{10y}{10}=\frac{19}{10}$$
$$y=1\frac{9}{10}$$

The solution is $1\frac{9}{10}$.

**79.** $4b-2(b+9)=8$

$$4b-2b-18=8$$
$$2b-18=8$$
$$2b-18+18=8+18$$
$$2b=26$$
$$\frac{2b}{2}=\frac{26}{2}$$
$$b=13$$

The solution is 13.

**81.** $3x+5(x-2)=10$

$$3x+5x-10=10$$
$$8x-10=10$$
$$8x-10+10=10+10$$
$$8x=20$$
$$\frac{8x}{8}=\frac{20}{8}$$
$$x=\frac{5}{2}=2\frac{1}{2}$$

The solution is $2\frac{1}{2}$.

**83.** $3x+4(x+2)=2(x+9)$

$$3x+4x+8=2x+18$$
$$7x+8=2x+18$$
$$7x-2x+8=2x-2x+18$$
$$5x+8=18$$
$$5x+8-8=18-8$$
$$5x=10$$
$$\frac{5x}{10}=\frac{10}{5}$$
$$x=2$$

The solution is 2.

**85.** $2d-3(d-4)=2(d+6)$

$$2d-3d+12=2d+12$$
$$-d+12=2d+12$$
$$-d-2d+12=2d-2d+12$$
$$-3d+12=12$$
$$-3d+12-12=12-12$$
$$-3d=0$$
$$\frac{-3d}{-3}=\frac{0}{-3}$$
$$d=0$$

The solution is 0.

**87.** $7-2(x-3)=3(x-1)$

$$7-2x+6=3x-3$$
$$-2x+13=3x-3$$
$$-2x-3x+13=3x-3x-3$$
$$-5x+13=-3$$

© 2013 Cengage Learning. All Rights Reserved. May not be scanned, copied or duplicated, or posted to a publicly accessible website, in whole or in part.

$$-5x+13-13=-3-13$$

$$-5x=-16$$

$$\frac{-5x}{-5}=\frac{-16}{-5}$$

$$x=3\frac{1}{5}$$

The solution is $3\frac{1}{5}$.

**89.** $6x-2(x-3)=11(x-2)$

$$6x-2x+6=11x-22$$

$$4x+6=11x-22$$

$$4x-11x+6=11x-11x-22$$

$$-7x+6=-22$$

$$-7x+6-6=-22-6$$

$$-7x=-28$$

$$\frac{-7x}{-7}=\frac{-28}{-7}$$

$$x=4$$

The solution is 4.

**91.** $6c-3(c+1)=5(c+2)$

$$6c-3c-3=5c+10$$

$$3c-3=5c+10$$

$$3c-5c-3=5c-5c+10$$

$$-2c-3=10$$

$$-2c-3+3=10+3$$

$$-2c=13$$

$$\frac{-2c}{-2}=\frac{13}{-2}$$

$$c=-6\frac{1}{2}$$

The solution is $-6\frac{1}{2}$.

**93.** $7-(x+1)=3(x+3)$

$$7-x-1=3x+9$$

$$-x+6=3x+9$$

$$-x-3x+6=3x-3x+9$$

$$-4x+6=9$$

$$-4x+6-6=9-6$$

$$-4x=3$$

$$\frac{-4x}{-4}=\frac{3}{-4}$$

$$x=-\frac{3}{4}$$

The solution is $-\frac{3}{4}$.

**95.** $2x-3(x+4)=2(x-5)$

$$2x-3x-12=2x-10$$

$$-x-12=2x-10$$

$$-x-2x-12=2x-2x-10$$

$$-3x-12=-10$$

$$-3x-12+12=-10+12$$

$$-3x=2$$

$$\frac{-3x}{-3}=\frac{2}{-3}$$

$$x=-\frac{2}{3}$$

The solution is $-\frac{2}{3}$.

**97.** $x+5(x-4)=3(x-8)-5$

$$x+5x-20=3x-24-5$$

$$6x-20=3x-29$$

$$6x-3x-20=3x-3x-29$$

© 2013 Cengage Learning. All Rights Reserved. May not be scanned, copied or duplicated, or posted to a publicly accessible website, in whole or in part.

$$3x - 20 = -29$$
$$3x - 20 + 20 = -29 + 20$$
$$3x = -9$$
$$\frac{3x}{3} = \frac{-9}{3}$$
$$x = -3$$

The solution is $-3$.

**99.** $9b - 3(b - 4) = 13 + 2(b - 3)$

$$9b - 3b + 12 = 13 + 2b - 6$$
$$6b + 12 = 2b + 7$$
$$6b - 2b + 12 = 2b - 2b + 7$$
$$4b + 12 = 7$$
$$4b + 12 - 12 = 7 - 12$$
$$4b = -5$$
$$\frac{4b}{4} = \frac{-5}{4}$$
$$b = -1\frac{1}{4}$$

The solution is $-1\frac{1}{4}$.

**101.** $3(x - 4) + 3x = 7 - 2(x - 1)$

$$3x - 12 + 3x = 7 - 2x + 2$$
$$6x - 12 = -2x + 9$$
$$6x + 2x - 12 = -2x + 2x + 9$$
$$8x - 12 = 9$$
$$8x - 12 + 12 = 9 + 12$$
$$8x = 21$$
$$\frac{8x}{8} = \frac{21}{8}$$
$$x = 2\frac{5}{8}$$

The solution is $2\frac{5}{8}$.

**103.**
$$3.67x - 5.3(x - 1.932) = 6.99$$
$$3.67x - 5.3x + 10.2396 = 6.99$$
$$-1.63x + 10.2396 = 6.99$$
$$-1.63x + 10.2396 - 10.2396 = 6.99 - 10.2396$$
$$-1.63x = -3.2496$$
$$\frac{-1.63x}{-1.63} = \frac{-3.2496}{-1.63}$$
$$x \approx 1.9936196$$

The solution is 1.99.

## Applying the Concepts

**105.**
$$2x - 2 = 4x + 6$$
$$2x - 4x - 2 = 4x - 4x + 6$$
$$-2x - 2 = 6$$
$$-2x - 2 + 2 = 6 + 2$$
$$-2x = 8$$
$$x = -4$$

Then $3x^2 = 3(-4)^2 = 48$.

**107.** Many beginning algebra students do not differentiate between an equation that has no solution and an equation whose solution is zero. Students should explain that zero is a (real) number and that the solution of the equation $2x + 3 = 3$ is the (real) number zero. However, there is no solution to the equation $x = x + 1$ because there is no (real) number that is equal to itself plus 1.

© 2013 Cengage Learning. All Rights Reserved. May not be scanned, copied or duplicated, or posted to a publicly accessible website, in whole or in part.

## Section 11.5

### Objective A Exercises

**1.** $y - 9$

**3.** $z + 3$

**5.** $\frac{2}{3}n + n$

**7.** $\frac{m}{m-3}$

**9.** $9(x + 4)$

**11.** $x - \frac{x}{2}$

**13.** $\frac{z-3}{z}$

**15.** $2(t + 6)$

**17.** $\frac{x}{9+x}$

**19.** $3(b + 6)$

**21a.** 3 more than twice $x$

**b.** Twice the sum of $x$ and 3

**22a.** The quotient of twice $x$ and 7

**b.** The quotient of 2 plus $x$ and 7

### Objective B Exercises

**23.** The *square* of a number

The unknown number: $x$

$x^2$

**25.** A number *divided* by twenty

The unknown number: $x$

$\frac{x}{20}$

**27.** Four *times* some number

The unknown number: $x$

$4x$

**29.** Three-fourths *of* a number

The unknown number: $x$

$\frac{3}{4}x$

**31.** Four *increased* by some number

The unknown number: $x$

$4 + x$

**33.** The *difference between* five *times* a number and the number

The unknown number: $x$

Five times the number: $5x$

$5x - x$

**35.** The *product* of a number and two *more than* the number

The unknown number: $x$

Two more than the number: $x + 2$

$x(x + 2)$

**37.** Seven *times* the *total* of a number and eight

The unknown number: $x$

The total of the number and eight: $x + 8$

$7(x + 8)$

**39.** The *square* of a number *plus* the *product* of three and the number

The unknown number: $x$

The square of the number: $x^2$

The product of three and the number: $3x$

$x^2 + 3x$

© 2013 Cengage Learning. All Rights Reserved. May not be scanned, copied or duplicated, or posted to a publicly accessible website, in whole or in part.

**41.** The *sum* of three *more than* a number and *one-half* of the number

The unknown number: $x$

Three more than the number: $x + 3$

One-half of the number: $\frac{1}{2}x$

$(x+3)+\frac{1}{2}x$

**43.** No

## Applying the Concepts

**45.** Students will provide different explanations of how variables are used. Look for the idea that a variable is used to represent a number that is unknown or a number that can change, or vary.

**47.** $\frac{1}{2}x$ : number of carbon atoms

$\frac{1}{2}x$ : number of oxygen atoms

# Section 11.6

## Objective A Exercises

**1.** The unknown number: $x$

$$\begin{aligned} x+7&=12 \\ x+7-7&=12-7 \\ x&=5 \end{aligned}$$

The number is 5.

**3.** The unknown number: $x$

$$\begin{aligned} 3x&=18 \\ \frac{3x}{3}&=\frac{18}{3} \\ x&=6 \end{aligned}$$

The number is 6.

**5.** The unknown number: $x$

$$\begin{aligned} x+5&=3 \\ x+5-5&=3-5 \\ x&=-2 \end{aligned}$$

The number is –2.

**7.** The unknown number: $x$

$$\begin{aligned} 6x&=14 \\ \frac{6x}{6}&=\frac{14}{6} \\ x&=\frac{7}{3}=2\frac{1}{3} \end{aligned}$$

The number is $2\frac{1}{3}$.

**9.** The unknown number: $x$

$$\begin{aligned} \frac{5}{6}x&=15 \\ \frac{6}{5}\cdot\frac{5}{6}x&=\frac{6}{5}\cdot 15 \\ x&=18 \end{aligned}$$

The number is 18.

**11.** The unknown number: $x$

$$\begin{aligned} 3x+4&=8 \\ 3x+4-4&=8-4 \\ 3x&=4 \\ \frac{3x}{3}&=\frac{4}{3} \\ x&=\frac{4}{3}=1\frac{1}{3} \end{aligned}$$

The number is $1\frac{1}{3}$.

© 2013 Cengage Learning. All Rights Reserved. May not be scanned, copied or duplicated, or posted to a publicly accessible website, in whole or in part.

**13.** The unknown number: $x$

$$\begin{aligned} \frac{1}{4}x - 7 &= 9 \\ \frac{1}{4}x - 7 + 7 &= 9 + 7 \\ \frac{1}{4}x &= 16 \\ 4 \cdot \frac{1}{4}x &= 4 \cdot 16 \\ x &= 64 \end{aligned}$$

The number is 64.

**15.** The unknown number: $x$

$$\begin{aligned} \frac{x}{9} &= 14 \\ 9 \cdot \frac{x}{9} &= 9 \cdot 14 \\ x &= 126 \end{aligned}$$

The number is 126.

**17.** The unknown number: $x$

$$\begin{aligned} \frac{x}{4} - 6 &= -2 \\ \frac{x}{4} - 6 + 6 &= -2 + 6 \\ \frac{x}{4} &= 4 \\ 4 \cdot \frac{x}{4} &= 4 \cdot 4 \\ x &= 16 \end{aligned}$$

The number is 16.

**19.** The unknown number: $x$

$$\begin{aligned} 7 - 2x &= 13 \\ 7 - 7 - 2x &= 13 - 7 \\ -2x &= 6 \\ \frac{-2x}{-2} &= \frac{6}{-2} \\ x &= -3 \end{aligned}$$

The number is –3.

**21.** The unknown number: $x$

$$\begin{aligned} 9 - \frac{x}{2} &= 5 \\ 9 - 9 - \frac{x}{2} &= 5 - 9 \\ -\frac{x}{2} &= -4 \\ (-2)\left(-\frac{x}{2}\right) &= (-2)(-4) \\ x &= 8 \end{aligned}$$

The number is 8.

**23.** The unknown number: $x$

$$\begin{aligned} \frac{3}{5}x + 8 &= 2 \\ \frac{3}{5}x + 8 - 8 &= 2 - 8 \\ \frac{3}{5}x &= -6 \\ \frac{5}{3} \cdot \frac{3}{5}x &= \frac{5}{3} \cdot (-6) \\ x &= -10 \end{aligned}$$

The number is –10.

**25.** The unknown number: $x$

$$\begin{aligned} \frac{x}{4.18} - 7.92 &= 12.52 \\ \frac{x}{4.18} - 7.92 + 7.92 &= 12.52 + 7.92 \\ \frac{x}{4.18} &= 20.44 \\ 4.18 \cdot \frac{x}{4.18} &= 4.18(20.44) \\ x &= 85.4392 \end{aligned}$$

The number is 85.4392.

© 2013 Cengage Learning. All Rights Reserved. May not be scanned, copied or duplicated, or posted to a publicly accessible website, in whole or in part.

**27.** No

## Objective B Exercises

**29.** The amount the of the certified pharmacy technician's annual salary.

**31.** **Strategy** To find the annual salary, write and solve and equation using $C$ to represent the annual salary of a certified pharmacy technician.

**Solution**

| | | |
|---|---|---|
| \$33,475 | is | \$4260 million more than the salary of a certified pharmacy technician. |

$$33{,}475 = 4260 + C$$
$$33{,}475 - 4260 = 4260 - 4260 + C$$
$$29{,}215 = C$$

The certified pharmacy technician makes \$29,215 a year.

$$230{,}200 = M - 6300$$
$$230{,}200 + 6300 = M - 6300 + 6300$$
$$236{,}500 = M$$

The median price of a house in 2010was \$236,500.

**33.** **Strategy** To find Ethan's height, write and solve an equation using $L$ to represent Ethan's height.

**Solution**

| | | |
|---|---|---|
| 38 in. | is | 3.5 in. taller than Ethan. |

$$38 = L + 3.5$$
$$38 - 3.5 = L + 3.5 - 3.5$$
$$34.5 = L$$

Ethan is 34.5 in. tall.

**35.** **Strategy** To current, write and solve an equation using $W$ as the current weight.

**Solution**

| | | |
|---|---|---|
| 162 | is | $\frac{2}{3}$ of his current weight. |

$$162 = \frac{2}{3}W$$
$$\frac{3}{2} \cdot 162 = \frac{3}{2} \cdot \frac{2}{3}W$$
$$243 = W$$

The current weight is 243 lb.

© 2013 Cengage Learning. All Rights Reserved. May not be scanned, copied or duplicated, or posted to a publicly accessible website, in whole or in part.

**37. Strategy** To find the number of hours, write and solve an equation using $h$ to represent the number of hours infants sleep each day.

**Solution**

| 9.5 h | is | three-fourths the number of hours infants sleep. |
|---|---|---|

$$9.5 = \frac{3}{4}h$$
$$\frac{4}{3}\cdot 9.5 = \frac{4}{3}\cdot\frac{3}{4}h$$
$$12.7 \approx h$$

Infants aged 3 months to 11 months sleep an average of 12.7 h each day.

$$1360 = \frac{1}{4}S$$
$$4\cdot 1360 = 4\cdot\frac{1}{4}S$$
$$5440 = S$$

The family's monthly income is \$5440.

**39. Strategy** To find the cost of the calculator 5 years ago, write and solve an equation using $C$ to represent the cost 5 years ago.

**Solution**

| \$72 | is | three-fourths of the cost 5 years ago. |
|---|---|---|

$$72 = \frac{3}{4}C$$
$$\frac{4}{3}\cdot 72 = \frac{4}{3}\cdot\frac{3}{4}C$$
$$96 = C$$

The cost of the calculator 5 years ago was \$96.

**41. Strategy** To find the recommended daily allowance of sodium:

- Write and solve an equation using $x$ to represent the daily allowance of sodium.
- Convert the milligrams to grams.

**Solution**

| 8% of the daily recommended allowance | is | 200 mg. |
|---|---|---|

$$8\%\cdot x = 200$$
$$0.08x = 200$$
$$\frac{0.08x}{0.08} = \frac{200}{0.08}$$
$$x = 2{,}500$$

2,500 mg = 2.5g

The recommended daily allowance of sodium is 2.5 g.

© 2013 Cengage Learning. All Rights Reserved. May not be scanned, copied or duplicated, or posted to a publicly accessible website, in whole or in part.

**43. Strategy** To find the number of hot dogs, write and solve an equation using $x$ to represent the number of hot dogs Americans consume annually.

**Solution**

| 7 billion | is | 35% of the number consumed annually. |
|---|---|---|

$$7 = 35\% \cdot x$$
$$7 = 0.35x$$
$$\frac{7}{0.35} = \frac{0.35}{0.35}x$$
$$20 = x$$

Americans consume 20 billion hot dogs annually.

**45. Strategy** To find the number of emergency room visits, write and solve an equation using $E$ to represent the number emergency room visits.

**Solution**

| 42.4 million | represents | 34.3% of all emergency room visits in the U.S. |
|---|---|---|

$$42,400,000 = 34.3\% \times E$$
$$42,400,000 = 0.343E$$
$$\frac{42,400,000}{0.343} = \frac{0.343E}{0.343}$$
$$123,600,000 \approx E$$

There were 123,600,000 emergency room visits.

Percent × base = amount

$$P \times 295 = 9.8$$
$$295P = 9.8$$
$$\frac{295P}{295} = \frac{9.8}{295}$$
$$P \approx 0.0332$$

The percent is 3.3%.

**47. Strategy** To find the height, write and solve an equation using $H$ to represent the height over 5 ft.

**Solution**

| 73 | is | The sum of 50 and 2.3 kg per inch over 5 ft. |
|---|---|---|

$$73 = 50 + 2.3H$$
$$73 - 50 = 50 - 50 + 2.3H$$
$$23 = 2.3H$$
$$\frac{23}{2.3} = \frac{23H}{2.3}$$
$$10 = H$$

The height is 10 in. over 5 ft.

The height is 5 ft 10 in.

© 2013 Cengage Learning. All Rights Reserved. May not be scanned, copied or duplicated, or posted to a publicly accessible website, in whole or in part.

**49. Strategy** To find the number of vacation days, write and solve an equation using $d$ to represent the number of vacation days U.S. workers take per year.

**Solution**

| 42 days | is | 3 more than three times the number of vacation days taken by U.S. workers. |
|---|---|---|

$$42 = 3d + 3$$
$$42 - 3 = 3d + 3 - 3$$
$$39 = 3d$$
$$\frac{39}{3} = \frac{3d}{3}$$
$$13 = d$$

U.S. workers take an average of 13 days of vacation each year.

$$417 = 8w + 25$$
$$417 - 25 = 8w + 25 - 25$$
$$392 = 8w$$
$$\frac{392}{8} = \frac{8w}{8}$$
$$49 = w$$

49 women have flown into space.

**51. Strategy** To find the total sales for the month, write and solve an equation using $T$ to represent the total sales.

**Solution**

| The base monthly salary of \$600 plus an 8.25% commission on total sales | is | \$4109.55. |
|---|---|---|

$$600 + 0.0825T = 4109.55$$
$$600 - 600 + 0.0825T = 4109.55 - 600$$
$$0.0825T = 3509.55$$
$$\frac{0.0825T}{0.0825} = \frac{3509.55}{0.0825}$$
$$T = 42,540$$

The total sales for the month were \$42,540.

© 2013 Cengage Learning. All Rights Reserved. May not be scanned, copied or duplicated, or posted to a publicly accessible website, in whole or in part.

# Chapter 11 Concept Review

**1.** To evaluate a variable expression, replace the variable or variables with numbers and then simplify the resulting numerical expression.

**2.** To add like terms, add the numerical coefficients. The variable part stays the same. For example, $6x + 7x = 13x$.

**3.** To simplify a variable expression containing parentheses, use the Distributive Property to remove the parentheses from the variable expression. Then combine like terms.

**4.** A solution of an equation is a number that, when substituted for the variable, results in a true equation. 6 is a solution is $x + 3 = 9$ because 6 + 3 = 9.

**5.** To check the solution to an equation, substitute the solution into the original equation. Evaluate the resulting numerical expressions. Compare the results. If the results are the same, the given umber is a solution. If the results are not the same, the given number is not a solution.

**6.** The Multiplication Property of Equations states that both sides of an equation can be multiplied by the same nonzero number without changing the solution of the equation.

**7.** The Addition Property of Equations states that the same number or variable expression can be added to each side of an equation without changing the solution of the equation.

**8.** To solve the equation $5x - 4 = 26$, apply both the Addition Property of Equations and the Multiplication Property of Equations.

**9.** After you substitute a number or numbers into a formula, solve the formula by using the Distributive Property if there are parentheses to remove. Then use the Addition and Multiplication Properties of Equations to rewrite the equation in the form *variable = constant* or *constant = variable.*

**10.** To isolate the variable in the equation $5x - 3 = 10 - 8x$, first add $8x$ to each side of the equation so that there is only one variable term. The result is $13x - 3 = 10$. Then add 3 to both sides of the equation so that there is only one constant term. The result is $13x = 13$. Next divide each side of the equation by the coefficient of $x$, 13. The result is $x$ = 1. The variable is alone on the left side of the equation. The constant on the right side of the equation is the solution. The solution is 1.

**11.** Some mathematical terms that translate into addition are *more than, the sum of, the total of,* and *increased by.*

**12.** Some mathematical terms that translate into "equals" are *is, is equal to, amounts to,* and *represents.*

© 2013 Cengage Learning. All Rights Reserved. May not be scanned, copied or duplicated, or posted to a publicly accessible website, in whole or in part.

## Chapter 11 Review Exercises

**1.** $-2(a-b) = -2[a+(-b)]$

$= -2(a) + (-2)(-b)$

$= -2a + 2b$

**2.** $3x - 2 = -8$

| $3(-2) - 2$ | $-8$ |
|---|---|
| $-6 - 2$ | $-8$ |
| $-6 + (-2)$ | $-8$ |

$-8 = -8$

Yes, –2 is a solution.

**3.**
$$\begin{aligned} x - 3 &= -7 \\ x - 3 + 3 &= -7 + 3 \\ x &= -4 \end{aligned}$$

The solution is $-4$.

**4.**
$$\begin{aligned} -2x + 5 &= -9 \\ -2x + 5 - 5 &= -9 - 5 \\ -2x &= -14 \\ \frac{-2x}{-2} &= \frac{-14}{-2} \\ x &= 7 \end{aligned}$$

The solution is 7.

**5.** $a^2 - 3b = 2^2 - 3(-3)$

$= 4 + 9 = 13$

**6.**
$$\begin{aligned} -3x &= 27 \\ \frac{-3x}{-3} &= \frac{27}{-3} \\ x &= -9 \end{aligned}$$

The solution is $-9$.

**7.**
$$\begin{aligned} \frac{2}{3}x + 3 &= -9 \\ \frac{2}{3}x + 3 - 3 &= -9 - 3 \\ \frac{2}{3}x &= -12 \\ \frac{3}{2} \cdot \frac{2}{3}x &= \frac{3}{2}(-12) \\ x &= -18 \end{aligned}$$

The solution is $-18$.

**8.** $3x - 2(3x-2) = 3x + (-2)[3x + (-2)]$

$= 3x + (-2)(3x) + (-2)(-2)$

$= 3x + (-6x) + 4$

$= -3x + 4$

**9.**
$$\begin{aligned} 6x - 9 &= -3x + 36 \\ 6x + 3x - 9 &= -3x + 3x + 36 \\ 9x - 9 &= 36 \\ 9x - 9 + 9 &= 36 + 9 \\ 9x &= 45 \\ \frac{9x}{9} &= \frac{45}{9} \\ x &= 5 \end{aligned}$$

The solution is 5.

**10.**
$$\begin{aligned} x + 3 &= -2 \\ x + 3 - 3 &= -2 - 3 \\ x &= -5 \end{aligned}$$

The solution is $-5$.

**11.** $3x - 5 = -10$

| $3(5) - 5$ | $-10$ |
|---|---|
| $15 - 5$ | $-10$ |
| $15 + (-5)$ | $-10$ |

$10 \neq -10$

No, 5 is not a solution.

**12.** $a^2 - (b \div c) = (-2)^2 - [8 \div (-4)]$

$= 4 - (-2) = 6$

**13.**
$$\begin{aligned} 3(x-2) + 2 &= 11 \\ 3x - 6 + 2 &= 11 \\ 3x - 4 &= 11 \\ 3x - 4 + 4 &= 11 + 4 \\ 3x &= 15 \\ \frac{3x}{3} &= \frac{15}{3} \\ x &= 5 \end{aligned}$$

The solution is 5.

© 2013 Cengage Learning. All Rights Reserved. May not be scanned, copied or duplicated, or posted to a publicly accessible website, in whole or in part.

**14.**
$$\begin{aligned} 35 - 3x &= 5 \\ 35 - 35 - 3x &= 5 - 35 \\ -3x &= -30 \\ \frac{-3x}{-3} &= \frac{-30}{-3} \\ x &= 10 \end{aligned}$$

The solution is 10.

**15.** $6bc - 7bc + 2bc - 5bc$
$$\begin{aligned} &= 6bc + (-7)bc + 2bc + (-5)bc \\ &= (-1)bc + 2bc + (-5)bc \\ &= 1bc + (-5)bc \\ &= -4bc \end{aligned}$$

**16.**
$$\begin{aligned} 7 - 3x &= 2 - 5x \\ 7 - 3x + 5x &= 2 - 5x + 5x \\ 7 + 2x &= 2 \\ 7 - 7 + 2x &= 2 - 7 \\ 2x &= -5 \\ \frac{2x}{2} &= \frac{-5}{2} \\ x &= \frac{-5}{2} = -2\frac{1}{2} \end{aligned}$$

The solution is $-2\frac{1}{2}$.

**17.**
$$\begin{aligned} -\frac{3}{8}x &= -\frac{15}{32} \\ -\frac{8}{3}\left(-\frac{3}{8}x\right) &= \left(-\frac{8}{3}\right)\left(-\frac{15}{32}\right) \\ x &= \frac{5}{4} = 1\frac{1}{4} \end{aligned}$$

The solution is $1\frac{1}{4}$.

**18.** $\frac{1}{2}x^2 - \frac{1}{3}x^2 + \frac{1}{5}x^2 + 2x^2$
$$\begin{aligned} &= \frac{1}{2}x^2 + \left(-\frac{1}{3}\right)x^2 + \frac{1}{5}x2 + 2x^2 \\ &= \frac{3}{6}x^2 + \left(-\frac{2}{6}\right)x^2 + \frac{1}{5}x^2 + 2x^2 \\ &= \frac{1}{6}x^2 + \frac{1}{5}x^2 + 2x^2 \\ &= \frac{5}{30}x^2 + \frac{6}{30}x^2 + 2x^2 \\ &= \frac{11}{30}x^2 + 2x^2 \\ &= \frac{11}{30}x^2 + \frac{60}{30}x^2 \\ &= \frac{71}{30}x^2 \end{aligned}$$

**19.** $5x - 3(1 - 2x) = 4(2x - 1)$
$$\begin{aligned} 5x - 3 + 6x &= 8x - 4 \\ 11x - 3 &= 8x - 4 \\ 11x - 8x - 3 &= 8x - 8x - 4 \\ 3x - 3 &= -4 \\ 3x - 3 + 3 &= -4 + 3 \\ 3x &= -1 \\ \frac{3x}{3} &= \frac{-1}{3} \\ x &= -\frac{1}{3} \end{aligned}$$

The solution is $-\frac{1}{3}$.

**20.**
$$\begin{aligned} \frac{5}{6}x - 4 &= 5 \\ \frac{5}{6}x - 4 + 4 &= 5 + 4 \\ \frac{5}{6}x &= 9 \\ \frac{6}{5}\cdot\frac{5}{6}x &= \frac{6}{5}\cdot 9 \\ x &= \frac{54}{5} = 10\frac{4}{5} \end{aligned}$$

The solution is $10\frac{4}{5}$.

© 2013 Cengage Learning. All Rights Reserved. May not be scanned, copied or duplicated, or posted to a publicly accessible website, in whole or in part.

**21. Strategy** To find the cost, replace $S$ and $R$ formula by the given values and solve for $C$.

**Solution**

$$\begin{aligned} S &= C + R \cdot C \\ 28.62 &= C + 35\%C \\ 28.62 &= C + 0.35C \\ 28.62 &= 1.35C \\ \frac{28.62}{1.35} &= \frac{1.35C}{1.35} \\ 21.20 &= C \end{aligned}$$

The cost was \$21.20.

**22. Strategy** To find the Celsius temperature, replace the variable $F$ in the formula by the given value and solve for $C$.

**Solution**

$$\begin{aligned} F &= 1.8C + 32 \\ 100 &= 1.8C + 32 \\ 100 - 32 &= 1.8C + 32 - 32 \\ 68 &= 1.8C \\ 37.8 &\approx C \end{aligned}$$

The temperature is 37.8°C.

**23.** The *total* of $n$ and the *quotient* of $n$ and 5

The unknown number: $n$

The quotient of $n$ and 5: $\frac{n}{5}$

$n + \frac{n}{5}$

**24.** The *sum* of five more than a number and one-third *of* the number

The unknown number: $n$

Five more than the number: $n + 5$

One-third of the number: $\frac{1}{3}n$

$(n + 5) + \frac{1}{3}n$

**25.** The unknown number: $x$

$$\begin{aligned} 9 - 2x &= 5 \\ 9 - 9 - 2x &= 5 - 9 \\ -2x &= -4 \\ \frac{-2x}{-2} &= \frac{-4}{-2} \\ x &= 2 \end{aligned}$$

The number is 2.

**26.** The unknown number: $p$

$$\begin{aligned} 5p &= 50 \\ \frac{5p}{5} &= \frac{50}{5} \\ p &= 10 \end{aligned}$$

The number is 10.

**27. Strategy** To find the regular price, write and solve an equation using $R$ to represent the regular price.

**Solution**

| \$1276 | is | 80% of the regular price. |
|---|---|---|

$$\begin{aligned} 1276 &= 80\% \cdot R \\ 1276 &= 0.80R \\ \frac{1276}{0.80} &= \frac{0.80R}{0.80} \\ 1595 &= R \end{aligned}$$

The regular price of the defibrillator is \$1595.

**28. Strategy** Let $x$ represent the weight prior to the loss. Then $0.15x$ is the decrease weight. Previous weight less $0.15x$ is 187.

© 2013 Cengage Learning. All Rights Reserved. May not be scanned, copied or duplicated, or posted to a publicly accessible website, in whole or in part.

**Solution**

| 187 | is | weight less 15% of weight. |
|---|---|---|

$$187 = x - 0.15x$$
$$187 = 0.85x$$
$$\frac{187}{0.85} = \frac{0.85x}{0.85}$$
$$220 = x$$

The patient's weight was 220 lb prior to the weight loss.

## Chapter 11 Test

**1.**
$$\frac{x}{5} - 12 = 7$$
$$\frac{x}{5} - 12 + 12 = 7 + 12$$
$$\frac{x}{5} = 19$$
$$5 \cdot \frac{x}{5} = 5 \cdot 19$$
$$x = 95$$

The solution is 95.

**2.**
$$x - 12 = 14$$
$$x - 12 + 12 = 14 + 12$$
$$x = 26$$

The solution is 26.

**3.**
$$\begin{aligned} 3y - 2x - 7y - 9x &= 3y + (-2x) + (-7y) + (-9x) \\ &= 3y + (-7y) + (-2x) + (-9x) \\ &= -4y + (-2x) + (-9x) \\ &= -4y + (-11x) \\ &= -4y - 11x = -11x - 4y \end{aligned}$$

**4.**
$$8 - 3x = 2x - 8$$
$$8 - 3x - 2x = 2x - 2x - 8$$
$$8 - 5x = -8$$
$$8 - 8 - 5x = -8 - 8$$
$$-5x = -16$$
$$\frac{-5x}{5} = \frac{-16}{-5}$$
$$x = \frac{16}{5} = 3\frac{1}{5}$$

The solution is $3\frac{1}{5}$.

**5.**
$$3x - 12 = -18$$
$$3x - 12 + 12 = -18 + 12$$
$$3x = -6$$
$$\frac{3x}{3} = \frac{-6}{3}$$
$$x = -2$$

The solution is $-2$.

**6.**
$$\begin{aligned} c^2 - (2a + b^2) &= (-2)^2 - \left[2(3) + (-6)^2\right] \\ &= 4 - (6 + 36) \\ &= 4 - (42) \\ &= 4 + (-42) = -38 \end{aligned}$$

**7.**

| $x^2 + 3x - 7$ | $= 3x - 2$ |
|---|---|
| $3^2 + 3(3) - 7$ | $3(3) - 2$ |
| $9 + 9 - 7$ | $9 - 2$ |
| $18 - 7$ | $7$ |

$$11 \neq 7$$

No, 3 is not a solution.

© 2013 Cengage Learning. All Rights Reserved. May not be scanned, copied or duplicated, or posted to a publicly accessible website, in whole or in part.

**8.** $9 - 8ab - 6ab = 9 - 14ab = -14ab + 9$

**9.** 
$$\begin{aligned} -5x &= 14 \\ \frac{-5x}{-5} &= \frac{14}{-5} \\ x &= -2\frac{4}{5} \end{aligned}$$

The solution is $-2\frac{4}{5}$.

**10.** 
$$\begin{aligned} 3y + 5(y-3) + 8 &= 3y + 5[y + (-3)] + 8 \\ &= 3y + 5y + 5(-3) + 8 \\ &= 8y + (-15) + 8 \\ &= 8y + (-7) \\ &= 8y - 7 \end{aligned}$$

**11.** 
$$\begin{aligned} 3x - 4(x-2) &= 8 \\ 3x - 4x + 8 &= 8 \\ -x + 8 &= 8 \\ -x + 8 - 8 &= 8 - 8 \\ -x &= 0 \\ (-1)(-x) &= (-1)0 \\ x &= 0 \end{aligned}$$

The solution is 0.

**12.** 
$$\begin{aligned} 5 &= 3 - 4x \\ 5 - 3 &= 3 - 3 - 4x \\ 2 &= -4x \\ \frac{2}{-4} &= \frac{-4x}{-4} \\ -\frac{1}{2} &= x \end{aligned}$$

The solution is $-\frac{1}{2}$.

**13.** 
$$\begin{aligned} \frac{x^2}{y} - \frac{y2}{x} &= \frac{3^2}{-2} - \frac{(-2)^2}{3} \\ &= \frac{9}{-2} - \frac{4}{3} \\ &= \frac{-27}{6} - \frac{8}{6} \\ &= \frac{-35}{6} = -5\frac{5}{6} \end{aligned}$$

**14.** 
$$\begin{aligned} \frac{5}{8}x &= -10 \\ \frac{8}{5} \cdot \frac{5}{8}x &= \frac{8}{5}(-10) \\ x &= -16 \end{aligned}$$

The solution is $-16$.

**15.** 
$$\begin{aligned} y - 4y + 3 &= 12 \\ -3y + 3 &= 12 \\ -3y + 3 - 3 &= 12 - 3 \\ -3y &= 9 \\ \frac{-3y}{-3} &= \frac{9}{-3} \\ y &= -3 \end{aligned}$$

The solution is $-3$.

**16.** 
$$\begin{aligned} 2x + 4(x-3) &= 5x - 1 \\ 2x + 4x - 12 &= 5x - 1 \\ 6x - 12 &= 5x - 1 \\ 6x - 5x - 12 &= 5x - 5x - 1 \\ x - 12 &= -1 \\ x - 12 + 12 &= -1 + 12 \\ x &= 11 \end{aligned}$$

The solution is 11.

**17.** **Strategy** To find the monthly payment, replace the variables $L$ and $N$ in the formula by the given values and solve for $P$.

**Solution**
$$\begin{aligned} L &= P \cdot N \\ 6600 &= P \cdot 48 \\ \frac{6600}{48} &= \frac{48P}{48} \\ 137.50 &= P \end{aligned}$$

The monthly payment is \$137.50.

**18.** **Strategy** To find the height, replace the variables $L$ in the formula by the given value and solve for $H$.

**Solution**
$$\begin{aligned} H &= 1.9L + 32 \\ H &= 1.9 \times 18.9 + 32 \\ H &= 35.91 + 32 \\ H &\approx 67.9 \end{aligned}$$

The man's height was 67.9 in..

© 2013 Cengage Learning. All Rights Reserved. May not be scanned, copied or duplicated, or posted to a publicly accessible website, in whole or in part.

**19. Strategy** To find the time, replace the variables $V$ and $V_0$ in the formula by the given values and solve for $t$.

**Solution**

$$V = V_0 + 32t$$
$$392 = 24 + 32t$$
$$392 - 24 = 24 - 24 + 32t$$
$$368 = 32t$$
$$\frac{368}{32} = \frac{32t}{32}$$
$$11.5 = t$$

The object will fall for 11.5 s.

**20.** The *sum* of $x$ and one-third of $x$

The unknown number: $x$

One-third of $x$: $\frac{1}{3}x$

$x + \frac{1}{3}x$

**21.** Five *times* the *sum* of a number and three

The unknown number: $x$

The sum of a number and three: $x + 3$

$5(x + 3)$

**22.** The unknown number: $x$

$$2x - 3 = 7$$
$$2x - 3 + 3 = 7 + 3$$
$$2x = 10$$
$$\frac{2x}{2} = \frac{10}{2}$$
$$x = 5$$

The number is 5.

**23.** The unknown number: $w$

$$5 + 3w = w - 2$$
$$5 + 3w - w = w - w - 2$$
$$5 + 2w = -2$$
$$5 - 5 + 2w = -2 - 5$$
$$2w = -7$$
$$\frac{2w}{2} = \frac{-7}{2}$$
$$w = -3\frac{1}{2}$$

The number is $-3\frac{1}{2}$.

© 2013 Cengage Learning. All Rights Reserved. May not be scanned, copied or duplicated, or posted to a publicly accessible website, in whole or in part.

**24. Strategy** To find Santos's total sales for the month, write and solve an equation using $T$ to represent the total sales.

**Solution**

| $3600 | is | the sum of a base monthly salary of $1200 and a 6% commission on total sales. |
|---|---|---|

$$3600 = 1200 + 0.06T$$
$$3600 - 1200 = 1200 - 1200 + 0.06T$$
$$2400 = 0.06T$$
$$\frac{2400}{0.06} = \frac{0.06T}{0.06}$$
$$40{,}000 = T$$

Santos's total sales for the month were $40,000.

**25. Strategy** To find the number of in. over 5 feet, write and solve an equation using $h$ to represent the number of in.

**Solution**

| 57 | is | sum of 45.5 and 2.3 kg per inch over 5 ft. |
|---|---|---|

$$57 = 45.5 + 2.3h$$
$$57 - 45.5 = 45.5 - 45.5 + 2.3h$$
$$11.5 = 2.3h$$
$$\frac{11.5}{2.3} = \frac{2.3h}{2.3}$$
$$5 = h$$

The woman is 5 in. over 5 ft.

The woman is 5 ft 5 in.

## Cumulative Review Exercises

**1.** $6^2 - (18 - 6) \div 4 + 8 = 36 - (12) \div 4 + 8$
$= 36 - 3 + 8$
$= 33 + 8 = 41$

**2.**
$$3\frac{1}{6} = 3\frac{5}{30} = 2\frac{35}{30}$$
$$-1\frac{7}{15} = 1\frac{14}{30} = 1\frac{14}{30}$$
$$1\frac{21}{30} = 1\frac{7}{10}$$

**3.** $\left(\frac{3}{8} - \frac{1}{4}\right) \div \frac{3}{4} + \frac{4}{9} = \left(\frac{3}{8} - \frac{2}{8}\right) \div \frac{3}{4} + \frac{4}{9}$
$$= \frac{1}{8} \div \frac{3}{4} + \frac{4}{9}$$
$$= \frac{1}{8} \times \frac{4}{3} + \frac{4}{9}$$
$$= \frac{1}{6} + \frac{4}{9}$$
$$= \frac{3}{18} + \frac{8}{18} = \frac{11}{18}$$

© 2013 Cengage Learning. All Rights Reserved. May not be scanned, copied or duplicated, or posted to a publicly accessible website, in whole or in part.

**4.**
$$\begin{array}{r} 9.67 \\ \times\ 0.0049 \\ \hline 8703 \\ 3868\phantom{0} \\ \hline 0.047383 \end{array}$$

**5.** $\dfrac{\$182}{20\text{h}} = \$9.10/\text{h}$

**6.**
$$\frac{2}{3} = \frac{n}{40}$$
$$2 \times 40 = 3 \cdot n$$
$$80 = 3 \cdot n$$
$$80 \div 3 = n$$
$$26.67 \approx n$$

**7.** $5\frac{1}{3}\% = \frac{16}{3} \times \frac{1}{100} = \frac{16}{300} = \frac{4}{75}$

**8.** Percent × base = amount
$$n \times 30 = 42$$
$$n = 42 \div 30$$
$$n = 1.40 = 140\%$$

**9.** Percent × base = amount
$$125\% \times n = 8$$
$$1.25 \times n = 8$$
$$n = 8 \div 1.25 = 6.4$$

**10.**
$$\begin{array}{r} 3 \text{ ft } 9 \text{ in.} \\ \times \qquad\quad 5 \\ \hline 15 \text{ ft } 45 \text{ in.} \end{array} = 18 \text{ ft } 9 \text{ in.}$$

**11.** $1\frac{3}{8} \text{ lb} = \frac{11}{8} \cancel{\text{lb}} \times \frac{16 \text{ oz}}{1 \cancel{\text{lb}}} = \frac{11 \cdot 16 \text{ oz}}{8} = 22 \text{ oz}$

**12.** 282 mg = 0.282g

**13.** $-2 + 5 + (-8) + 4 = 3 + (-8) + 4$
$$= -5 + 4 = -1$$

**14.** 13 – (–6) = 13 + 6 = 19

**15.** $(-2)^2 - (-8) \div (3-5)^2 = (-2)^2 - (-8) \div (-2)^2$
$$= 4 - (-8) \div 4$$
$$= 4 - (-2) = 4 + 2 = 6$$

**16.** $3ab - 2ac = 3(-2)(6) - 2(-2)(-3)$
$$= -36 - 12 = -36 + (-12) = -48$$

**17.** $3z - 2x + 5z - 8x = 3z + (-2x) + 5z + (-8x)$
$$= 3z + 5z + (-2x) + (-8x)$$
$$= 8z + (-10x)$$
$$= 8z - 10x = -10x + 8z$$

**18.** $6y - 3(y-5) + 8 = 6y + (-3)[y + (-5)] + 8$
$$= 6y + (-3)y + (-3)(-5) + 8$$
$$= 6y + (-3y) + 15 + 8$$
$$-3y + 23$$

**19.**
$$2x - 5 = -7$$
$$2x - 5 + 5 = -7 + 5$$
$$2x = -2$$
$$2x = -2$$
$$\frac{2x}{2} = \frac{-2}{2}$$
$$x = -1$$

The solution is $-1$.

**20.** $7x - 3(x-5) = -10$
$$7x - 3x + 15 = -10$$
$$4x + 15 = -10$$
$$4x + 15 - 15 = -10 - 15$$
$$4x = -25$$
$$\frac{4x}{4} = \frac{-25}{4}$$
$$x = -6\frac{1}{4}$$

The solution is $-6\frac{1}{4}$.

**21.**
$$-\frac{2}{3}x = 5$$
$$\left(-\frac{3}{2}\right)\left(-\frac{2}{3}\right)x = -\frac{3}{2} \cdot 5$$
$$x = -\frac{15}{2} = -7\frac{1}{2}$$

The solution is $-7\frac{1}{2}$.

© 2013 Cengage Learning. All Rights Reserved. May not be scanned, copied or duplicated, or posted to a publicly accessible website, in whole or in part.

**22.** $\frac{x}{3} - 5 = -12$

$$\frac{x}{3} - 5 + 5 = -12 + 5$$

$$\frac{x}{3} = -7$$

$$3 \cdot \frac{x}{3} = 3(-7)$$

$$x = -21$$

The solution is $-21$.

**23. Strategy** To find the percent of the students who received an A grade, solve the basic percent equation for percent.

**Solution** Percent · base = amount

$$n \cdot 34 = 6$$

$$n = 6 \div 34$$

$$n \approx 0.176 = 17.6\%$$

The percent is 17.6%.

**24. Strategy** To find the price:

- Find the amount of the markup by solving the basic percent equation for amount. The base is \$28.50 and the percent is 40%.
- Add the amount of the markup to the cost.

**Solution** $0.40 \times 28.50 = n$

$11.40 = n$

$$\begin{array}{r} 28.50 \\ +11.40 \\ \hline 39.90 \end{array}$$

The price of the hair and skin multinutrient is \$39.90.

**25a. Strategy** To find the discount subtract the sale price (\$369) from the regular price (\$450).

**Solution** 450 – 369 = 81

The discount is \$81.

**b. Strategy** To find the discount rate, write and solve the basic percent equation for percent. The base is the regular price and the amount is the discount.

**Solution** Percent × base = amount

$$n \times 450 = 81$$

$$n = 81 \div 450$$

$$n = 0.18$$

The discount rate is 18%.

**26. Strategy** To find the simple interest due, multiply the principal and rate and time (in years).

**Solution**

$$\text{Interest} = 80{,}000 \times 11\% \times \frac{4}{12}$$

$$= 80{,}000 \times 0.11 \times \frac{4}{12}$$

$$\approx 2933.33$$

The simple interest due on the loan is \$2933.33.

**27. Strategy** To find the amount, write and solve a basic percent equation using $f$ to represent the number of first time donors. The base is 16 million and the percent is 31%.

Percent × base = amount

$$31\% \cdot 16 = f$$

$$0.31 \cdot 16 = f$$

$$4.96 = f$$

There were 4.96 million donors.

**28. Strategy** To calculate the probability:

- Count the number of possible outcomes.
- Count the number of favorable outcomes.
- Use the probability formula.

**Solution** There are 16 possible outcomes. There are 2 favorable outcomes: (3, 4), (4, 3).

© 2013 Cengage Learning. All Rights Reserved. May not be scanned, copied or duplicated, or posted to a publicly accessible website, in whole or in part.

$$\text{Probability} = \frac{2}{16} = \frac{1}{8}$$

The probability is $\frac{1}{8}$ that the sum of the upward faces on the two dice is 7.

**29. Strategy** To find the total sales, replace the variables *M*, *R*, and *B* in the formula with the given values and solve for *S*.

**Solution**

$$\begin{aligned} M &= S \cdot R + B \\ 3400 &= S \cdot 0.08 + 800 \\ 3400 - 800 &= S \cdot 0.08 + 800 - 800 \\ 2600 &= S \cdot 0.08 \\ \frac{2600}{0.08} &= \frac{S \cdot 0.08}{0.08} \\ 32,500 &= S \end{aligned}$$

The total sales were \$32,500.

**30.** The unknown number: $x$

$$\begin{aligned} 8x - 3 &= 3 + 5x \\ 8x - 5x - 3 &= 3 + 5x - 5x \\ 3x - 3 &= 3 \\ 3x - 3 + 3 &= 3 + 3 \\ 3x &= 6 \\ \frac{3x}{3} &= \frac{6}{3} \\ x &= 2 \end{aligned}$$

The number is 2.

© 2013 Cengage Learning. All Rights Reserved. May not be scanned, copied or duplicated, or posted to a publicly accessible website, in whole or in part.

## Final Exam

**1.**
$$\begin{array}{r} \overset{9}{\phantom{0}}\;\;\overset{10}{\phantom{0}} \\ 0\,1\,\not{0}\,10\;\;8\,\not{0}\,14 \\ \not{1}\not{0}\not{0},\not{9}\not{1}\not{4} \\ -97,655 \\ \hline 3\,259 \end{array}$$

**2.**
$$\begin{array}{r} 53 \\ 657\overline{)34,821} \\ -3285 \\ \hline 1971 \\ -1971 \\ \hline 0 \end{array}$$

**3.**
$$\begin{array}{r} \overset{9}{8}\not{10}\;\;\overset{9}{1}\not{0}\overset{9}{1}\not{0}11 \\ \not{9}\not{0},\not{0}\not{0}\not{1} \\ 27,796 \\ \hline 60,205 \end{array}$$

**4.**
$$\begin{aligned} 3^2\cdot(5-3)^2\div 3+4 &= 3^2\cdot(2)^2\div 3+4 \\ &= 9\cdot 4\div 3+4 \\ &= 36\div 3+4 \\ &= 12+4 \\ &= 16 \end{aligned}$$

**5.**

| | 2 | 3 |
|---|---|---|
| 9 = | | (3 · 3) |
| 12 = | 2 · 2 | 3 |
| 16 = | (2 · 2 · 2 · 2) | |

LCM = 2 · 2 · 2 · 2 · 3 · 3 = 144

**6.** $\frac{3}{8}+\frac{5}{6}+\frac{1}{5}=\frac{45}{120}+\frac{100}{120}+\frac{24}{120}=\frac{169}{120}=1\frac{49}{120}$

**7.**
$$\begin{array}{r} 7\frac{5}{12}=7\frac{20}{48}=6\frac{68}{48} \\ -3\frac{13}{16}=3\frac{39}{48}=3\frac{39}{48} \\ \hline 3\frac{29}{48} \end{array}$$

**8.** $3\frac{5}{8}\times 1\frac{5}{7}=\frac{29}{8}\times\frac{12}{7}=\frac{29\cdot \overset{3}{\not{12}}}{\underset{2}{\not{8}}\cdot 7}=\frac{87}{14}=6\frac{3}{14}$

**9.** $1\frac{2}{3}\div 3\frac{3}{4}=\frac{5}{3}\div\frac{15}{4}=\frac{5}{3}\times\frac{4}{15}=\frac{5\times 4}{3\times 15}=\frac{20}{45}=\frac{4}{9}$

**10.**
$$\begin{aligned} \left(\frac{2}{3}\right)^3\left(\frac{3}{4}\right)^2 &= \left(\frac{2}{3}\cdot\frac{2}{3}\cdot\frac{2}{3}\right)\left(\frac{3}{4}\cdot\frac{3}{4}\right)=\left(\frac{8}{27}\right)\left(\frac{9}{16}\right) \\ &= \frac{72}{432}=\frac{1}{6} \end{aligned}$$

**11.**
$$\begin{aligned} \left(\frac{2}{3}\right)^2\div\left(\frac{3}{4}+\frac{1}{3}\right)-\frac{1}{3} &= \left(\frac{2}{3}\right)^2\div\left(\frac{9}{12}+\frac{4}{12}\right)-\frac{1}{3} \\ &= \frac{4}{9}\div\frac{13}{12}-\frac{1}{3} \\ &= \frac{4}{\underset{3}{\not{9}}}\times\frac{\overset{4}{\not{12}}}{13}-\frac{1}{3} \\ &= \frac{16}{39}-\frac{1}{3} \\ &= \frac{16}{39}-\frac{13}{39}=\frac{3}{39}=\frac{1}{13} \end{aligned}$$

**12.**
$$\begin{array}{r} {\scriptstyle 2\;3\;\;1}\phantom{00} \\ 4.972\phantom{0} \\ 28.6\phantom{000} \\ 1.88\phantom{00} \\ +\,128.725 \\ \hline 164.177 \end{array}$$

**13.**
$$\begin{array}{r} 2.97 \\ \times\;0.0094 \\ \hline 1188 \\ 2673\phantom{0} \\ \hline 0.027918 \end{array}$$

**14.**
$$\begin{array}{r} 0.687 \approx 0.69 \\ 0.062.\overline{)0.042.600} \\ -372 \\ \hline 540 \\ -496 \\ \hline 440 \\ -434 \\ \hline 6 \end{array}$$

**15.** $0.45=\frac{45}{100}=\frac{9}{20}$

**16.** $\frac{323.4\text{ mi}}{13.2\text{ gal}}=24.5\text{ mi/gal}$

© 2013 Cengage Learning. All Rights Reserved. May not be scanned, copied or duplicated, or posted to a publicly accessible website, in whole or in part.

**17.** $$\frac{12}{35}=\frac{n}{160}$$
$$12\times 160 = n\times 35$$
$$1920 = n\times 35$$
$$1920\div 35 = n$$
$$54.9\approx n$$

**18.** $22\frac{1}{2}\% = \frac{45}{2}\times\frac{1}{100}=\frac{45}{200}=\frac{9}{40}$

**19.** $1.35 = 1.35\times 100\% = 135\%$

**20.** $\frac{5}{4}=\frac{5}{4}\times 100\% = \frac{500}{4}\% = 125\%$

**21.** Percent × base = amount
$$120\% \times 30 = n$$
$$1.2\times 30 = n$$
$$36 = n$$

**22.** Percent × base = amount
$$n\times 9 = 12$$
$$n = 12\div 9 = 1\frac{1}{3} = 133\frac{1}{3}\%$$

**23.** Percent × base = amount
$$60\% \times n = 42$$
$$0.60\times n = 42$$
$$n = 42\div 0.60 = 70$$

**24.** $1\frac{2}{3}\text{ ft} = \frac{5}{3}\text{ ft} = \frac{5}{3}\,\cancel{\text{ft}}\times\frac{12\text{ in.}}{1\,\cancel{\text{ft}}} = 20\text{ in.}$

**25.**
$$\begin{array}{rl} 3\text{ ft }2\text{ in.} = & 2\text{ ft }14\text{ in.} \\ -1\text{ ft }10\text{ in.} = & 1\text{ ft }10\text{ in.} \\ \hline & 1\text{ ft }\ 4\text{ in.}\end{array}$$

**26.** $40\text{ oz} = 40\,\cancel{\text{oz}}\times\frac{1\text{ lb}}{16\,\cancel{\text{oz}}} = \frac{40}{16}\text{ lb} = 2.5\text{ lb}$

**27.**
$$\begin{array}{r} 3\text{ lb }12\text{ oz} \\ +2\text{ lb }10\text{ oz} \\ \hline 5\text{ lb }22\text{ oz} = 6\text{ lb }6\text{ oz}\end{array}$$

**28.** $18\text{ pt} = 18\,\cancel{\text{pt}}\times\frac{1\,\cancel{\text{qt}}}{2\,\cancel{\text{pt}}}\times\frac{1\text{ gal}}{4\,\cancel{\text{qt}}} = \frac{18\text{ gal}}{8} = 2.25\text{ gal}$

**29.**
$$\begin{array}{r} 1\text{ gal }3\text{ qt} \\ 3\overline{)5\text{ gal }1\text{ qt}} \\ -3\text{ gal} \\ \hline 2\text{ gal} = 8\text{ qt} \\ 9\text{ qt} \\ -9\text{ qt} \\ \hline 0 \end{array}$$

**30.** 2.48 m = 248 cm

**31.** 4 m 62 cm = 4 m+ 0.62 m = 4.62 m

**32.** 1 kg 614 g =1 kg + 0.614 kg = 1.614 kg

**33.** 2 L 67 ml = 2000 ml + 67 ml = 2067 ml

**34.** $55\text{ mi}\approx 55\text{ mi}\times\frac{1.61\text{ km}}{1\text{ mi}}\approx 88.55\text{ km}$

**35.** **Strategy** To find the number of calories from carbohydrates, write and solve a basic percent equation using $C$ to represent the carbohydrates. The base is 1800 and the percent is 55%.

**Solution** Percent × base = amount
$$55\%\times 1800 = C$$
$$0.55\times 1800 = C$$
$$990 = C$$

There should be 990 calories from carbohydrates.

**36.** The number is less than 10. Move the decimal point 8 places to the right. The exponent on 10 is –8.

$0.0000000679 = 6.79\times 10^{-8}$

**37.** **Strategy** To find the dilution rate as a percent, change $\frac{1}{5}$ to a percent.

**Solution** $\frac{1}{5} = 0.20 = 20\%$

The dilution rate is 20%.

© 2013 Cengage Learning. All Rights Reserved. May not be scanned, copied or duplicated, or posted to a publicly accessible website, in whole or in part.

**38. Strategy** To find the original cost, write and solve a basic percent equation using $C$ to represent the original cost. The percent is 80% and the amount is \$1500.

$$\text{Percent} \times \text{base} = \text{amount}$$
$$80\% \times C = 1500$$
$$0.80C = 1500$$
$$\frac{0.80C}{0.80} = \frac{1500}{0.80}$$
$$C = 1875$$

The original cost was \$1875.

**39. Strategy** To find the unit rate, write and simplify a ratio.

**Solution** $\dfrac{1500 \text{ milliliters}}{12 \text{ hours}} = \dfrac{125 \text{ milliliters}}{1 \text{ hour}}$

The infusion rage is 125 ml/h.

**40.** $-2 + 8 + (-10) = 6 + (-10) = -4$

**41.** $-30 - (-15) = -30 + 15 = -15$

**42.** $2\frac{1}{2} \times -\frac{1}{5} = \frac{5}{2} \times \frac{-1}{5} = -\frac{1}{2}$

**43.** $-1\frac{3}{8} \div 5\frac{1}{2} = \frac{-11}{8} \div \frac{11}{2} = \frac{-11}{8} \times \frac{2}{11} = \frac{-1}{4} = -\frac{1}{4}$

**44.**
$$\begin{aligned}(-4)^2 \div (1-3)^2 - (-2) &= (-4)^2 \div (-2)^2 - (-2)\\ &= 16 \div 4 - (-2)\\ &= 4 - (-2)\\ &= 4 + 2\\ &= 6\end{aligned}$$

**45.**
$$\begin{aligned}2x - 3(x-4) + 5 &= 2x + (-3)[x + (-4)] + 5\\ &= 2x + (-3)x + (-3)(-4) + 5\\ &= 2x + (-3)x + 12 + 5\\ &= -x + 12 + 5\\ &= -x + 17\end{aligned}$$

**46.**
$$\frac{2}{3}x = -12$$
$$\frac{3}{2} \cdot \frac{2}{3}x = \frac{3}{2} \cdot (-12)$$
$$x = -18$$

The solution is $-18$.

**47.**
$$3x - 5 = 10$$
$$3x - 5 + 5 = 10 + 5$$
$$3x = 15$$
$$\frac{3x}{3} = \frac{15}{3}$$
$$x = 5$$

The solution is 5.

**48.**
$$8 - 3x = x + 4$$
$$8 - 3x - x = x - x + 4$$
$$8 - 4x = 4$$
$$8 - 8 - 4x = 4 - 8$$
$$-4x = -4$$
$$\frac{-4x}{-4} = \frac{-4}{-4}$$
$$x = 1$$

The solution is 1.

**49. Strategy** To find your new balance, subtract the check amounts (\$321.88 and \$34.23) and add the amount of the deposit (\$443.56).

**Solution**

$$\begin{array}{r} 872.48\\ \underline{-321.88}\\ 550.60\\ \underline{-34.23}\\ 516.37\\ \underline{+443.56}\\ 959.93\end{array}$$

Your new balance is \$959.93.

© 2013 Cengage Learning. All Rights Reserved. May not be scanned, copied or duplicated, or posted to a publicly accessible website, in whole or in part.

**50. Strategy** To find the amount of salt, write and solve a proportion.

**Solution**
$$\frac{1.5 \text{ mg of salt}}{100 \text{ ml of solution}} = \frac{x \text{ mg of salt}}{500 \text{ ml}}$$
$$100 \times x = 1.5 \times 500$$
$$100x = 750$$
$$\frac{100x}{100} = \frac{750}{100}$$
$$x = 7.5$$
7.5 mg of salt are needed.

**51. Strategy** To find inflation rate:
- subtract the original cost ($15.99) from the new cost ($18.99) to find the increase.
- Divide the increase by the original cost ($15.99) and express as a decimal.

**Solution** $18.99 - 15.99 = 3.00$
$$\frac{3.00}{15.99} \approx 0.188 = 18.8\%$$
The inflation rate is 18.8%.

**52. Strategy** To find the mean income for the 4 months, add the incomes and divide the sum by the number of incomes (4).

**Solution**
$$\begin{array}{r} 4320 \\ 3572 \\ 2864 \\ +\ 4420 \\ \hline 15{,}176 \end{array} \qquad 4\overline{)15{,}176} = 3794$$
The mean income is $3794.

**53. Strategy** To find the simple interest due, multiply the principal ($120,000) by the interest rate by the time (in years).

**Solution**
$$\text{Interest} = 120{,}000 \times 8\% \times \frac{9}{12}$$
$$= 120{,}000 \times 0.08 \times \frac{9}{12}$$
$$= 7200$$
The simple interest due is $7200.

**54. Strategy** To calculate the probability:
- Count the number of possible outcomes.
- Count the number of favorable outcomes.
- Use the probability formula.

**Solution** There are 36 possible outcomes. There are 12 favorable outcomes: (1, 2), (2, 1), (1, 5), (5, 1), (2, 4), (4, 2),(3, 3), (3, 6), (6, 3), (4, 5), (5, 4), (6, 6).
$$\text{Probability} = \frac{12}{36} = \frac{1}{3}$$
The probability is $\frac{1}{3}$ that the sum of the dots on upward faces of the two dice is divisible by 3.

**55. Strategy** To find the percent:
- Read the graph and find the death count of China.
- Read the circle graph and find the death count of the other three countries.
- Find the sum of the death counts by adding the four death counts.
- Solve the basic percent equation for percent. The base is the sum of the four death counts and the amount is the death count of China.

© 2013 Cengage Learning. All Rights Reserved. May not be scanned, copied or duplicated, or posted to a publicly accessible website, in whole or in part.

**Solution**

| | |
|---|---|
| China: | 1300 thousand |
| Japan: | 1100 thousand |
| USSR: | 13,600 thousand |
| Germany: | + 3300 thousand |
| | 19,300 thousand |

Percent × base = amount

$$n \times 19{,}300 = 1300$$
$$n = 1300 \div 19{,}300$$
$$n \approx 0.067$$

China has 6.7% of the death count of the four countries.

**56. Strategy** To find units needed:

- Convert 3200 g to kg.
- Write and solve a proportion.

**Solution** 3200 g = 3.2 kg

$$\frac{25 \text{ units}}{\text{kg}} = \frac{x \text{ units}}{3.2 \text{ kg}}$$
$$x = 25 \times 3.2$$
$$x = 80$$

The dose is 80 units.

**57. Strategy** To find the mother's height, write and solve an equation using $h$ to represent the number of inches. Convert the answer to ft and in.

**Solution** [46 in.] is [$\frac{2}{3}$ mother's height]

**Solution**

$$46 = \frac{2}{3}h$$
$$\frac{3}{2} \cdot 46 = \frac{3}{2} \cdot \frac{2}{3}h$$
$$69 = h$$

$$69 \text{ in.} = 69 \text{ in.} \times \frac{1 \text{ ft}}{12 \text{ in.}}$$

5 ft 9 in.

$$12\overline{)69}$$
$$\underline{60}$$
$$9$$

The mother is 5 ft 9 in.

**58. Strategy** To find the dosage:

- Convert 0.5 mg to mcg.
- Write and solve a proportion.

**Solution** 0.5 mg = 500 mcg

$$\frac{100 \text{ mcg}}{\text{ml}} = \frac{500 \text{ mcg}}{x \text{ ml}}$$
$$500 = 100 \cdot x$$
$$\frac{500}{100} = \frac{100x}{100}$$
$$5 = x$$

The dose is 5 ml.

**59. Strategy** To find the patient's height in ft and in., convert 73 in. to ft and in.

**Solution**

$$73 \text{ in.} = 73 \text{ ~~in.~~} \times \frac{1 \text{ ft}}{12 \text{ ~~in.~~}}$$

6 ft 1 in.

$$12\overline{)73}$$
$$\underline{72}$$
$$1$$

The patient is 6 ft 1 in.

**60.** The unknown number: $n$

$$\frac{n}{2} - 5 = 3$$
$$\frac{n}{2} - 5 + 5 = 3 + 5$$
$$\frac{n}{2} = 8$$
$$2 \cdot \frac{n}{2} = 2 \cdot 8$$
$$n = 16$$

The number is 16.

© 2013 Cengage Learning. All Rights Reserved. May not be scanned, copied or duplicated, or posted to a publicly accessible website, in whole or in part.

Made in United States
Orlando, FL
04 November 2026

90205879R00151